T0313898

Cleft lip and palate management

A comprehensive atlas

Cleft lip and palate management

A comprehensive atlas

Edited by

Ricardo D. Bennun, MD, MS, PHD

Director, Cleft Lip/Palate Program
Asociacion PIEL & Maimonides University
Buenos Aires, Argentina

Julia F. Harfin, DDS, PHD

Professor and Chairman, Orthodontics Department
Maimonides University
Buenos Aires, Argentina

George K. B. Sándor, MD, DDS, PHD, DR. HABIL

Oral and Maxillofacial, Plastic and Craniofacial Surgeon
Professor of Tissue Engineering, Professor of Oral and Maxillofacial Surgery
University of Oulu, Oulu University Hospital
Oulu, Finland;
Director of Research
BioMediTech
University of Tampere
Tampere, Finland

David Genecov, MD, FACS, FAAP

International Craniofacial Institute
Cleft Lip & Palate Treatment Center
Dallas, TX, USA

WILEY Blackwell

Copyright © 2016 by John Wiley & Sons, Inc. All rights reserved

Published by John Wiley & Sons, Inc., Hoboken, New Jersey
Published simultaneously in Canada

No part of this publication may be reproduced, stored in a retrieval system, or transmitted in any form or by any means, electronic, mechanical, photocopying, recording, scanning, or otherwise, except as permitted under Section 107 or 108 of the 1976 United States Copyright Act, without either the prior written permission of the Publisher, or authorization through payment of the appropriate per-copy fee to the Copyright Clearance Center, Inc., 222 Rosewood Drive, Danvers, MA 01923, (978) 750-8400, fax (978) 750-4470, or on the web at www.copyright.com. Requests to the Publisher for permission should be addressed to the Permissions Department, John Wiley & Sons, Inc., 111 River Street, Hoboken, NJ 07030, (201) 748-6011, fax (201) 748-6008, or online at http://www.wiley.com/go/permission.

The contents of this work are intended to further general scientific research, understanding, and discussion only and are not intended and should not be relied upon as recommending or promoting a specific method, diagnosis, or treatment by health science practitioners for any particular patient. The publisher and the author make no representations or warranties with respect to the accuracy or completeness of the contents of this work and specifically disclaim all warranties, including without limitation any implied warranties of fitness for a particular purpose. In view of ongoing research, equipment modifications, changes in governmental regulations, and the constant flow of information relating to the use of medicines, equipment, and devices, the reader is urged to review and evaluate the information provided in the package insert or instructions for each medicine, equipment, or device for, among other things, any changes in the instructions or indication of usage and for added warnings and precautions. Readers should consult with a specialist where appropriate. The fact that an organization or Website is referred to in this work as a citation and/or a potential source of further information does not mean that the author or the publisher endorses the information the organization or Website may provide or recommendations it may make. Further, readers should be aware that Internet Websites listed in this work may have changed or disappeared between when this work was written and when it is read. No warranty may be created or extended by any promotional statements for this work. Neither the publisher nor the author shall be liable for any damages arising herefrom.

For general information on our other products and services or for technical support, please contact our Customer Care Department within the United States at (800) 762-2974, outside the United States at (317) 572-3993 or fax (317) 572-4002.

Wiley also publishes its books in a variety of electronic formats. Some content that appears in print may not be available in electronic formats. For more information about Wiley products, visit our web site at www.wiley.com.

Library of Congress Cataloging-in-Publication Data:

Cleft lip and palate management : a comprehensive atlas/edited by Ricardo D. Bennun, Julia F. Harfin, George K.B. Sándor, David Genecov.
       p. ; cm.
  Includes bibliographical references and index.
  ISBN 978-1-118-60754-1 (cloth: alk. paper)
  I. Bennun, Ricardo D., editor. II. Harfin, Julia F. de, editor. III. Sándor, George K. B., editor. IV. Genecov, David, editor.
  [DNLM: 1. Cleft Lip–surgery–Atlases. 2. Cleft Palate–surgery–Atlases. 3. Cleft Lip–diagnosis–Atlases. 4. Cleft Palate–diagnosis–Atlases. 5. Oral Surgical Procedures–methods–Atlases. 6. Reconstructive Surgical Procedures–methods–Atlases. WV 17]
  RD524
  617.5′22059–dc23

                                        2015026543

Printed in Singapore

10 9 8 7 6 5 4 3 2 1

Contents

List of contributors

Luis Monasterio Aljaro, MD, Fundacion Gantz, Santiago de Chile

María Bevilacqua, MD Anesthesiologist Asociacion PIEL, Buenos Aires, Argentina

Michael H. Carstens, MD, FACS, Clinical Associate Professor of Plastic Surgery, Saint Louis University; Profesor de Cirugía Plástica (Honoris Causa), Universidad Nacional Autonoma de Nicaragua, Leon, Nicaragua; Attending Surgeon, Hospital Metropolitano Vivian Pellas Managua, Nicaragua

Vanesa Casadio, PhD, Speech Therapist Asociacion PIEL, Buenos Aires, Argentina

Agustina Vila Echagüe, MD, PhD, Dermatologist Asociacion PIEL, Buenos Aires, Argentina

Virpi Harila, DDS, PhD, Oulu University, Finland

Tuomo Heikkinen, DDS, PhD, Oulu University, Finland

Analia Langsam, DMD, Pediatric Dentist Asociacion PIEL, Buenos Aires, Argentina

Luis Moggi, MD Anesthesiologist Asociacion PIEL, Buenos Aires, Argentina

Pertti Pirttiniemi, DDS, PhD, Oulu University, Finland

Diofre Ponce, MD, Anesthesiologist Asociacion PIEL, Argentina

Suvi P. Tainijoki, Clinical Nurse Specialist, Oulu University Hospital, Oulu, Finland

Ville Vuollo, MSc, Oulu University, Finland

Leena P. Ylikontiola, MD, DDS, PhD, Oulu University, Finland

Preface

A nonsyndromic oral cleft delivery not only creates an emotional burden on the family and the medical team, but also compromises the physical and psychological development of the patient as well as disadvantaging their social insertion.

This affliction, characterized by misplaced central facial pieces, occurs on average in 1/800 live newborns. Added to the initial problems of feeding and suction are the encumbering complications in hearing.

The overwhelming complexity of the problems to be treated in an oral cleft patient induced the organization of the first interdisciplinary team by Cooper in Lancaster, Pennsylvania, in 1939.

Although the first references to oral cleft repair in the literature were written by Ambroise Paré and Gaspare Tagliacozzi in the sixteenth century, a large number of authors have published diverse techniques, using different skin incisions and a great variety of flaps, arguing for better cosmetic results.

In all aspects of plastic surgery, there is an equal measure of art and knowledge. However in the repair of the cleft lip, art seems to take the upper hand. In art, there is no excellence: you must go through knowledge, to reach a privileged level of achievement.

Unfavorable results in unilateral and bilateral cleft lip, nose, and palate repair are often easy to score, and probably less easy to prevent, but are really difficult to treat.

It is not the intention of this Atlas to report a historical revision; our aim is to transmit to you more than 20 years of practical experience from different teams working but connected throughout the world, showing both successful as well as unsuccessful results with the intention of avoiding unwanted sequels.

What we have attempted to do in this book is to try and deal with the more common problems, explain our point of view regarding their causation, and define their best possible management – mostly from our personal experiences over many years, and never forgetting Sir Harold Gillies' words: "Diagnose before you treat."

Meticulous documentation and follow-up are uniquely valid actions that have allowed us to choose and recommend some techniques over other less-effective procedures, and to discard many of them as being really dangerous.

Today, the accepted universal goal is to obtain excellent aesthetic and functional results during primary reconstruction of the lip and nose, and normal speech, in 85–90% of cases.

Using less aggressive techniques, conserving and respecting growth centers, innervations, and blood supply, will allow us to prevent the growth and development of facial alterations.

With the introduction of presurgical orthopedics, reconstructive surgery in cleft patients has entered a period of inductive surgery or regeneration of missing anatomic parts. This also coincides with two other phenomena currently observed in all surgical disciplines: (i) the simplification or minimization of surgery and (ii) recognition of the need for delivery of healthcare services at a lower cost.

Although we are aiming to outline principles, we feel that a problem as complex as the 45 variants of cleft presentation described in epidemiological research realized in Argentina cannot be solved using one technique. We need to know how the deformity occurs and what normal looks like. Only with normal as a guide can we repair the misplaced central facial pieces.

This book's intention is to provide a selection of the best procedures and resources performed by experienced surgeons that have shown the best results over the years. Milestones and difficulties are analyzed in this book in a step by step manner.

With regard to the large number of untoward sequels created by surgeons, the aim of this book will be to show the reader how to arrive at a normal appearance using the least invasive procedure. Post-surgical evaluation by the interdisciplinary team is transcendental to prevent hipoacusia, speech, and bite alterations.

Ensuring the safety of the patients must be the number one priority and the guiding force behind every treatment plan. In this way, we share Smile Train's Safety and Quality Protocol, together with over 400 cleft centers from 72 countries around the world as an important tool helping to advance the excellence of care for all cleft patients.

The authors also wish to show that it is possible to employ similar treatment protocols, in a number of different places in the world, with diametrically opposite cultural, social, and scientific insights. In recent years, our collaboration has even extended to molecular biologists and geneticists, who have done so much to shed light on the etiopathogenesis; and tissue engineering researchers who work for the future in tissue culturing.

Unquestionably the answers to cleft causation and its prevention are the goals of the future.

There are few surgeons who meet their patients before birth, as when the parents present the surgeon with an ultrasonic image of their unborn child. We are privileged to work with parents, as the geneticist attempts to help them answer the inevitable question, "Why?" and, with the help of the psychosocial team recruited to encourage the parents in their frustration and worry, to help them relish the joy of having brought a child into the world.

Ricardo D. Bennun, MD, MS, PhD

Acknowledgments

Our international project receives the human and scientific support of multidisciplinary teams from Buenos Aires, Argentina; Santiago de Chile; Oulu, Finland; and Dallas, USA.

We are indebted to our families, friends, patients, as well as our professors, institutions, and colleagues. Special thanks to our administrative staff and contributors for making our passion for this work a reality.

The present book represents a huge effort to condense experiences and suggestions. Our intention is to facilitate the multidisciplinary treatment of cleft patients, improve results, and prevent sequels. This work is aimed at young professionals in different places in the world dealing with different realities.

Our achievements would not be possible without the invaluable support of The Smile Train and The World of Children foundations.

The Editors

PART 1

Principles

CHAPTER 1

Mechanisms of cleft palate: developmental field analysis

Michael H. Carstens

Saint Louis University and Universidad Nacional Autonoma de Nicaragua, Nicaragua

The purpose of this chapter is to present concepts of cleft palate repair based on a single unifying concept: the embryology of the oronasopharynx. We shall begin with an in-depth discussion of how the bone and soft tissue structures are assembled, based upon the developmental field model. Next, we shall consider how this normal process is altered when a disruption of the neurovascular pedicle to an individual field results in a deficiency state such that the affected field is unable to fuse with its partner fields. Attention will also be give to the effect that such a deficiency state has on the subsequent development of the partner fields. Surgical procedures based on the embryologic model are designed to restore functional tissue relationships.

Craniofacial development: the Lego® model

The anatomic structures of the head and neck are assembled from tissue units known as *developmental fields*, each of which has a distinct neurovascular pedicle providing sensory and/or autonomic control and blood supply. Fields are often composite structures containing mesenchymal elements such as cartilage, bone, fascia, muscle and so on. They may have an associated epithelium such as skin or mucosa. Adjacent fields interact. Muscles with a primary attachment to bone or cartilage within one field may have a secondary attachment site in an adjacent field.

Fields develop in a strict spatio-temporal sequence. Congenital conditions that reduce the size or content of a field will affect subsequent growth. In the Pierre Robin sequence, the relative decrease in volume of the mandibular ramus leads to a posterior position of the chin and subsequent relationships of the infrahyoid musculature. The reduction of the frontal process of the premaxilla seen in the typical orofacial cleft causes a relative narrowing of the nasal fossa, malposition of the internal nasal valve, and respiratory dysfunction (Figure 1.1).

The anatomic defects seen in clefts of the hard and soft palate present as a spectrum involving several fields. Many cases involve deficiency states of the piriform fossa and/or premaxilla and soft tissues of the lip and nose. In other, rarer conditions, such as the Tessier 3 cleft, a cleft palate defect coincides with defects in seemingly unrelated anatomic zones, such as the inferior turbinate and medial maxillary wall. For this reason, it is necessary to have a comprehensive picture of the neurovascular anatomy of the oronasopharynx.

The zones of anatomic interest are all supplied by arterial axes running in parallel with the various sensory branches of V1 and V2. Development of the pedicles is a reciprocal process. Neuronal growth cones secrete vascular endothelial growth factor (VEGF) while the arterial growth cone secretes nerve growth factor (NGF). Like all cranial nerves, the trigeminal complex is constructed from neural crest, whereas the histologic composition of the arteries consists of a tubular conduit of endothelial cells made from paraxial mesoderm embraced by pericytes. These latter cells are contractile and control capillary permeability. Pericytes are ubiquitous throughout the human body (Figure 1.2). They are the precursor for mesenchymal stem cells. They also elaborate paracrine factors that are essential for survival of the vascular growth cone. Thus, we come to a very simple and powerful idea: dysfunction of a vascular growth cone will result in either a reduction of volume of mesenchymal structures within the target field, or the outright loss of the field itself. In the first case, the physical effect of the small field is to constrain subsequent growth of surrounding fields. If a frank tissue defect exists (i.e., a cleft) adjacent fields actually collapse into the site.

The reader will note here terminology that may be unfamiliar: it harkens back to those embryology lectures that we endured … an endless list of structures that morphed into a final result via mechanisms that were unknown. The molecular revolution transformed the science into developmental biology with a

Cleft Lip and Palate Management: A Comprehensive Atlas, First Edition. Edited by Ricardo D. Bennun, Julia F. Harfin, George K. B. Sándor, and David Genecov.
© 2016 John Wiley & Sons, Inc. Published 2016 by John Wiley & Sons, Inc.

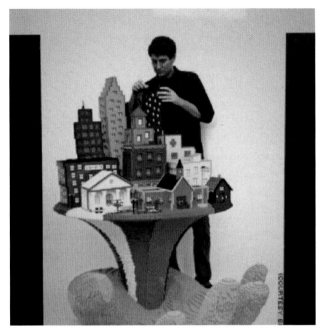

Figure 1.1 Craniofacial fields are composite blocks of tissue supplied by a specific neurovascular pedicle. Fields grow in relation to each other over time, each with a different volume and rate of growth. Deficiency or absence of a field results in collapse of adjacent partner fields. The leaning tower of Pisa is a classic example of what happens when a supporting field is absent – the entire complex is displaced and, if the upper stories of the tower were made of soft plastic, would become distorted as well. A "cleft" is really a condition of excess or deficiency in a given field that results in displacement and/or distortion of adjacent fields.

tight connection to genetics (these fields formerly co-existed in virtual isolation from each other). In the following section we shall consider the tissue composition of developmental fields, how they are arranged in the intermediate state as pharyngeal arches, and how, with growth-driven folding of the embryo, these fields become physically repositioned and interactive (Carlson, 2013; Gilbert, 2013).

The embryonic period lasts 8 weeks and is divided into 23 anatomic stages (see Figure 1.3). In the first three stages, the embryo is a rapidly dividing ball of cells. Stages 4–5 are all about survival as the embryo implants itself into the uterine wall and begins the process by which blood supply will come from the mother. The stage 4 embryo secretes fluid into its center, becoming a hollow blastocyst with a single layer of cells, the epiblast, becoming segregated to one side of the ball. Thus there is an inner cell mass (the future organism) and enveloping wall (the trophoblast) that will eventually form the extraembryonic structures, such as the placenta (O'Rahilly & Müller, 1996). The tightly-bound cells of the epiblast then become transiently "loose," allowing some of the epiblast cells to drop down below their previous plane, coalesce and form a new second layer, the *hypoblast*. By the end of stage 5, the hypoblast has proliferated and formed a lining layer around the inner wall of the trophoblast. The hypoblast now secretes a new

layer, extraembryonic mesoderm (EEM), interposed between it and the trophoblast. This geometry allows the EEM to surround the entire embryo and move into the zone of the future placenta. Since blood vessels are formed exclusively from mesoderm, the EEM becomes the source for the entire extraembryonic blood supply.

Stages 6–7 involve a transformation of the intraembryonic tissues into three layers (ectoderm, mesoderm, and endoderm) via a process called *gastrulation*: "the single most important event in the life of every organism." There are excellent videos of gastrulation available on YouTube. Note that at the completion of gastrulation, the hypoblast is pushed out of the way; it has no role in the formation of the organism *per se*. In point of fact, the epiblast contributes first to endoderm, then to mesoderm. When the gastrulation process is complete, the cells remaining behind on the surface are known as the ectoderm proper.

The concept of three germ layers is outmoded and inapplicable to understanding craniofacial development. For simplicity, let's leave the epithelial germ layers (ecto- and endoderm) behind and concentrate on mesoderm. This layer outside the head and neck is responsible for all striated muscles, bone, cartilage, brown fat (white fat is more complex), fascia, and the non-neural internal organs. Furthermore, as mesoderm fans out over the surface of the embryo, its identity becomes determined by the interplay of gene products expressed either from the midline (i.e., the neural tube) such as sonic hedgehog (SHH) and wingless (WNT) or from the peripheral epithelial surfaces of future skin (ectoderm) and mucosa (endoderm) such as BMP-4 (Carstens, 2000, 2002).

Depending upon location, mesoderm assumes three basic fates. *Paraxial mesoderm* (PAM) lies next to the neural tube. It becomes segmented into individual tissue blocks called *somites*, each one of which is developmentally related to the segment of the nervous system from which it derives its innervation. Somites construct the entire axial skeleton, related striated muscles, and the major axial arteries (aorta, carotids, etc.). *Intermediate mesoderm* (IM) is also segmentally organized; it forms the genito-urinary system. Finally, *lateral plate mesoderm* (LPM) forms the entire appendicular skeleton, the remainder of the arteries, smooth muscle, and the viscera (Carstens, 2008a, 2008b) (Figure 1.4).

Left out from this equation is the fourth germ layer, the *neural crest*. The vast majority of all facial soft tissues in the face and all the craniofacial membranous bones arise from neural crest. These cells substitute for mesoderm in the head. They also form the ensheathing Schwann cells of the peripheral nervous system and the entire autonomic nervous system.

During stages 8–9 *neurulation* takes place. First, a flat neural plate is formed; this then rolls up like a cigar to form the neural tube. Neural crest cells develop at the interface between the outlying ectoderm and the neural plate. These rapidly multiply and are distributed over the entire organism, immediately subjacent to the epithelia (ectoderm and endoderm) and throughout the

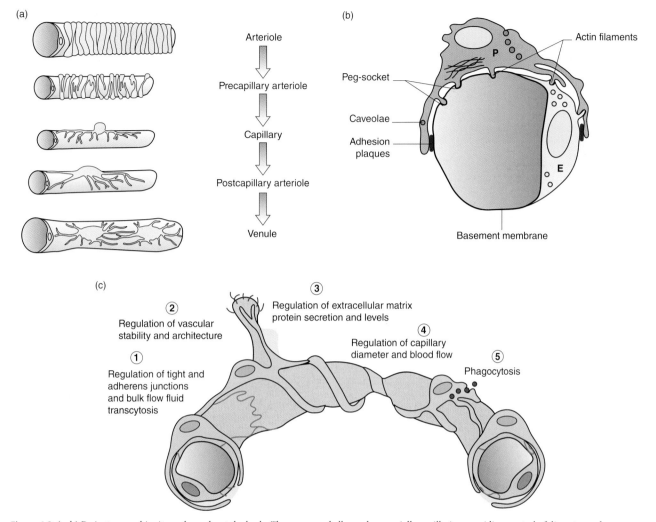

Figure 1.2 (a, b) Pericytes are ubiquitous throughout the body. They surround all vessels, especially capillaries, providing control of diameter and permeability. Pericytes have contractile fibers. They are interconnected, including between adjacent vessels. Pericytes may have a connection with neural crest, can detach under conditions of inflammation, are the source of white fat, and also give rise to all mesenchymal stem cells of the body. (c) Demonstrated are the multiple physiologic functions of pericytes.

mesoderm. Neural crest cells are critical for craniofacial development (Figure 1.5).

Stages 8–9 are also notable for the segmentation of the zone of paraxial mesoderm flanking the neural tube. PAM forms into distinct blocks called somites. There are names for their respective locations: 4 occipital, 8 cervical, 12 thoracic, 5 lumbar, 5 sacral, and 3–4 coccygeal. The appearance of the first three occipital somites alongside the hindbrain defines stage 9. *Somitogenesis* is a cranial-caudal process in which one somite appears approximately every 4 hours (Figure 1.6). However, there is an additional zone of PAM which lies cranial to the somites alongside the midbrain and forebrain in which the segmentation is incomplete, forming seven *somitomeres*. Somitomeres (Sms) have very limited developmental potential. They produce the striated muscles of the orbit and the first

three pharyngeal arches; Sm1 and Sm2 also contribute to the posterior wall of the orbit.

So what we have now is a critical mass of tissues that will mix together to form a series of five intermediate structures, the *pharyngeal arches*, each of which is innervated by a specific cranial nerve. These structures first develop at a stage when the embryo is still flat; at stage 9 the embryo begins a complex folding process. The first pharyngeal arch can be seen at this stage. It hangs downward like a sock filled with neural crest and PAM. At each stage thereafter a new pharyngeal arch makes its formal appearance. The process of making the five pharyngeal arches is thus complete by stage 14 (Figures 1.7 and 1.8). All pharyngeal arches are organized into distinct zones by a series of distal-less (Dlx) genes: proximal/distal, cranial/caudal, and medial/lateral. All arches have the same organizational pattern.

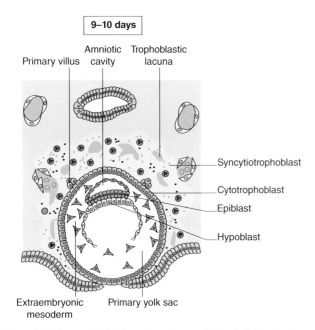

9–10 days

Primary villus
Amniotic cavity
Trophoblastic lacuna

Syncytiotrophoblast

Cytotrophoblast

Epiblast

Hypoblast

Extraembryonic mesoderm
Primary yolk sac

Figure 1.3 At stage 5, 9–10 days, the embryo is a hollow ball (blastocyt) consisting of the embryo proper surrounded by trophoblast (green) that will eventually make non-embryonic tissues such as the placenta. From the original inner cell mass a second layer of cells develops beneath. The embryo now has an epiblast (blue), and a hypoblast (yellow), also termed the primitive endoderm. Hypoblast spreads out to line the entire blastocyst cavity. It then secretes the primitive mesoderm (red) which will flow up into the future placenta and make the extra-embryonic circulation.

Arch 1 has a rostral maxillary zone innervated by V2 and a caudal mandibular zone supplied by V3. Muscles of mastication in the first arch all arise from somitomere 4. Arch 2 fuses with arch 1; it contains the muscles for facial expression. The

upper division of VII supplies facial muscles from somitomere 5 distributed over the maxillary zone while the lower division of VII innervates muscles from somitomere 6 distributed over the mandible (see Figure 1.9).

Embryonic folding driven largely by explosive brain growth causes the pharyngeal arches to swing upward into the adult position. They subsequently fuse. Growth of the vascular channels into the arches proceeds concomitant with penetration of the arches by cranial nerves from the brain. We will now briefly explore how the individual neurovascular pedicles associated with the nasopharynx and oropharynx are organized. This will give us insight into the manner in which the developmental fields are assembled (O'Rahilly & Müller, 1999).

The final configuration of craniofacial arteries is the result of a step-wise process by which primitive structures meld into more complex forms. Arteries are mesodermal structures, the earliest ones appear after gastrulation is complete. The forebrain and midbrain are supplied by a *primitive head plexus* while *primitive hindbrain channels* supply the remainder of the brain. The *dorsal aortae* run alongside the body axis and supply non-neural tissues. Anterior extensions of the dorsa aortae connect with one another anterior to the brain and to the oropharyngeal membrane, greater complexity is assumed. The arteries to the brain and spinal cord assume a segmental pattern to supply each developmental unit of the CNS, that is neuromeres. Each of the five pharyngeal arches is supplied by a segmental aortic arch artery connecting the primitive outflow tract with the paired dorsal aortae above. The fifth aortic arch artery atrophies with AA4 supplying both pharyngeal arch 4 and 5. AA6 is dedicated exclusively to the pulmonary circulation (Figures 1.10–1.12).

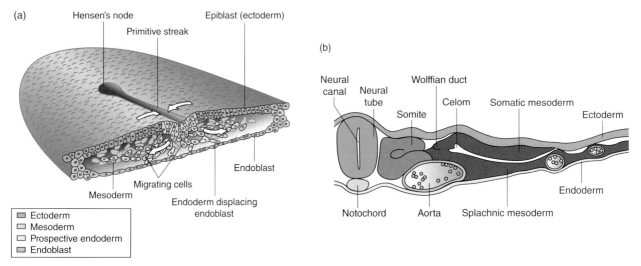

(a)
Hensen's node
Primitive streak
Epiblast (ectoderm)

Endoblast

Mesoderm
Migrating cells
Endoderm displacing endoblast

☐ Ectoderm
☐ Mesoderm
☐ Prospective endoderm
☐ Endoblast

(b)
Neural canal
Neural tube
Somite
Wolffian duct
Celom
Somatic mesoderm
Ectoderm

Endoderm

Notochord
Aorta
Splanchnic mesoderm

Figure 1.4 (a) Note here that the primitive endoderm/hypoblast (green) will be pushed out of the way by the definitive endoderm (yellow). Hypoblast thus has no biologic role in development other than to serve as a temporary layer. (b) Mesoderm will have specific roles depending upon its location in the embryo. This is because at each physical location a unique combination of gene products from ectoderm and endoderm act as signals to the mesoderm, "instructing" it as to its ontogenic fate. *Paraxial mesoderm* (red) forms: somites, dermis, striated muscle, the axial skeleton. *Intermediate mesoderm* (not seen) is a long thin rod of tissue extending along the axis of the embryo. It is neuromerically organized. It produces the entire genito-urinary system. *Lateral plate mesoderm* (purple) forms: the cardiovascular system, smooth muscle, the appendicular skeleton, and the mesenchyme for all internal organs.

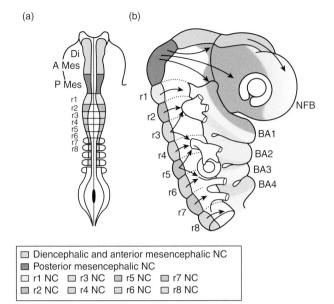

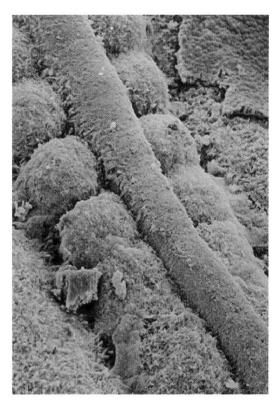

Figure 1.5 (a) Neuromeres are developmental units of the nervous system, the boundaries of which are established by unique combination of products from homeotic genes (Hox). In humans there are 38 Hox genes distributed over four chromosomes. Common to each is a 60 amino acid sequence that unlocks DNA. Hox genes code for the CNS as far forward as the midbrain/hindbrain junction. Recently discovered additional Hox-related genes code for the neuromeres of the midbrain and forebrain. Carlson BM. Human Embryology and Developmental Biology, 3rd edn. Reproduced with permission of Elsevier. (b) Neural crest at any given level of the CNS has exactly the same Hox code as the neuromere above which it originates. Color coding shows contributions as follows. PROSENCEPHALON (forebrain) = pink. Non-neural ectoderm (not truly neural crest) lies above prosomeres p5 and p6. P6 produces the nasopharyngeal mucosa supplied by V1. P5 produces the epidermis supplied by V1. Prosomeres p4-p1 are unclear but probably flow beneath p6 and p5 to produce (respectively) nasopharyngeal submucosa and dermis. MESENCEPHALON (midbrain) = red. M1 goes to membranous bone. M2 goes to meninges, orbit, and first arch. First arch contains m2, r1, r2, and r3; second arch contains r4 and r5; third arch has r5 and r6; fourth arch has r7 and r8. NB: each arch has a longitudinal axis with equal numbers of neuromeres represented on either side. The coordinates of the arches are determined by the distal-less (Dlx) system of genes.

Figure 1.6 Somitomeres and somites develop from paraxial mesoderm. Somitomeres are hollow balls with a somitocoele in the center; they are incompletely separated from each other, so mesenchyme can be shared. Somites are discrete units with epithelial boundaries. They have regional specializations for axial bone (sclerotome), muscle (myotome), and epaxial dermis (dermatome). Humans have 7 somitomeres and 39 somites. The process of somitogenesis in mammals takes approximately 4 hours per somite. Gilbert SF, *Developmental Biology*, 10th edn., Sinauer, 2014. Sinauer Associates, Inc.

Within the pharyngeal arches, the *aortic arch arteries* constitute primitive vascular cores. These rapidly involute, each one being replaced with a plexus, the confluence of which forms the external carotid system. At Carnegie stage 17 an entirely new system of *stapedial arteries* develops, the initial stem of which runs upward from internal carotid through the temporal bone. The timing of stapedial development precisely matches the emergence of the cranial nerves, each nerve serving as the template for a respective artery. These dural arteries connect externally to the external carotid system via the trigeminal ganglion. In the orbit the V1-related stapedial (StV1) plugs into the ophthalmic. The latter supplies the ocular apparatus while the former supplies all the periocular structures (muscle, fascia, bone, etc.). When the parent stem of stapedial involutes, the final anatomy takes shape: the dural arteries are now supplied

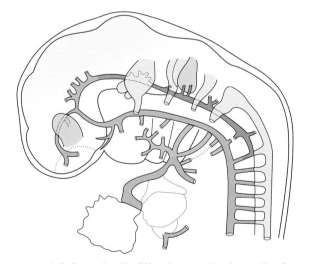

Figure 1.7 Only four arches (the fifth is diminuitive) and no sixth arch. Aortic arch arteries span the four arches, AA4 supplying pharyngeal arch 5. Arteries to the sixth "arch" are dedicated to pulmonary circulation. http://creatureandcreator.ca/. Reproduced with permission of Terry Picton. Last accessed December 2014.

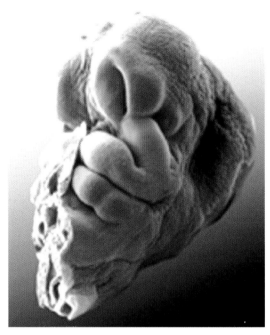

Figure 1.8 Note the longitudinal fissure in the first pharyngeal arch separating the maxillary (green) and mandibular (blue) fields. Each pharyngeal arch has a similar axis which is specified by the distal-less (Dlx) genes.

by the external carotid system. The ophthalmic is a hybrid; the original stem from the internal carotid is dedicated to the eye while StV1 serves the orbital structures exclusively (Figures 1.13 and 1.14).

The extension of the stapedial downward through the trigeminal ganglion gives it access to the distal extent of the external carotid system, to which it attaches just beyond the take-off of the facial artery. Those branches associated with StV2 supply the maxilla. Each of these is distributed through the pterygopalatine plexus while StV3 supplies the mandible.

Developmental fields of the naso-oropharynx containing membranous bones

We come now to the crucial concept. Each of the StV2 branches is responsible for supplying one or more fields within the maxilla. Thus, a reduction or knock-out in any one of these branches will create a tissue deficiency state (cleft). Each of the *Tessier cleft zones* contains specific bone and cartilagenous structures. Thus it is possible to use the reduction in size or absence in a marker structure to define the presence of a Tessier cleft.

- Internal medial nasal (StV1), Tessier zone 1: nasal bones and upper septum.
- External medial nasal (anterior ethmoid) (StV1), Tessier zone 1: distally these extend down through the columella and into the philtrum. Collaterals to central incisor.
- Internal lateral nasal (StV1), Tessier zone 3: upper turbinate and middle turbinate.
- External lateral nasal (StV1). Tessier zone 4: piriform fossa.
- Lacrimal (StV1), Tessier zone 9: lateral orbit – anastomoses with orbital branch of middle meningeal.
- Supraorbital (StV1), Tessier zone 10–11.
- Supratrochlear artery (StV1), Tessier zones 12–13.
- Medial nasopalatine (StV2), Tessier zone 2: lower septum, vomer, and premaxilla.
- Lateral nasopalatine (StV2), Tessier zone 3: inferior turbinate, medial maxillary wall, and the nasal mucosa of the secondary hard palate.
- Descending palatine (StV2), Tessier zone 3: palatine bone, oral mucosa of the secondary hard palate.
- Medial infraorbital (anterior alveolar) (StV2), Tessier zone 4: frontal process of maxilla, canine, anterior maxilla medial to the foramen.
- Lateral infraorbital artery (middle alveolar) (StV2), Tessier zone 5: premolars, anterior maxilla lateral to foramen.

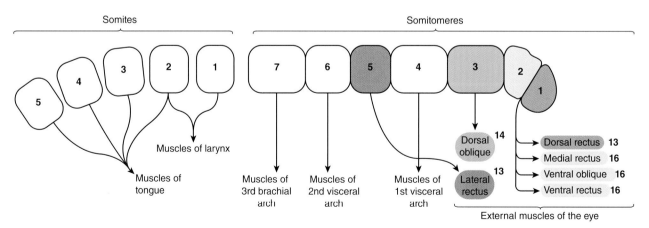

Figure 1.9 Mesoderm from the first seven somitomeres has a very limited role in craniofacial development. Somitomere 4 supplies the muscles of mastication. Somitomeres 5–6 supply the muscles of facial expression. Somitomere 7 supplies all muscles of the palate except the tensor. Adapted from Butler AB, Hodos W. *Comparative Vertebrate Neuroanatomy*, 2nd edn., Wiley-Liss, 2005. Reproduced with permission of John Wiley & Sons.

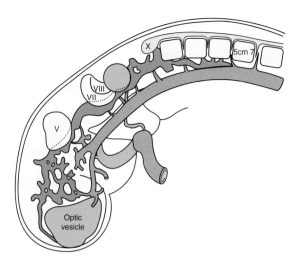

Figure 1.10 Dorsal aortae (purple), aortic arch arteries (green) with AA1 well developed and AA2 in formation, primitive internal carotid (red) connects via the trigeminal artery with the neural arcade consisting of head plexus covering forebrain and midbrain (pink) and the primitive hindbrain channels (pink). Four occipital somites are depicted.

- Posterior alveolar (StV2), Tessier zone 6: molars, posterior maxillary wall.
- Zygomatico - facial (StV2), Tessier zone 7: malar bone (lower zygoma).
- Zygomatico - temporal (StV2), Tessier zone 8: post-orbital bone (upper zygoma).
  (NB: Tessier zone 9 is the rarest cleft, most likely because of its dual blood supply – the anastomosis between the lacrimal and zygomatico-temporal.)

All of the above fields contain one or more membranous bones, *all of which are derived from neural crest*. (NB: in craniofacial development the only bones that are derived from mesoderm (lateral plate) are the basisphenoid, part of the temporal bone, and the occipital bone complex below the superior nuchal line. All remaining bones arise from neural crest.)

Developmental fields of the naso-oropharynx containing muscle

What about fields that are composed exclusively of muscle? This would include the muscles of the soft palate and pharynx. How do we categorize their blood supply? What could go wrong in development to produce the pathologies associated with cleft palate?

The physiology of speech depends upon muscles that are both intrinsic to the soft palate and those that are extrinsic to it. The following concepts are essential for understanding the developmental anatomy of this integrated muscle system.

(1) Craniofacial muscles arise from paraxial mesoderm (PAM).
(2) PAM is segmentally organized into 7 somitomeres and 35 somites. The process of mesoderm segmentation takes place

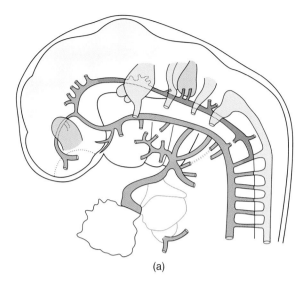

(a)

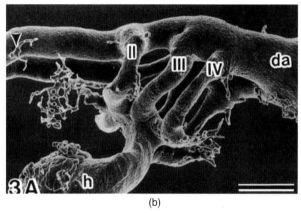

(b)

Figure 1.11 (a) shows the internal carotid artery has extended up to the forebrain and midbrain; it has segmental branches. PHCs have morphed into longitudinal neural arteries (still pink). These will later on move to the midline and fuse to form the basilar system. Paired segmental branches from the dorsal aortae supply the cervical somites and spinal cord. These will later break down and form a new secondary vertical axis, the vertebral artery which will, in turn, anastomose with the segmentalized basilar trunk. (b) shows four aortic arch arteries connecting the outlet tract with the dorsal aortae. The arrowhead is the primitive trigeminal. The pharyngeal arch remnants form a plexus that will morph into the external carotid system. Hiruma T. Formation of the pharyngeal arch arteries in the chick embryo. Observations of corrosion casts by scanning electron microscopy. *Anat Embryol* 1995; 191:415–424. Reproduced with permission of Springer Science and Business Media.

during stages 7–8 and proceeds in a cranio-caudal direction. Each segment will be supplied by a designated motor nerve.
(3) Craniofacial mesenchyme is predominantly neural crest, not mesoderm. From stages 9 to 14 this mesenchyme becomes itself segmented into five pharyngeal arches.
(4) Located in the core of each arch is an *aortic arch artery* that spans from the cardiac outflow tract located below the future pharynx to the dorsal aorta lying above the pharynx. The fifth aortic arch artery involutes and the fourth takes over the supply for the structures of both pharyngeal arches 4 and 5.

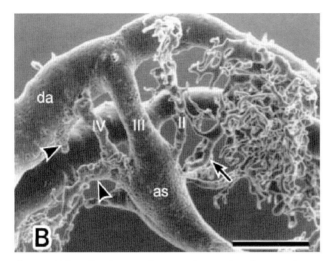

Figure 1.12 Scanning electron microscopy shows embryo in reversed position (head to right). At this stage the pharyngeal arch plexus is very dense. Just caudal to the fourth aortic arch artery, arrowheads indicate the stumps of the involuting fifth aortic arch artery. AA4 will subsequently supply both pharyngeal arches 4 and 5. There is no sixth pharyngeal arch in mammals (in fish, yes). The artery assigned to this mesnchyme, AA6, will be incorporated into the pulmonary circulation. Hiruma T. Formation of the pharyngeal arch arteries in the chick embryo. Observations of corrosion casts by scanning electron microscopy. *Anat Embryol* 1995; 191:415–424. Reproduced with permission of Springer Science and Business Media.

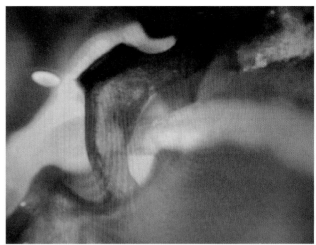

Figure 1.14 The stapedial system develops at stage 17 precisely when the cranial nerves emerge. The stem ascends through the tympanic cavity, goes intracranial, and follows the intracranial sensory nerves throughout the dura. A forward branch to the trigeminal ganglion picks up intracrancial V1 and gains access to the orbit where it supplies all extraocular structures. From the trigeminal ganglion a branch goes extracranial to connect to the maxillary system as the middle meningeal. From the typanic cavity a branch tracks extracranial following chorda tympani until it connects with the external carotid system. When the stem involutes, all the branches of stapedial survive on anastomoses with other systems, such as the opthalmic from the internal carotid, the external carotid distal to facial artery to form the internal maxillary, and multiple connections with other branches of the external carotid system, such as occipital. Huang C-H, Hu DK. Noggin heterozygyous mice: an animal model for congenital conductive hearing loss in humans. *Hum Mol Genet* 2008; 17(6):844–853. Reproduced with permission of Oxford University Press.

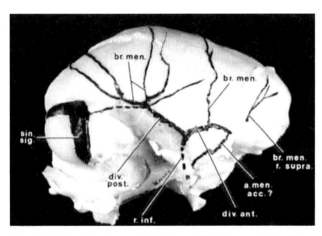

Figure 1.13 Dural arteries are all derivatives of the intracranial stapedial system. Upon involution of the stem these all form anastomoses with branches of the internal and external carotid systems. Diamond MK. Homologies of the stapedial artery in humans, with a reconstruction of the primitive stapedial artery configuration in euprimates. *Am J Phys Anthro* 1991; 84:433–462. Reproduced with permission of John Wiley & Sons.

(5) Despite textbook dogma, there is no sixth pharyngeal arch. The sixth aortic arch artery becomes incorporated into the pulmonary circulation.

(6) The muscles that develop within the pharyngeal arches originate from paraxial mesoderm that becomes physically incorporated into the arch system. Hypoplasia or aplasia of palate musculature can occur from an intrinsic defect of the

mesoderm or from a failure of the arterial axis that supplies it. Such defects can be isolated to a single muscle or can be more global as in hemi-palate.

Craniofacial mesoderm assigned to the orbit and to the first three pharyngeal arches comes from seven somitomeres (Sm). These are incompletely separated balls of mesoderm with a hollow center. The first three somitomeres produce the extraocular muscles (Figure 1.15). The remaining somitomeres are assigned as follows. Sm4 gives rise to the muscles of mastication in the first pharyngeal arch; these are innervated by the Vth cranial nerve. Sm5 and Sm6 produce the muscles of facial expression in the second phayrngeal arch; these are innervated by the VIIth cranial nerve. Sm7 contains the muscles of the soft palate; in contrast to dogma, these are innervated by the IXth cranial nerve *via the Xth cranial nerve*, the vagus. Somites are completely separate from one another. Somites 1 and 2 provide the muscles of phonation in the fourth and fifth pharyngeal arches; these are supplied by the Xth cranial nerve. Mesoderm from S1–S4 that is not incorporated into the pharyngeal arches produces the muscles of the tongue, the sternocleidomastoid, and the trapezius.

The pharyngeal arch system is transient; so too are the aortic arch arteries that originally supplied each pharyngeal arch. These break down, reorganize, and eventually are connected

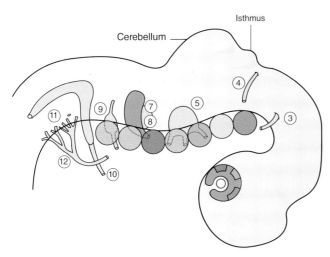

Figure 1.15 The pathways of extraocular muscles from somitomeres 1, 2, 3, and 5 to their insertion sites on the sclera are depicted.

to the carotid; thus is formed the external carotid artery and all its derivatives serving the pharyngeal arch structures of the face – but not the maxilla. Recall that the V2-associated stapedial artery system forms an anastomosis distal to the facial artery and to the superficial temporal artery – thus is born the system of arteries emanating from the pterygo-palatine fossa that supplies the maxilla and inferior oro-nasopharynx. These are responsible for the bone-bearing fields of the maxilla.

Let us look at the arterial axes that supply the soft palate. The *primary axis of the soft palate* is the ascending pharyngeal artery. It supplies the most primitive muscles, that is those that develop first, but are last to be affected. The absence of a soft palate is a survivable condition; not so the absence of pharyngeal muscles. The *palatal branch* of ascending pharyngeal supplies the palatoglossus. The *pharyngeal branch* of the ascending pharyngeal supplies the superior constrictor, middle constrictor, salpingopharyngeus, and stylopharyngeus, and palatopharyngeus. These are all important for swallowing; the first two constrict the pharynx while the latter two function as elevators of the pharynx. The *secondary axes of the soft palate* are: the *descending* (a.k.a. greater) *palatine branch* of the StV2 distal internal maxillary artery and the *ascending palatine branch* of the facial artery. These axes supply the more recent additions to the soft palate: levator veli palatini, tensor veli palatini, and uvulus. The first two have attachments to the tympanic tube while uvulus relates to the posterior spine of the palatine bone.

Where do these muscles originate? Tensor veli palatini arises from somitomere 4; it is supplied by the Vth cranial nerve. Levator veli palatini arises from somitomere 7; it is supplied – with controversy – by cranial nerve IX vs. the cranial portion of the spinal accessory nerve: cranial nerve XI. All of the pharyngeal muscles under consideration here are supplied by the cranial portion of spinal accessory nerve: cranial nerve XI. The reason for the overlap between cranial nerves

IX and XI is that they are in register with the same zone of the brain stem; their nuclei simply represent two parallel columns reflecting different functions. The constrictors are likely to arise from somites 2 and 3; their motor supply is cranial nerve XI. Stylopharyngeus relates to the second arch and therefore is likely to arise from somitomere 5 (or 6). Salpingopharyngeus relates to the portion of the tympanic tube that is developmentally related to the third arch; thus it likely comes from somitomere 7.

Knowing the above facts, we can make some general statements about muscle pathologies in cleft palate. All defects of the hard palate, either primary (the premaxilla), from the incisive foramen forward, or secondary, from the incisive foramen backward, involve deficiencies in membranous bone. These are readily diagnosed by physical examination and 3D CT scanning. Such bone defects involve one or more arterial axes of the StV2 stapedial system supplying the maxilla. The nucleus of V2 resides within the second rhombomere of the hindbrain (r2). Thus defects of the maxillary complex represent deficiencies in the population of neural crest cells arising from that segment of the neural fold in genetic register with r2. Strictly by logic a bone defect occurs when something is intrinsically wrong with the r2 mesenchymal population or there is defective formation of a neurovascular axis supplying a portion of the r2 population. The latter mechanism is more specific; it explains isolated bone defects at later stages in development rather than a global failure of neural crest mesenchyme in the first arch.

Mandibular defects associated with cleft palate, as in the Pierre Robin sequence, can be diagnosed in a similar way. Defects involving any developmental zone of the mandible involve one or more arterial axes of the StV3 stapedial system. The nucleus of V3 resides within the third rhombomere of the hindbrain (r3). Thus, defects of the mandibular complex represent deficiencies in the population of neural crest cells arising from that segment of the neural fold in genetic register with r3. Tensor veli palatini is the sole palate muscle belonging to the first arch; it comes from somitomere Sm4 (which also bears the muscles of mastication). For this reason, any form of cleft palate involving TVP implies a more proximal "hit" to the StV2–StV3 system or a more global involvement of first arch neural crest.

Summary of neural crest and mesodermal derivatives that contribute to cleft palate

- r0/r1 = bone fields from stapedial V1: perpendicular plate of the ethmoid, septum, columella, prolabium.
- r2 = bone fields from stapedial V2: vomer, premaxilla, palatal shelf, inferior turbinate.
- r3 = bone fields from stapedial V3: mandible.
- r5 = neural crest to arterial wall of ascending palatine branch of facial > soft palate muscles.

- r7 = neural crest to arterial wall of ascending pharyngeal to soft palate/pharynx muscles.
- Sm4 = mesoderm of tensor veli palatini.
- Sm7 = mesoderm of levator veli palatini, palatoglossus, palatopharyngeus, uvulus.

Mechanisms of developmental field failure

Now that we have an idea of the various neurovascular axes, let us consider a first mechanism of failure, *alteration of function of the growth cone*. Because growth of the axes proceeds outward, the earlier in time the failure occurs the more structures will be affected. For example, the premaxilla is the terminal field for the medial nasopalatine axis. It has three sub-fields: the central incisor, lateral incisor, and the frontal process of the premaxilla (which lies tucked beneath the frontal process of the maxilla). Any perturbation of the nasopalatine axis will show up first as a deformation in the inferolateral rim of the piriform fossa. Next the lateral incisor and its bony housing are affected. Finally, a total loss of premaxilla can occur (Figure 1.16).

A simplifying concept involves failure of the vascular growth cone (Figures 1.17 and 1.18). The growth cone of the artery consists of an endothelial tip sprout that produces PDGF-*B* which is chemoattractive for pericytes and positive for the receptor PDGFR*B*. These cells distribute themselves along the abluminal wall of the vessel along which they secrete cytoplasmic processes.

We turn our attention to the specific anatomic variations of cleft palate. We postulate that fusion of these mesenchymal tissue units (*partner fields*) requires that they be physically positioned relative to each other within a *critical contact distance*. If the tissue volume of one of the fields is reduced, and the critical contact distance is exceeded, fusion will not occur and a cleft will result. A second mechanism involves the *alteration of fusion potential of the epithelial surface*. The stability of the epithelium is controlled by sonic hedgehog (SHH). As long as this is active, the epithelial surface will be incapable of fusion. SHH is itself inhibited by BMP-4 of the underlying mesenchyme. The total amount of BMP-4 produced by a field is proportional to its mesenchymal volume. Thus, any reduction in BMP-4 production will promote the stability of the epithelial surface and prevent its fusion.

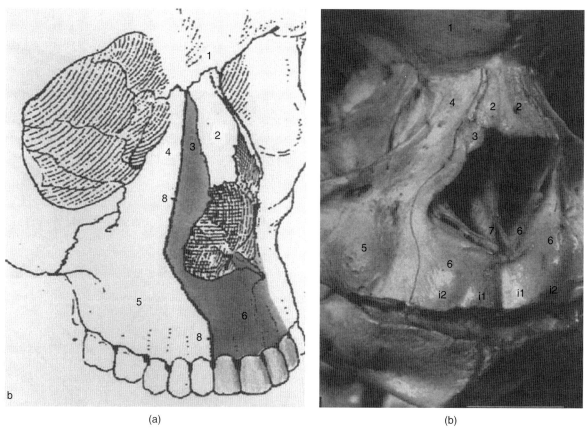

(a)   (b)

Figure 1.16 The alveolar walls of the premaxilla (PMx) are supplied by medial nasopalatine artery; the labial alveolar wall receives collateral supply from the medial infraorbital. Premaxilla has three subfields: the medial incisor, lateral incisor, and the frontal process. Since the frontal process is the most distal, it is always affected first in deficiency states. Bartezko K, Jacob M. A re-evaluation of the premaxillary bone in humans. *Anat Embryol* 2004; 207:417–437. Reproduced with permission of Springer Science and Business Media.

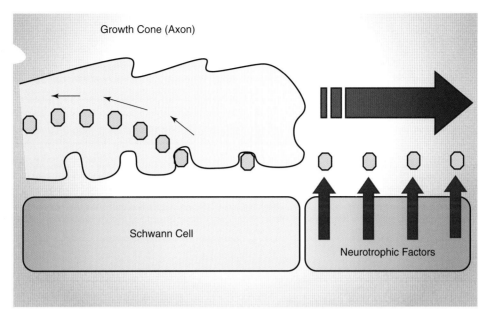

Figure 1.17 Schwann cells pick up nutrients and growth factors from the environment and transmit them back into the axon. NGF (nerve growth factor) produced by the pericytes promotes growth of the neural axis in register with the vascular axis. Adapted from: May F et al. Nerve replacement strategeis for cavernous nerves. *Europ Urol* 2005; 48:372–378.

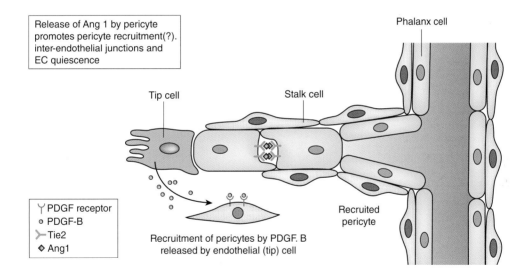

Figure 1.18 Vascular endothelial growth factor (VEGF) produced by the nerve cone causes outgrowth of endothelial cells from a vascular axis. These endothelial cells form the core of the new vessel or they add on to an existing vessel to elongate it. But stabilization of the new vessel by pericytes is now required. Tip cells produce PDGF-Beta that recruits pericytes to come alongside the endothelial axis and stabilize it. Adapted from: Quaegebeur A, Lange C, Carmeliet P. The neurovascular link in health and disease: molecular mechanisms and therapeutic implications. *Neuron* 2011; 71:406–424. Reproduced with permission of Elsevier.

Fusion of the palate is bi-directional, proceeding both forward and backward from the incisive foramen. Closure of the primary palate involves interaction between the alveolar processes of the premaxilla (medial nasopalatine artery) and the canine-bearing mesial maxilla (lateral nasopalatine artery). In addition, the frontal process of premaxilla fuses with the overlying frontal process of the maxilla. This latter structure is supplied by the medial branch of the infraorbital and belongs to the Tessier cleft zone 4.

Fusion of the secondary hard palate takes place concomitantly. It involves union between the vomer and the horizontal palatal shelf. The vomer is the proximal tissue field along the medial nasopalatine shelf. Its partner field, the horizontal palatine shelf, is actually supplied by two distinct neurovascular axes: lateral nasopalatine on the nasal side and greater palatine artery on the oral side. Sinus formation within the horizontal shelf has been previously reported. *All sinuses represent the separation of adjacent fields from one another.*

It is useful to think of field development as a flow of mesenchyme into a geometric space. Flow into the palatal shelf appears to follow an anterior-to-posterior gradient. Thus, insufficiency will always manifest itself in the "newest" zone, that is, posteriorly. The fusion process of the secondary hard palate is anterior-to-posterior.

Cleft palate: analysis by zones

Tessier cleft zone 14: a misleading concept

The zone does not exist. This was a *trompe l'oeil* for Tessier. The fontal bone is not singular; it is two halves which fuse in the midline. Each hemi-frontal bone is a bilaminar structure with four develomental fields, all of which are organized around four StV1 neurovascular axes. Zones 13 and 12 are supplied by the supraorbital externally and internally these zones are supported by the medial meningeal flowing over the ethmoid plate. Zones 11 and 10 are supplied externally by the supraorbital, while internally the lacrimal supplies the lateral orbital. Development of the frontal bone takes place by the membranous ossification of the neural crest which migrates from rhombomere 0 (zones 13–12) and from rhombomere 1 (zones 11–10). This ectomesenchyme follows a pathway alongside the midbrain and forebrain, forward over the orbit and downward to form the nasal process. This mesenchyme is the source of the dura and dermis within which the membranous bone fields develop. The

neural crest populates and pushes forward a unique ectodermal envelope which is described below (Figure 1.19).

The epidermis of the zones overlying the forehead and nose is likewise unique. As the r0/r1 neural crest flows forward it tracks beneath the overlying *non-neural ectoderm* to produce the skin of the V1 region. Non-neural ectoderm (NNE) is a layer of tissue overlying the prosencephalon (forebrain). NNE acts like ectoderm; it is in genetic register with the six underlying prosomeres of the forebrain (p1–p6). The interaction between the r0/r1 beneath the NNE covering the most rostral prosomeres, p5 and p6, produces frontonasal skin, a structure radically different from the remainder of facial skin and body. (NB: The reader will recall that the source of dermis of all head and neck skin down to the level of C2 is not mesodermal, but neural crest.) For this reason, in frontonasal dysplasia the skin appears different in thickness and consistency.

Closure of the frontal bone zones takes place by a process of *apoptosis*, a controlled breakdown of tissue that allows the frontal fields to move forward into the midline. Of course, the driving force for this is the medialization of the orbits, a process that is dictated by the growth pattern of the brain and the anterior cranial base. The ethmoid complex is interposed between the orbits. Failure of apoptosis in the ethmoid zones will lead to hypertelorisim. Since the ethmoid is a bilateral structure, such hypertelorism can be unilateral or bilateral. Probably the apoptosis process required of the frontal bone is subject to whatever degree of apoptosis is taking place in the ethmoid complex.

Midline pathologies can manifest as a simple excess of tissue or as a fusion failure or cleft (sic). For this reason, it appeared to Tessier as if this were truly an autonomous zone. Recall that the pituitary sits in a cavity between two bones: the anterior neural crest presphenoid and a posterior mesodermal post-sphenoid

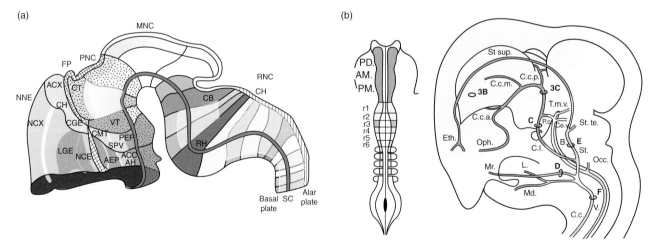

Figure 1.19 (a) Non-neural ectoderm overlying prosomeres p5 (blue) and p6 (red) is not formally neural crest; it is responsible for the frontonasal epidermis. Frontonasal dermis results from sub-epidermal forward flow of more posterior neural crest. (b) Note neural crest contributions to craniofacial arterial systems. Etchevers HC, Couly G, Le Douarin NM. Morphogenesis of the branchial vascular sector. *Trends Cardiovasc Med* 2002; 12(7):299–306. Reproduced with permission of Elsevier.

(basisphenoid). The former has a sinus while the latter is solid. Fusion failures extending backward into the sphenoid have a biologic limit to viability. Failure of apoptosis in the midline of zone 13 also leads to a residual excess of mesenchyme in the midline; this is normal orbital approximation and results in hypertelorism.

Medialization can also be altered by the presence of an encephalocoele that can seek out a field failure between any of the zones to achieve an extracranial position and thereby block the closure. The escape routes of encephalocoeles are well documented, be they forward through the frontal bone zones, in the midline or in paramedian positions.

Neuroembryologic simplification of zones 1 and zone 13/zone 2 and zone 12

Tessier originally perceived that a fundamental difference existed between clefts (states of mesenchymal deficiency and/or excess) involving the maxilla and those involving the orbit. At the time, neuroembryology of the area was not recognized. In our correspondence, Tessier was impressed by the correlation between his findings and the regional sensory neuroanatomy (Flores-Sarnat, *et al.*, 2007). The structures of the nose are unique in that the topology of the fields supplied by the neurovascular axes of StV1 and StV2 is not one of simple planar separation, rather these fields are *interlocking*. This makes the interpretation of congenital field defects difficult. The best way to keep things straight is for us to consider these zones by their neuroanatomy, with 1–2 supplied by StV2 axes while those of zones 13 and 12 are supplied STV1 axes. For this reason, we are going to violate the traditional way of describing Tessier

clefts in this region. In the end, as he himself commented, the observations will be clearer (Ewings and Carstens, 2009).

Tessier cleft zone 1

Zone 1 consists of the structures in the midline of the nose and mouth, the paried vomer and perpendicular ethmoid bones. The nasal cavity is supplied by two neurovascular pedicles: StV2 medial nasopalatine axis, and StV1 internal medial nasal axis. The medial zone of dorsal nasal skin and nasal bones are supplied by the StV1 external medial nasal axis (Figures 1.20 and 1.21).

Paired medial nasopalatine arteries supply paired vomerine bones. Occasionally, these bones may fail to fuse. Alternatively, the intervomerine space may allow for the descent of a tumor or encephalocoele into the oral cavity. Such situations require concomitant pathology of the perpendicular plates of the ethmoid. In the routine case, a deficiency of vomerine mesenchyme will impair the inhibition of sonic hedgehog (SHH) and thus the epithelial surface of that vomer front-to-back fusion process with the palatal shelf. If the palatal shelf is normal the cleft will be narrow (Figure 1.22). In the minimal state, the palate cleft is very posterior, at the posterior nasal spine, but as the degree of vomer deficiency increases, the palate cleft will extend forward until it reaches the incisive foramen.

When a minimal vomerine deficiency exists in isolation, the width of the palate cleft will be fairly narrow and uniform. The vomer develops in posterior-to-anterior sequence; as it does so, it descends from front to back into the palatal plane like a scimitar. Thus, the most vulnerable zone of the vomer is posterior

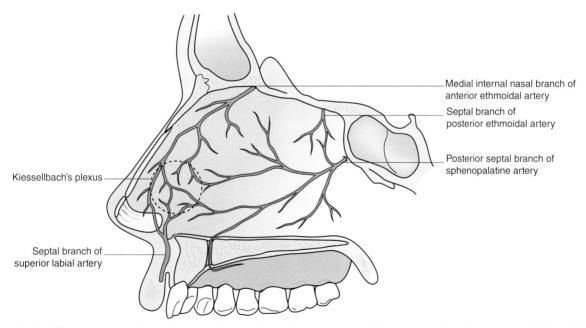

Figure 1.20 The obliquely-oriented midline of the septum is a vascular interface zone between StV1 posterior and anterior ethmoid and StV2 medial nasopalatine arteries.

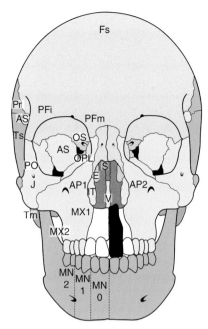

Figure 1.21 The piriform rim is unaffected. Lateral incisors are intact because of collateral blood flow from the medial infraorbital and greater palatine arteries. Loss of the central incisor, narrow midline cleft from the deficient vomer can be either in the palatal plane or elevated above it.

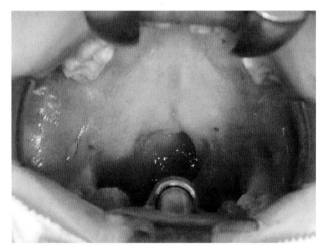

Figure 1.22 The vomer cleft.

and inferior. Vomerine-based palate clefts can start as a posterior notch in which the vomer is literally lifted upward and away from the palatal plane. If the cleft runs all the way to the incisive foramen, compromise of the arterial supply to the ipsilateral premaxilla is likely. The differential diagnosis of these clefts depends on whether the palatal shelf is uninvolved or involved because, in the latter situation, the cleft is wider with the posterior aspect more deficient (wider cleft). Bilateral vomer pathology in the absence of all other field defects results in a bilateral cleft palate that is narrow and can potentially run forward to the

incisive foramen. Note that since the vomer is a narrow structure, changes in width of the palatal cleft are due to additional involvement of the palatal shelf based on the StV2 greater palatine artery and/or (rarely) lateral nasopalatine artery.

Tessier cleft zone 13

Zone 13 consists of the midline structures of the cranial base and of the forehead up to, but not including, the eyebrow. It interdigitates with zone 1 because it shares common arterial axes supplying both structures of the upper nasal cavity and the medial external nasal soft tissues of the nose.

Let's begin with the internal upper medial structures of the nasal cavity, the perpendicular plates of the ethmoid and septum. These are supplied by the posterior and anterior ethmoid arteries. The StV1 posterior ethmoid arises within the orbit, enters the posterior air cells and then does two things: (i) it tracks upward through the cribriform plate and the presphenoid to gain access to the dura mater as the meningeal branch supplying the meninges over the ethmoid complex; and (ii) it enters the nasal cavity to supply the perpendicular plate of the ethmoid and the posterior superior septum.

Defects in the posterior ethmoid axis can selectively influence hypertrophy or distrophy of the ethmoid complex and consequent ethmoid-based hyper/hypotelorism. A vertical deficiency of the perpendicular plate of the ethmoid causes a *high arched palate* in which case the vomer has successfully fused with the palatal shelves (Figure 1.23). In severe cases, a small ethmoid can retract a normal vomer so far upward out of the palatal plane that fusion is impossible, thereby leading to a midline cleft palate with foreshortening of the vomer. Diagnosis of the latter condition depends upon the physical size of the vomer discerned either by inspection or using a 3D CT scan.

The StV1 anterior ethmoid artery enters from the orbits to supply the anterior and middle ethmoid air cells and thence proceeds to supply the frontal sinus. It has three destinies.

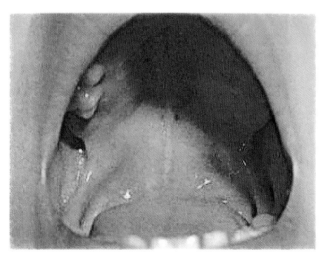

Figure 1.23 High arched palate. Deficient ethmoid can lift a normal vomer upward and create a barrel-shaped vault.

(1) It tracks upward through the cribiform plate to supply the dura underlying zones 13 and 12.

(2) Internal nasal branches descend medially over the anterior superior septum and laterally to supply the superior and middle turbinate. Defects in this axis explain upsilateral ethmoid hypertropy and hypotrophy and consequent changes in orbital position and/or dystopias. They also can explain warping or absence of the septum.

(3) The anterior ethmoid supplies the nasal bone from its internal surface. A defect here can cause absence of the nasal bone. The artery emerges between the nasal bone and the upper lateral cartilage to run forward and downward. A defect in this part of the axis causes the nasal skin cleft noted by Tessier in zone 1. Its terminus follows along the upper and caudal border of the septum to supply columella and prolabium. Defects in this part of the axis are responsible for rare cases of absent columella, with or without affectation of the prolabium. Note that the prolabium is generally autonomous as it gets a collateral supply from a branch of medial nasaopalatine that penetrates through the premaxilla to enter the prolabium from below.

The intracranial anatomy of zone 13 is of great importance. The StV1 ethmoid branch of the anterior ethmoid can lead via its medial dural branches to hypertrophy of the anterior cranial fossa between the midline and the medial border of the cribriform plate, that is the olfactory groove. This enlarges the cribriform plate medial to the ethmoid labyrinth. The result is hypertelorism. A defect in the field borders allows for the escape of an encephalocoele into the nose. The StV1 medial branch of the supratrochlear artery supplies the external frontal skin running from the midline to the medial border of the eyebrow. The skin overlying a deficiency site can atrophy while that over a zone of osseous excess may be dysplastic. The eyebrow is *not* involved.

Tessier cleft zone 2

Zone 2 (Figure 1.24) consists of relatively simplistic oral components, the premaxilla and the internal (lingual) lamina of the alveolus housing the central and lateral incisors. These structures are supplied by the StV2 medial nasopalatine artery. The external (labial) alveolar lamina housing the medial and lateral incisors is supplied by the StV2 medial infraorbital. It also helps support the frontal process of the maxilla. Note that the internal (lingual) lamina of the alveolus housing the lateral incisor territory has an additional collateral supply from the StV2 greater palatine. This explains the great variability in nature seen in the presence or absence of the lateral incisor. On the other hand, the frontal process of the premaxilla appears to be uniquely dependent on the medial sphenopalatine. Because bone is the most distal element of the premaxilla it is the most vulnerable part of the premaxilla.

The cleft process, when the medial nasopalatine is involved, affects the premaxilla in a very predictable sequence. The frontal process is always involved, even in the most trivial of clefts; this

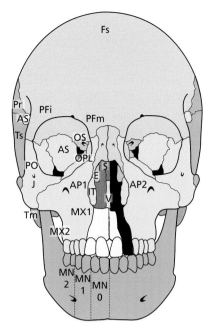

Figure 1.24 Piriform defect plus loss of the lateral incisor. Probable deficiency in greater palatine field explaining the width of the cleft.

causes a deformity of the piriform fossa. At the lateral incisor zone, an external groove will appear in the alveolus. Further deficiency causes the loss of the lateral incisor. If, for any reason, the most distal aspect of the lateral nasopalatine or that of the greater palatine are affected, the back wall of the alveolus fails to develop and a full-thickness defect of the primary palate ensues. The sequence is always the same: from the incisive surface cephalad and from labial to lingual (Figures 1.25 and 1.26).

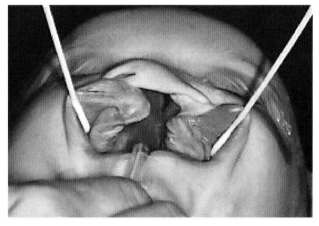

Figure 1.25 Cleft lip/cleft palate. Common pathology involving ipsilateral vomer and premaxilla with reduction in the contralateral palatal shelf. The anterior head of nasalis should be inserted into the lateral incisor field but occupies a position beneath the skin of the nostril sill. The posterior head of nasalis, normally inserted at the canine field, falls into the piriform fossa.

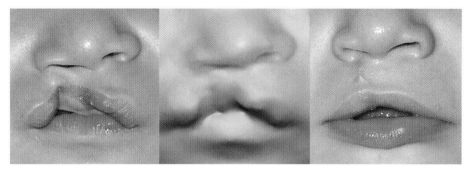

Figure 1.26 Minimal cleft lip. Note that the forme fruste has all the features of a complete cleft: depressed nostril floor and malposition of nasalis. The greater the degree of mesenchymal deficiency, the less BMP-4 is produced. This in turn, maintains SHH in the epithelium at high levels, thus preventing fusion.

Tessier zone 12

Zone 12 is analogous to zone 13. It consists of intracranial and extracranial structures and extranasal structures. The intracranial part of zone 12 corresponds to the internal lamina of the frontal bone overlying the frontal sinus. The anatomy of the dural arterial supply here is uncertain but may involve contributions from the intraorbital part of the ophthalmic artery or of its branches through the anterior ethmoid. Excess tissue here can enlarge the sinus. This in turn can lead to orbital dystopia (Tessier *et al.*, 1977).

These are all supplied by the terminal branch of the ophthalmic artery; this gives rise to two branches: the StV1 medial branch of supratrochlear artery supplies the frontal bone and the StV1 infratrochlear artery (dorsal nasal artery) supplies the lateral nasal wall. The medial supratrochlear supplies the external lamina of the frontal bone and the forehead. Excess in this zone can enlarge the frontal sinus; the glabella can be flat. Deficiencies cause cutaneous defects such as coloboma or notch in the medial 1/3 of the brow. Inferiorly, the infratrochlear axis supplies the lacrimal sac. There are two descending branches: one runs along the nasal dorsum while the other follows along the lateral nasal wall. This latter is involved in cleft zone 11. Deficiency of zone 11 shows up most commonly as a mild vertical deficiency of nasal skin. The lacrimal system is unaffected. The formation of the nostril involves induction of soft tissues by the nasal placode. When this process is interrupted, the result is either a proboscis or the outright loss of the structure altogether, a condition called hemi-nose. It is of note that the proboscis, when present, descends from the lacrimal zone. Clefts involving the infratrochlear axis are associated with absence of a recognizable lacrimal apparatus (Figure 1.27).

Tessier cleft zone 3

Zone 3 consists of the inferior turbinate and the corresponding lateral nasal wall, the palatal shelf, and the palatine bone. Blood supply to the lateral nasal wall comes from the StV2 lateral nasopalatine artery, including the nasal mucoperiosteum of the palatal shelf while the StV2 descending palatine artery supplies via the greater palatine artery the oral mucoperiosteum of the palatal shelf and via the lesser palatine artery the palatine bone proper (Figures 1.28 and 1.29).

A variety of cleft palate presentations can occur in this zone. The palatine bone has a horizontal shelf that develops from lateral to medial and from anterior to posterior. Isolated defects in this bone field range from a simple midline notch to complete elimination of the bone. Because the lesser palatine artery is responsible for the tensor veli palatini, this muscle may be affected as well. But the major blood supply to the muscles in the soft palate is the ascending palatine artery from the cervical division of the facial artery and the external carotid derivative.

The greater palatine artery sweeps forward to supply the lingual mucoperiosteum of the alveolus as well as the oral mucoperiosteum of the hard palate. The bone field develops from front-to-back and from lateral-to-medial. Since the closure pattern of the hard palate to the vomer follows the same vectors, an anterior mesenchymal defect will interrupt the "zipper" mechanism from that spot backwards. On the other hand, if the mesenchymal defect occurs further posteriorly in the hard palate field, palate closure will exist anteriorly, while a cleft appears posteriorly.

Tessier cleft zone 11

This zone consists of the frontal process of the maxilla. It involves the lacrimal groove and the lacrimal segment of the medial lower eyelid. Palate clefts of zone 3 are frequently associated with zone 11 pathology. The arterial axis of zone 11 is the StV1 lateral branch of the infratrochlear artery. For this reason, zone 11 clefts destroy the lacrimal apparatus – which remains intact in other cleft zones. There is marked foreshortening of the lateral nasal skin.

Cleft palate associated with mandibular deficiency states

Development of the mandible is similar in plan and execution to that of the maxilla, especially when one considers the anatomy of the alveolar apparatus. In both cases, dental units based upon neural crest blastema occupy a space between two intervening membranous bone units. Running through the membranous bone is either the superior alveolar artery or the

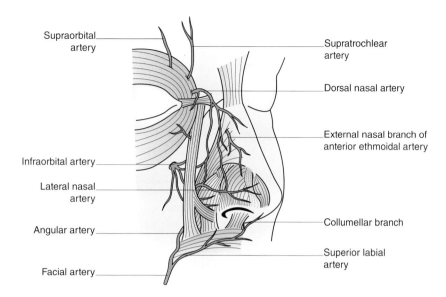

Figure 1.27 Zones of the nose. The infratrochlear artery emerges just above the medial canthus and divides into two branches, the more medial dorsal nasal artery defines the soft tissues of the paramedian nasal dorsum, zone 12. The lateral branch supplies zone 11 and overlies the lacrimal system; it anastomes with the angular branch of facial artery (external carotid system).

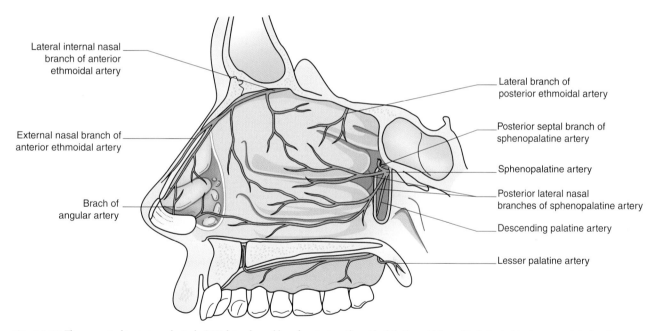

Figure 1.28 The upper turbinate is exclusively StV1 lateral nasal br. of posterior ethmoid while the middle and inferior turbinates are an interface between lateral nasal br. of anterior ethmoid and lateral nasopalatine. Knock-out of the latter axis (as in a zone 3 cleft) wipes out the entire inferior lateral nasal wall with exposure of the sinus to the oral cavity and loss of the ipsilateral palatal shelf.

inferior alveolar artery. The external (buccolabial) lamina of the maxilla supplied by the medial and lateral branches of infraorbital artery cover respectively the incisor/canine zone and the premolar zone while the external branch of superior alveolar artery supplies the molar zone. The internal (lingual) zone is supplied by the medial nasopalatine artery to the incisors while the greater palatine artery supplies all remaining dental zones. The external (buccolabial) lamina of mandibular alveolus is supplied by, posteriorly, the mylohyoid artery and, anteriorly, the submental branch of the facial. The internal (lingual) lamina

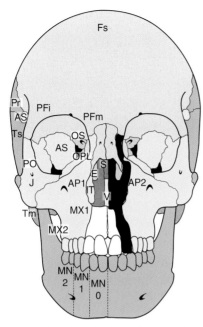

Figure 1.29 Entire piriform fossa dysplastic/absent. Knock-out of maxillary sinus. Lacrimal system uninvolved.

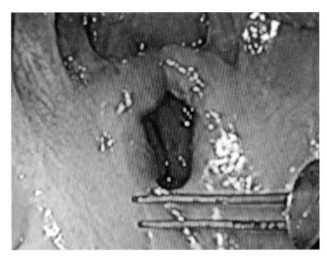

Figure 1.30 Arches at stage 14 and 17. Electrodes stimulating tensor veli palatini. Note ipsilateral closure of the soft palate at the level of the alveolus.

of mandibular alveolus is supplied by the lingual artery. Thus we see a commonality of bone units supporting the dentition.

The mandible has a third zone, the ramus, which is not part of the original embryonic dentary bone. It fact, its evolutionary history is quite distinct. Not surprisingly, the ramus has an entirely different blood supply. Here we find the source of nearly all dentofacial anomalies involving the mandible. Most importantly, for our purposes, is the situation of cleft palate involving the Pierre Robin anomalad. This entity involves contributions from the first and third arches since the muscle blastema of the palate arise from somitomeres 4 and 7. Associated problems with the fourth arch have also been documented. Retropositioning of the tongue and its potential interference with bony palate shelf development is one possibility. Another possibility is that a similarity in genetic programming exists between the ramus of the mandible and the palatal shelves themselves.

Soft palate defects: isolated vs. combined

Diagnosis: the simplest solution is direct testing of individual muscles using a muscle stimulator such as that available from Integra Life Sciences (Figure 1.30).

Any defect affecting the StV2 components of the hard palate (horizontal palatine shelf, palatine bone) is related to the first pharyngeal arch and therefore has the potential to affect the sole muscle arising from somitomere 4: tensor veli palatini (TVP). Because this muscle relates to the cartilagenous lateral wall of the pharyngotympanic tube it is associated with opening the tube to equalize air pressure, as in swallowing and yawning. First arch pathology affecting the wall of the lateral tube and TVP may explain the relationship seen in unilateral clefts between ipsilateral muscle function and middle ear disease.

Although the developmental fields of the third pharyngeal arch do not contribute membranous bone components to the palate, the cartilagenous medial wall of the pharyngotympanic tube is a third arch derivative. Levator veli palatini arises from somitomere 7 and, when dysfunctional, diminished elevation of the soft palate can be observed. In many cases of microtia, third arch pathology is present. These patients present almost uniformly with a characteristic dampening of physiologic soft palate lift ipsilateral to the microtia.

Failure of midline fusion of the soft palate presents in a posterior-to-anterior gradient. The "cleft" is simply a mesenchymal deficiency – including a reduction in mucosal surface area, with the oral side being more affected than the nasal side. The final muscle pair to form in the soft palate is uvulus. Thus, the first manifestation of the third arch pathology is a midline notch separating these two muscles. As the defect worsens, the levator is affected and the soft palate cleft extends forward toward the posterior nasal spine. Reduction/absence of the helix seen in microtia patients is a manifestation of third arch deficiency. Such patients frequently will demonstrate levator weakness even in the absence of a cleft palate. The combination of third arch with first arch is diagnosed by dysfunction of the tensor vali palatini and/or other osseous deficiency.

Speech problems associated with velopharyngeal insufficiency and/or dysfunction in the absence of cleft palate are not infrequent. Once again, the key to diagnosis is to recognize the existence of individual muscle defects, involving partial or global deficiencies of soft palate muscle. These also include dysfunction of the superior and/or middle constrictor.

Blood supply to the soft palate involves several vessels. The lesser palatine artery from the descending palatine supplies the mucosa. The muscles of the soft palate are supplied by the ascending palatine branch of the cervical division of the facial artery. The ascending pharyngeal artery, proper to the third pharyngeal arch, can also supply the muscles of the palate but its primary target is the superior and inferior constrictors of the pharynx. Isolated defects in the constrictors should be part of the differential diagnosis of non-cleft velopharyngeal insufficiency.

Summary

This chapter has reviewed the developmental anatomy of the oronasopharynx. We have examined the various components that make the mesenchymal structures of the palate. The concept of fields – each with a specific neurovascular axis, each containing neural crest originating from a specific neuromere, each susceptible to failure of formation vs. disruption based upon a growth cone dysfunction – has been presented in detail.

The surgical implications of developmental fields encourage all those concerned with pediatric craniofacial anomalies to work toward a better understanding of the basic mechanisms underlying the complex problems. Surgical solutions based upon a sound embryologic basis with respect for correct field boundaries offer the best chance for the achievement of harmonious growth and correct function (Carstens, 2008c).

References

Carlson, B. M. (2013) *Human Embryology and Molecular Biology*, 5 edn. Philadelphia, PA: Elsevier.

Carstens, M. H. (2000) Spectrum of minimal cleft revisited. *J Craniofac Surg* **11**(3):270–294.

Carstens, M. H. (2002) Development of the facial midline. *J Craniofac Surg* **13**(1):129–187.

Carstens, M. H. (2008a) Neural tube programming and the pathogenesis of craniofacial clefts, part I: the neuromeric organization of the head and neck. *Handb Clin Neurol* **87**:247–276.

Carstens, M. H. (2008b) Neural tube programming and the pathogenesis of craniofacial clefts, part 2: mesenchyme, pharyngeal arches, developmental fields, and the assembly of the human face. *Handb Clin Neurol* **87**:277–339.

Carstens, M. H. (2008c) Developmental field reassignment in unilateral cleft lip: Reconstruction of the premaxilla. In: Losee, J.E., Kirschner, R.E. (eds) *Comprehensive Cleft Care, chapter 15*. New York, NY: McGraw-Hill Medical.

Ewings, E. L. and Carstens, M. H. (2009) Neuroembryology and functional anatomy of craniofacial clefts. *Indian J Plast Surg* October Suppl. S19–S34.

Flores-Sarnat, L., Sarnat, H. B., Hahn, J. S, *et al.* (2007) Axes and gradients of the neural tube form a genetic classification of nervous system malformations. *Handb Clin Neurol* **83**:3–11.

Gilbert, S. (2013) *Developmental Biology*, 10 edn. Sunderland, MA: Sinauer Associates Inc.

O'Rahilly, R. and Müller, F. (1996) *Human Embryology and Teratology*. New York, NY: Wiley Liss.

O'Rahilly, R. and Müller, F. (1999) *The Embryonic Human Brain: An Atlas of Developmental Stages*. New York, NY: Wiley Liss.

Tessier, P., Hervouet, F., Lekieffre, M., *et al.* (1977) *Plastic Surgery of the Orbit and Eyelids*. Translated by S. Anthony Wolfe. Paris: Masson (distributed by Year Book Medical Publishers).

CHAPTER 2

Tissue engineering and regenerative medicine: evolving applications towards cleft lip and palate surgery

George K. B. Sándor

Tissue Engineering, University of Oulu, and Institute of Biosciences and Medical Technology, University of Tampere, Finland

Introduction

Tissue engineering was defined in 1993 as an interdisciplinary field of research that applies both the principles of engineering and the processes and phenomena of the life sciences toward the development of biological substitutes that restore, maintain, or improve tissue function (Langer & Vacanti, 1993). In contrast to the classic biomaterials approach, tissue engineering is based on the understanding of tissue formation and regeneration, and aims to induce new functional tissues, rather than just to implant new spare parts. One possible avenue to improve function is to use the reserve of stem cells in the body of an individual to regenerate missing or damaged structures (Sándor, 2013). The lateral thinking stimulated by the possibilities offered by tissue engineering and stem cells has enormous potential. Stem cells may allow regenerative treatment of myocardial infarction tissue (Hare et al., 2009; Panfilov et al., 2013), and may have application in Crohn's disease (Mannon, 2011), the management of recalcitrant graft versus host disease (Kebriaei et al., 2009; Prasad et al., 2011) and other pediatric conditions (Zheng et al., 2013). This chapter explores the possible use of stem cells in the context of cleft lip and palate reconstruction.

Bone as a target tissue for regeneration

Cleft defects by their very nature are associated with missing tissue, whether it is bone, cartilage, muscle, mucosa, or skin and its adnexal structures. As a target tissue, bone is a good candidate to begin tissue engineering efforts. Bone has a low basal metabolic rate and has the capacity to regenerate rather than repair itself with scar tissue (Sándor & Suuronen, 2008).

Bone reconstruction is required when there are defects in bone, or if bone is absent with missing adjacent soft tissue components. There are numerous causes of bone defects. Congenital bony defects in the cranio-maxillofacial skeleton can arise as a result of perturbations of development, as in cleft lip and palate (Carmichael & Sándor, 2008) (Figure 2.1). Ablative surgery, where segments of bone are removed or resected to treat various cysts, tumors, and infections may produce large bony defects (Sándor et al., 2008) (Figure 2.2). Large bony defects may result from accidental injury when tissue may have been traumatically avulsed (Sándor & Carmichael, 2008). Combined mucosal, osseous, and even cartilaginous defects can be reconstructed using flaps and bone grafts, or hopefully, in the future, with alloplastic biomaterials such as bone graft substitutes or even using cell therapy with tissue engineered constructs (Sándor & Suuronen, 2008). The healing of such complicated wounds always relies on the vascularity of the surrounding tissues (Fok et al., 2008; Brown et al., 1988).

Intramembranous versus endochondral bones

The head and neck are favored areas for bony regeneration as the cephalo-cervical blood supply is far more generous than the blood supply to the limbs and axial skeleton. Bone in the head and neck is generally formed by intramembranous ossification, without the need for cartilaginous precursors. This is unlike the more hypoxic environments of the weight-bearing long bones and the bones of the axial skeleton which require an additional step in endochondral ossification. Bones of the head and neck with the exception of the mandible do not require a cartilaginous template. All long bones and bones of the axial skeleton require the endochondral process with the exception of the scapula.

Cleft Lip and Palate Management: A Comprehensive Atlas, First Edition. Edited by Ricardo D. Bennun, Julia F. Harfin, George K. B. Sándor, and David Genecov.
© 2016 John Wiley & Sons, Inc. Published 2016 by John Wiley & Sons, Inc.

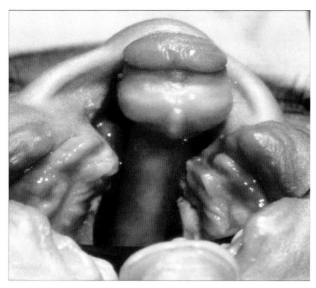

Figure 2.1 Bilateral complete cleft lip and palate deformity with missing bone, cartilage, muscle, mucosa, and skin.

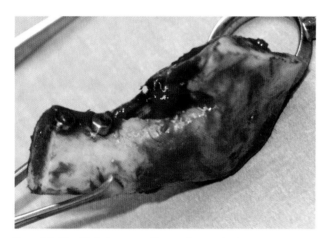

Figure 2.2 Mandibulectomy resection specimen to treat recurrent ameloblastoma. Ablative surgery is one significant cause of cranio-maxillofacial bony defects.

The clinical advances in tissue engineering using cell therapy (Sándor & Suuronen, 2008; Mesimäki *et al.*, 2009; Thesleff *et al.*, 2011; Sándor *et al.*, 2013; Wolff *et al.*, 2013; Sándor *et al.* 2014) have been made in those bones formed by the process of intramembranous ossification. This is due to the enriched blood supply found in the head and neck and the lack of complex loading resulting from larger magnitudes of forces. The difference between the cranio-maxillofacial milieu and the orthopedic context lies in the differences between endochondral versus intramembranous origins, blood supply, and the order of magnitude of forces sustained in axial loading. This chapter focuses on the reconstruction of cranio-maxillofacial bones formed by intramembranous ossification, in part to serve as a future stepping stone toward understanding the complex problems faced by long bones in the axial skeleton.

Bone tissue engineering principles

The reconstruction of a specific bone defect must follow logical and sound surgical principles. This author employs the concept of the reconstructive surgical ladder (Sándor *et al.*, 2010), in which techniques having a step-wise increasing complexity are used with a strong preference for the simplest possible procedure at the outset. The missing tissues are identified including covering mucosa or skin, muscle, bone, cartilage, nerve, and blood vessels. Then efforts ensue to replace missing tissue elements with similar or like tissue. For example in the mouth, at the hard palate, surgeons would ideally aim to replace missing palatal mucosa with keratinized attached mucosa rather than totally dissimilar non-keratinized unattached alveolar mucosa.

Then flaps containing the missing tissue elements can be planned using a hierarchy, with the simplest technique being considered first (Sándor *et al.*, 2012):
(1) Local soft tissue grafts (free gingival grafts).
(2) Local flaps (buccal advancement flaps, local pedicled flaps).
(3) Regional flaps (tongue flaps).
(4) Bone grafts harvested from intra-oral sources (ramus, chin, zygoma).
(5) Bone grafts harvested from extra-oral sources (iliac crest, tibia).
(6) Distant pedicled flaps (delto-pectoral, sternocleidomastoid, pectoralis flaps).
(7) Distant microvascular flaps (fibula, deep circumflex iliac artery (DCIA) flap, latisimus dorsi, rectus abdominis, scapula).
(8) Tissue engineered constructs consisting of resorbable alloplastic scaffold materials combined with growth factors or cell signaling molecules and mesenchymal stem cells. While autologous adult stem cells are used clinically at the present time, these autologous stem cells could be replaced by allogeneic stem cells in the future (Prasad *et al.*, 2011).

Reconstruction of membranous osseous defects in the cranio-maxillofacial skeleton represents one of the most challenging tasks to the reconstructive surgeon and encompasses the paradigm of tissue engineering (Figure 2.3). While significant advances have been made with bone substitutes, autogenous bone still remains the gold standard in the reconstruction of bone defects (Figure 2.4) (Sándor *et al.*, 2011; Janssen *et al.*,

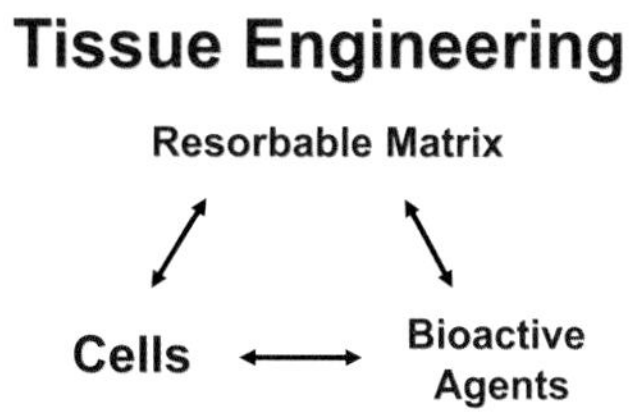

Tissue Engineering

Resorbable Matrix

Cells ⟷ Bioactive Agents

Figure 2.3 The tissue engineering triad illustrating the interplay between scaffolds or biomaterials, stem cells and signaling molecules or growth factors.

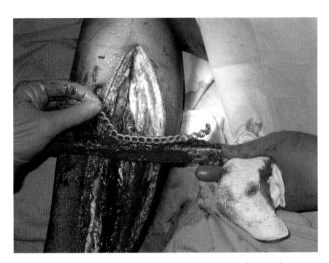

Figure 2.4 Vascularized fibula graft harvest being adapted to pre-bent reconstruction plate to replace missing mandibulectomy segment.

2014). To understand bone reconstruction, the surgeon must first fully understand bone healing and the healing of the surrounding soft tissues.

Types of bone healing

Inflammation, wound healing, vasculogenesis, and bone healing are closely intertwined. The three types of bone healing that have been described are: primary bone healing, secondary bone healing, and gap healing. The difference between these three actually depends on the pattern of fracture, the size of the osseous defect, and the rigidity of fixation. All three bone healing models give information about differences between bone regeneration both within non-grafted as well as grafted defects (Sándor *et al.*, 2012).

The milieu surrounding surgically or traumatically injured tissue is both hypoxic, with low oxygen partial pressures of 5–10 mmHg, as well as acidotic, with pH between 4 to 6. Acidosis and hypoxia are required for PMN and macrophage stimulation (Marx *et al.*, 1998). A proliferation phase begins with the healing by day 3 and can last up to 40 days following fracture. A reparative phase follows with the appearance of new blood vessels, collagen, and cells. Osteoprogenitor cells are then stimulated to proliferate and differentiate into active chondroblasts and osteoblasts, laying down large amounts of extracellular matrices, thereby forming a bridging callus.

During secondary bone healing chondroblasts lay down amorphous chondroitin sulfate matrices, then become chondrocytes, which eventually hypertrophy and die, leaving empty lacunae in a calcified matrix (Larmas & Sándor, 2013). These empty lacunae allow for vascular ingrowth resulting in a higher oxygen tension and normalized pH, which in turn favor the further differentiation of osteoblasts.

Those defects that are larger without any bony contact heal by gap healing, and if the defects are larger than critical size they may require bone grafts to allow the bony wound to regenerate

bone rather than produce a fibrous union or scar. Three essential processes are involved in the healing of bone grafts: osteogenesis, osteoinduction, and osteoconduction (Burchadt, 1983).

(1) Osteogenesis is defined as the formation of new bone using osteocompetent cells contained within bone tissue surrounding a defect or within a bone graft, and is dependent on Wnt-signaling pathways (Kim *et al.*, 2007; Leucht *et al.*, 2008).

(2) Osteoinduction is defined as bone formation that results from primitive mesenchymal cells in the recipient bed that have been stimulated to differentiate into bone forming cells by inductive proteins within the graft.

(3) Osteoconduction occurs by ingrowth of capillaries and osteoprogenitor cells from the recipient bed into and around the grafted material, eventually replacing the grafted scaffold with bone.

Cytokines and signaling molecules

Cell signaling molecules or growth factors important in bone healing include bone morphogenetic proteins (BMPs) (Wozney *et al.*, 1999) found in many species (Hu *et al.*, 2011). BMPs are small low molecular weight proteins of 19 to 30 kilo Daltons with a pH of 4.9 to 5.1 (Moghadam *et al.*, 2001; Schilephake, 2002). Some BMPs stimulate mesenchymal stem cells to differentiate into osteoblasts during development and during bone healing (Ducy *et al.*, 1997; Schmitt *et al.*, 1999). BMPs are present in most tissues and play an important role in remodeling of the adult skeleton. When osteoclasts resorb bone matrix, BMPs are released (Hu *et al.*, 2009a, b), initiating further recruitment and differentiation of stem cell precursors to form osteoblasts and ultimately the formation of new bone (Dragoo *et al.*, 2003).

BMP-7 or osteogenic protein-1 (OP-1) was first used in the craniofacial skeleton to treat a mandibular segmental defect in 2001 (Moghadam *et al.*, 2001). BMP-7 was later used to aid in the healing of a maxillary Lefort I osteotomy (Warnke & Coren, 2003). BMP-2 and BMP-7 are approved for human use. The recombinant human form, termed rhBMP, can be produced using Chinese hamster ovary (CHO) cell lines. Both laboratory and human studies using BMP have shown data with superior results in regenerating critical-sized defects (Moghadam *et al.*, 2001, 2004). Clokie and Sándor were the first to report the use of BMP-7 in human mandible resection defects (Figures 2.5a and 2.5b). They documented 10 cases of post-resection mandibular defects successfully reconstructed with BMP-7 (OP-1) in demineralized bone matrix (DBM) suspended in a reverse phase copolymer medium using poloxamer 407 (Figures 2.6a–6d). Uneventful postoperative courses were reported, with dental rehabilitation completed one year post-reconstruction (Clokie & Sándor, 2008).

Naming of growth factors

The relationship between the name of a particular growth factor and its actions may not always seem to be consistent. The name of a growth factor such as the BMPs would seem to imply that

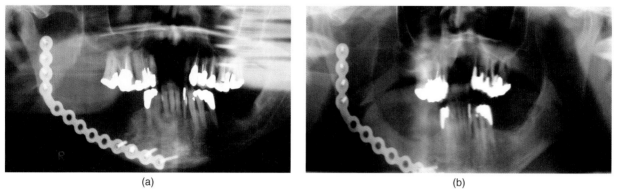

(a)   (b)

Figure 2.5 (a) First case in which BMP-7 was used together with demineralized bone matrix and poloxymer 407. The bioimplant is not visible immediately after implantation on this panoramic radiograph. (b) Panoramic radiograph of the same patient as in (a) showing bone formation restoring the continuity of the mandible one year post-surgery.

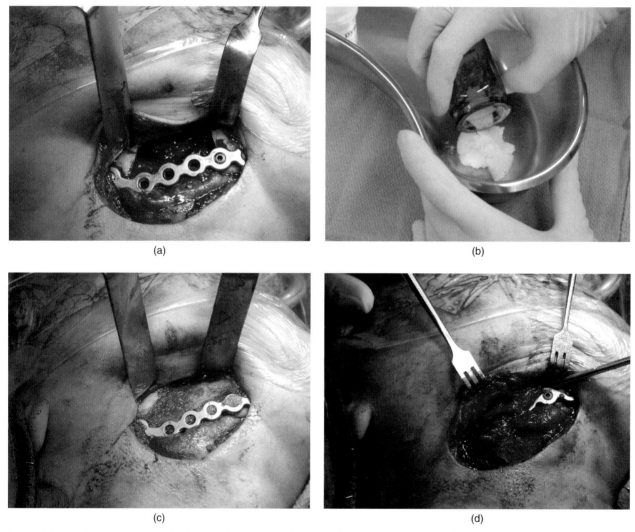

(a)   (b)

(c)   (d)

Figure 2.6 (a) Mandibulectomy defect following resection to treat ameloblastoma. (b) Putty made of demineralized bone matrix and reverse phase polxymer 407 being mixed with powder form of BMP-7. The reverse phase poloxymer will become hard at body temperature once implanted. (c) Putty is placed and adapted with finger pressure to the mandibular defect and left to set. (d) Bioimplant is placed into a well vascularized bed of muscle including mylohyoid and posterior belly of digastrico on its deep surface. On the lateral side the bioimplant is wrapped in the platysma and buccinators muscles.

their effect could be in the domain of bone regeneration or, in the case of vasculo-endothelial growth factor (VEGF), the effect would concern blood vessel formation. However, the effects of BMPs can be very specific during limb bud formation or far reaching in aspects of bone regeneration. When the various BMPs were discovered, their effects were thought to be osseous, but with time we have realized that the effects depend on the embryonic timing and anatomic location under discussion. Likewise, while VEGF has significant vasculogenic effects, it also effects osteoblast development, even though it is called VEGF. We cannot assume to know all the effects of a particular growth factor from its name alone.

Blood supply and overlying soft tissue

Establishment of a new blood supply is critical to wound healing (Bauer *et al.*, 2005). This is demonstrated most clearly in pathologic states where healing is compromised by diabetes, poor vascular supply, radiation, bisphosphonate exposure, and where the normal healing process becomes pathologic, such as in instances of heterotopic bone formation in response to surgery or trauma (Du Val *et al.*, 2007). In pathologic processes the need for the re-establishment of nutrient and oxygen supply to support regeneration and repair of the wound exceeds the maintenance needs of the tissue that will ultimately form. Vascular Endothelial Growth Factor (VEGF) is one growth factor involved in the recruitment, survival, and activity of endothelial cells, osteoblasts, and osteoclasts in wound healing (Bauer *et al.*, 2005; Midy & Plouet, 1994; Ferrara *et al.*, 2003; Deckers & Karperian, 2000; Ensig *et al.*, 2000; Niida *et al.*, 1999; Street *et al.*, 2000).

Soft tissue wound healing required to support bone healing is characterized by the following four phases (Sándor *et al.*, 2012):
(1) coagulation (immediate – 1 hour),
(2) inflammatory (1 hour – 3 days),
(3) proliferative (3 days – 21 days),
(4) remodeling (21 days onward).

Coagulation is characterized by endothelial damage and platelet activation resulting in the formation of a fibrin clot. Platelets release angiogenic cytokines including platelet-derived growth factor (PDGF) and transforming growth factor-beta (TGF-β).

Vasculoendothelial growth factor (VEGF) effects

Every tissue engineered construct is entirely dependent upon the vascular bed which surrounds it at the time of implantation (Figure 2.7). The growth factor VEGF has attracted a great deal of research attention because of its vasculogenic effects. Understanding VEGF is potentially very important for future tissue engineering efforts. This is not only so that exogenous VEGF can be added to a wound, but more importantly so that endogenous VEGF can be further harnessed in tissue engineering efforts.

As with other growth factors, VEGF is also released by monocytes, damaged keratinocytes, endothelial cells, and especially active macrophages in the wound (Byrne *et al.*, 2005; Sheikh

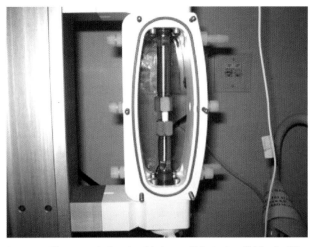

Figure 2.7 Bioreactor designed to fabricate cellularized scaffolds of solid resorbable blocks to replace segments of missing bone. The weakness of this approach is that the vitality of the bioimplant is entirely dependent upon the vascularity of the recipient bed and the chances of vascularizing granular implants is much greater than vascularizing even a porous block.

et al., 2000). VEGF acts on nearby capillaries to induce vascular leakage, supporting inflammation in physiologic and pathologic conditions by enhancing vascular permeability (Midy & Plouet, 1994). VEGF also attracts neutrophils and monocytes required for wound healing and likely also facilitates the formation of granulation tissue. The inflammatory phase is characterized by leukocyte migration, necessary for bacterial killing. VEGF release increases local leukocyte rolling by threefold and adhesion by fourfold, in addition to increasing vascular permeability, further facilitating inflammatory processes. Monocytes differentiate into macrophages, begin phagocytosis, and become important in releasing the cytokines necessary for subsequent healing and granulation tissue formation. VEGF is known to play a role in regulation of initiation and growth of new vascular structures (Midy & Plouet, 1994) as well as being necessary for endochondral ossification. Endothelial cells activated by VEGF initiate angiogenesis locally. Endothelial progenitors in bone marrow are also recruited to the wound to support vasculogensis. Together both processes supply the neovascularization required for granulation tissue formation (Byrne *et al.*, 2005), though angiogenesis dominates the process (Bauer *et al.*, 2005).

Absence of VEGF inhibits angiogenesis in wound healing, impairs the recruitment of cells necessary for normal bone development, and interferes with necessary cell to cell cytokine communication due to the absence of a developing vasculature. VEGF is important in bone repair and regeneration for similar reasons (Street *et al.*, 2000). The potent angiogenic activity of the blood clot that forms immediately after fracture has been attributed to VEGF.

In addition to stimulating and regulating angiogenesis, VEGF influences osteoblast differentiation and is involved in mineralization of the fracture callus (Schliephake, 2002; Barr *et al.*,

2008). Different growth factors influence wound and bone healing in a manner that is both distinct and synergistically interconnected (Barr *et al.*, 2010). VEGF is required in order for other factors to function, as is the case with BMP-2 or FGF-2-induced angiogenesis (Yeh & Lee, 1999). Inhibition of VEGF has been shown to block BMP-7 induction of osteoblast differentiation, and BMP-4-induced bone formation (Yeh & Lee, 1999).

Angiogenesis and osteogenesis

Angiogenesis is certainly important in soft tissue healing but it is also important for bone tissue differentiation, bone formation, maintenance, and remodeling. Vasculogenesis ensures the continued blood supply allowing for remodeling of bone to occur.

Bony wound healing, be it a fracture, a graft, or a defect requires stability and adequate blood supply. Bony wound healing relies on osteogenic progenitors from adjacent and distant bone marrow. Bone possesses limited potential for regeneration, yet this potential can be enhanced (Fok *et al.*, 2008; Jan *et al.* 2006, 2009, 2010). The periosteum is a key source of blood supply, especially in the cranio-maxillofacial skeleton. When it remains intact, the periosteum demonstrates the extensive microvasculature needed for bone healing and regeneration (Glowaki, 1998; Bourque *et al.*, 1992). Bone adjacent to a defect has limited capability for neovascularization and osteogenesis. The periosteum and, in the case of cranial defects, the pericranium and even the dura stimulates bone formation and neovascularization (Borque *et al.*, 1992).

Augmented angiogenesis in bony wounds and bone grafting application may improve graft survival, minimize resorption, and hopefully reduce reliance on autogenous graft, reduce the amount of autogenous graft required for a given defect, or ultimately enable entirely bio-engineered grafts. In addition, the ability to promote neo-angiogenesis could potentially prove very useful in the treatment and prevention of osteoradionecrosis and bisphosphonate related necrosis.

Since VEGF does not appear to drive osteoprogenitor cell differentiation but rather supports it, a combination therapy with BMPs may be ultimately required (Sándor & Suuronen, 2008). This type of combined treatment might lead to optimized wound healing. It is clear that endogenous VEGF is required for normal bone fracture healing, remodeling, osteoblast, and osteoclast activity (Street *et al.*, 2000). Such combination therapy or therapy with VEGF alone can only be entertained once all safety issues and concerns have been addressed (Figure 2.8).

Tissue engineering with BMPs

The constraints of both autogenous bone harvesting morbidity and allogeneic bone quality have stimulated researchers to focus on the fabrication of initially synthetic scaffolds that included new biomaterials and growth factors and later incorporated stem cells. One active factor responsible for the induction of bone was identified by Urist and named bone morphgenetic protein (BMP) (Urist *et al.*, 1983). BMP is regarded as a morphogen: a protein that replicates the embryonic induction of

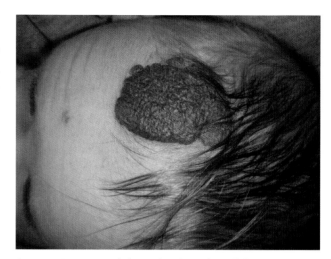

Figure 2.8 A concern with the combined use of growth factors together with adult mesenchymal stem cells is the theoretical possibility of the formation of a harmatoma, such as a hemangioma. While this has never happened, there is concern with the use of exogenous VEGF that this could result in such a hamartoma.

bone formation (Urist *et al.*, 1983). BMP can induce pluripotent mesenchymal stem cells to differentiate into bone forming osteoblasts. BMP-2, 4, and 7 have been shown to stimulate *de novo*, *in vitro*, and *in vivo* bone formation in various animal models (Khanna-Jain *et al.*, 2010a, b). Many BMPs have been isolated, and with the exception of BMP-1, they are all members of the Transforming Growth Factor β (TGF-β) superfamily (Clokie *et al.*, 2002). In the early 1990s the synthetic production of these proteins using recombinant technology was developed. In 2006, this led to the development of products such as OP-1 (BMP-7, Stryker, Allendale, New Jersey, USA) and Infuse (BMP-2, Medtronic, Fridley, Minnesota, USA), both of which are now available for clinical use. OP-1 is supplied as a simple powder and infuse has a collagen sponge carrier (Moghadam *et al.*, 2004; Barr *et al.*, 2010).

One of the greatest challenges to the clinical application of BMP has been the development of an acceptable carrier (Barr *et al.*, 2010). Clokie and Urist have explored the use of a reverse phase block poloxamer medium as a carrier for BMP with the first BMP bioimplant being successfully implanted in 1999 using poloxamer 407 (Clokie & Urist, 2000). Since that time, Clokie and Sándor have successfully reconstructed ten large human mandibular defects using bioimplants consisting of OP-1 (BMP-7; Stryker Biotech, Allendale, New Jersey, USA) and DynaGraft Putty (DBM in a reverse phased poloxamer medium, IsoTis, Irvine, California) (Clokie & Sándor, 2008).

The BMP bioimplant was created by manually mixing BMP-7 (OP-1; Stryker Biotech, Allendale, New Jersey, USA) with 10 cc of DBM in a reverse phased medium (DynaGRaft Putty, IsoTis, Irvine, California) and then molding it to form the shape of the resected segment of mandible (Figures 2.6a–6d). This was then inserted into the defect in the mandible and the pterygo-masseteric muscular sling surrounding the mandible was re-approximated to ensure complete muscular coverage of the bioimplant (Figure 2.6d). Patients were followed closely both clinically and radiographically and mandibular regeneration allowing successful dental implant restoration has been achieved (Clokie and Sándor 2008). All of these patients were reconstructed without the need to harvest any of the patient's own bone tissue. In the future biogels that allow sustained release of growth factors and other alloplastic implants that may allow the sequential release of combinations of growth factors will be of interest.

Disadvantages in using BMP clinically must include the cost. Recombinant BMP is extremely expensive. Investigators are searching for new technologies to provide less expensive rhBMP using transgenic sources. BMP is used in supraphysiologic concentrations. In nature BMP is found in nanogram quantities in bone whereas BMP is used in milligram quantities in clinical application. When used clinically patients exposed to BMP have remarkable postoperative edema beyond the normal expected amount of swelling.

In cell cultures, BMP on its own or in combination with other growth factors has failed to produce meaningful differences in osteoblastic differentiation (Khanna-Jain *et al.*, 2010a, b; Kyllönen *et al.*, 2013a, b). In fact, an osteogenic medium containing dexamethasone, glycerophosphate, and ascorbic acid has been more effective with regards to osteogenic differentiation than any of the tested BMPs (Kyllönen *et al.*, 2013a). Future biomaterials with the capability of sustained release of the components of osteogenic medium will be of great interest.

The effects of BMPs are considered less impressive due to the lack of predictable and even demonstrable effects at the cell culture level. The postoperative swelling associated with BMP use is disconcerting. While there is concern about the dosing of BMPs being extremely supraphysiologic, BMPs are in clinical usage. It may be that not all wounds require BMP. The more vascular the wound, the less the need for BMP. Stem cells may obviate or at least lessen the need for BMP in bone regeneration.

Tissue engineering with stem cells and growth factors combined

This chapter has discussed the use of allogeneic, alloplastic materials and growth factors. The addition of pluripotent mesenchymal stem cells (MSCs) has the promise of reconstructing larger bone defects with more predictable results. Cell therapy in this context has the goal of minimizing donor site morbidity by using easily harvested MSCs from autogenous subcutaneous fat.

Interdependency exists between adipogenesis, the formation of fat tissue from stem cells, and osteogenesis, the formation of bone from its stem cell precursors (Gimble, 2006). Adipose-derived adult mesenchymal stem cells may be useful in future bone regeneration and tissue engineering efforts using autogenous adipose-derived stem cells, growth factors, and resorbable.

Tissue engineering efforts require vital collaboration between cell biologists, biochemists, material scientists, engineers, and

Tissue Engineering

Resorbable Scaffold

Stem Cells ⟷ Culture Media

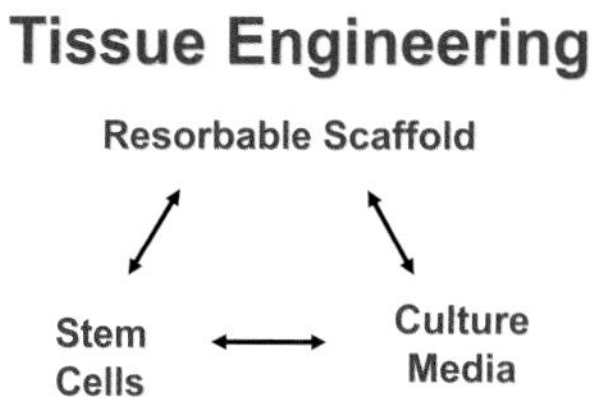

Figure 2.9 The more current *ex vivo* tissue engineering triad illustrating the interplay between resorbable scaffolds or biomaterials, stem cells, and culture media.

clinicians. In order to understand the complex role of the various components of tissue engineering, one can consider an equilateral triangle where stem cells, resorbable scaffolds, and bioactive molecules such as growth factors continuously interact with each other (Figure 2.3). It is the understanding of the nature of the interactions between these three key components on which tissue engineering is built (Sándor & Suuronen, 2008). The lack of effect of growth factors at the cell culture level has caused a focus toward manipulating the culture media in which the stem cells are expanded in efforts to promote osteogenic differentiation (Waselau *et al.*, 2012; Kyllönen *et al.*, 2013a, b) in *ex vivo* tissue engineering scenarios (Figure 2.9).

Stem cell sources

The source of cells for tissue engineering depends on the structure that is to be replaced. Human embryonic stem cells (hESC) are pluripotent stem cells isolated from the inner mass of human blastocysts. While these cells have great potential due to their differentiation capacity, there are problems that must be solved prior to their clinical use in tissue engineering. The problems with hESCs include culturing hESC without exposure to animal proteins, avoidance of teratoma development, and immune rejection by the recipient host (Grinnemo *et al.*, 2008). While there are possibilities with induced pleuripotent stem cells (iPSCs) and umbilical cord blood derivatives, for the present time autologous adult stem cells are used clinically. Whereas teratoma formation is a theoretical concern with hESCs, one possible concern with the combined use of growth factors together with adult mesenchymal stem cells is the theoretically possible formation of a harmatoma, such as a hemangioma (Figure 2.8). While this has never happened, there is concern with the use of exogenous VEGF that this could result in such a hamartoma.

Those autologous cells with the lowest morbidity in harvesting and those which still retain a degree of pluripotentiality would be the most advantageous in the tissue engineering of bone, for example. One source of mesenchymal stem cells (MSC) for bone regeneration is from adipose tissue which will provide adipose-derived stem cells (ASCs). This should not be surprising as there is an interder-relationship between adipogenesis and osteogenesis as seen in the bone marrow space (Gimble *et al.*, 2006). Certainly the harvesting of autogenous adipose tissue is not morbid (Figure 2.10) and may even be

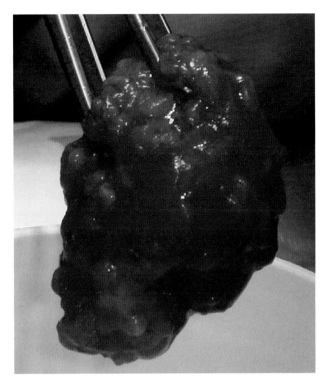

Figure 2.10 Fat can be harvested from the anterior abdominal wall using an open approach through a pre-exiting scar if one exists or through a peri-umbilical incision. Source: Wolff 2013. Permission granted to reproduce figure by *Annals of Maxillofacial Surgery*.

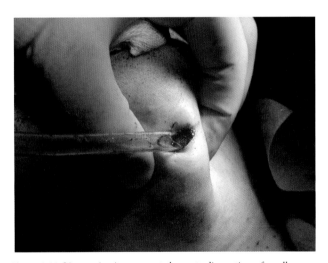

Figure 2.11 Liposuction is one way to harvest adipose tissue for cell culturing and tissue engineering applications.

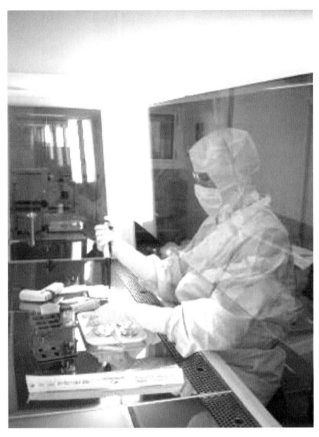

Figure 2.12 The harvested fat is transported from the operating room to GMP clean room facilities for separation of adipose stem cells and *ex vivo* expansion.

advantageous for some if liposuction were used as the harvesting method (Figure 2.11). Adipose-derived stem cells may be a hybrid source of cells that may provide material for both osteogenesis and vasculogenesis (Figure 2.12). Such autologous fat has been used for lipofilling of breast tissue in plastic surgery (Peltoniemi *et al.*, 2013). Bone marrow aspirates are another source of mesenchymal stem cells. Although many of these cells are already growing in a bone lineage, their harvesting by bone marrow aspiration may be considerably more morbid than the simple harvesting of subcutaneous fat. While autologous adult stem cells are used clinically at the present time, these autologous stem cells may be replaced by allogeneic stem cells in the future, which would decrease individual processing costs and totally obviate the need for donor site defects and pain. There is evidence that allogenic mesenchymal stem cells may moderate the immune response sufficiently to allow treatment of autoimmune conditions such as graft versus host disease (Prasad *et al.*, 2011). The behavior of allogenic ASCs needs to be studied further in the context of bone tissue engineering.

The osteogenic differentiation potential of autogenous ASCs with β-TCP has been shown *in vitro* (Waselau *et al.*, 2012; Sándor *et al.*, 2013; Wolff *et al.*, 2013; Sándor *et al.*, 2014). Stem cells should strongly express (70–90% of the cells) cell surface markers CD73, CD90, and CD105 that are typical mesenchymal cell markers. The expression of hematopoietic and endothelial markers CD14, CD19, CD34, CD45-RO, HLA-DR, CD3, CD11a, CD54, CD80, and CD86 should be moderate (<70%) or preferably low (<10%).

Another source of stem cells for cranio-maxillofacial reconstruction might be dental stem cells. Dental stem cells from dental follicle tissue, dental pulp or from apical papilla cells can be harvested and differentiated towards bone (Khanna-Jain *et al.* 2010a, b, 2012a, b). These cells may have a special relationship with cranio-maxillofacial membranous bone due to their mutual neural crest affected derivations (Larmas & Sándor, 2013).

Stimulation of stem cells

Using the tissue engineering model, autogenous ASCs could be harvested from a patient having a liposuction procedure and used to seed a resorbable scaffold (Suuronen & Asiakainen, 2004) that was made using CAD/CAM technology (Wolff *et al.*, 2013) to the precise dimensions of a missing segment of bone, for example. The seeded cells could be stimulated by physical means using vibration (Tirkkonen *et al.*, 2011), magnetic, galvanic, ultrasound or laser stimulation, along with hypoxic or hyperoxic gradients (Sándor *et al.* 2010) or growth factors such as TGF-β1 (Clokie & Bell, 2003) or the BMPs (Hu *et al.*, 2005) to guide the differentiation and growth of the cells.

Once adipose tissue has been harvested from the subcutaneous tissue of the anterior abdominal wall, the tissue is transported to the cell culture facility (Figure 2.12). The fat tissue is processed *ex vivo* in the laboratory and ASCs are separated and expanded over the next three to five weeks (Figure 2.13). The expanded ASCs are then seeded onto a resorbable granular scaffold, such as bioactive glass or β-tri-calcium phosphate (β-TCP), and are reimplanted into the defect to be treated three to four weeks following harvesting of the fat (Figures 2.14 and 2.15). one such combination product, RegeOS™ (BioMediTech, Tampere, Finland), containing ASCs resorbable scaffolds, and in certain cases BMP-2, has been in controled clinical usage (Figures 2.16 to 2.18). The mechanism of action is thought to be accelerated bone wound healing due to the synergy of the combination of ASCs, β-TCP, or BAG scaffolds and possibly BMP-2.

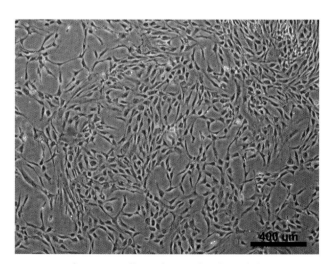

Figure 2.13 Adipose stem cells in culture ready to be seeded onto resorbable granular scaffold materials such as bioactive glass or β-TCP.

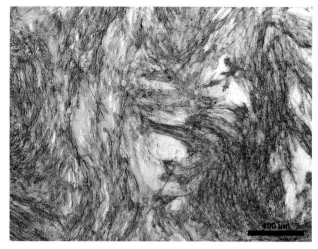

Figure 2.14 Alkaline phosphatase positive staining is an indication of cellular differentiation in an osteogenic pathway and is used as one pre-implantation test to determine the viability of a given population of ASCs. Source: Wolff 2013. Permission granted to reproduce figure by *Annals of Maxillofacial Surgery*.

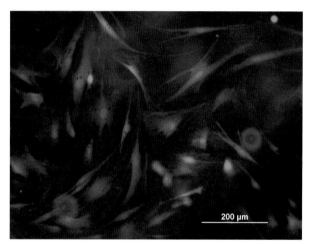

Figure 2.15 Live/dead staining showing vital green colored adipose stem cells attached onto a scaffold.

Scaffolds

In some cases the surface configuration of a particular scaffold may stimulate stem cells to differentiate in a desired direction. Bioactive glasses (BAG), for example, are known to cause mesenchymal stem cells to differentiate into osteoblasts (Haimi *et al.*, 2009). Future tissue engineering efforts will use such surface interactions of biomaterials and stem cells to guide cellular differentiation towards the desired tissue to be regenerated. Titanium or other metals will give way to resorbable biomaterials, even though titanium is so well tolerated by bone. One formidable challenge for resorbable polymers is to fabricate them to the exact shapes required in a particular reconstruction using CAD/CAM techniques without changing the properties of the resorbable biomaterial.

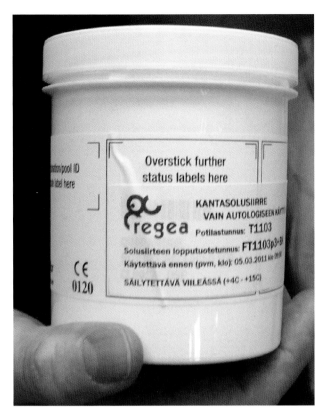

Figure 2.16 ASC seeded scaffolds are double packed into two sterile containers, one inside the other, and are ready for transport.

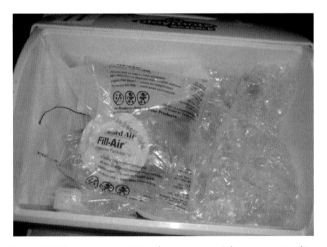

Figure 2.17 During transportation the temperature is kept constant and is documented and controlled.

Simple configurations of polymers already in widespread use as sutures, such as polylactate, polyglycolate, and caprolactones, will be modified to match their physical characteristics with loading requirements of the reconstructed bones and desired degradation profiles. Hybrid biomaterials using combinations of resorbable polymers and BAG, for example, may be used to

guide cellular differentiation with the goal of more immediate functional loading. Biomaterials also need to have optimal porosity to allow cellular seeding that penetrates well beyond just the surface of the scaffold. The pores should also interconnect to allow the establishment of vascular and lymphatic channels.

Surgeons must carefully plan surgical procedures using resorbable biomaterial scaffolds. The biomaterial must match the loading requirements of the bony wound and this can be tested in advance by finite element analysis (Avery *et al.*, 2013). Granular materials provide no load bearing possibilities, for example, even though they maximize surface area to allow tissue ingrowth and resorption of the biomaterial. Surgeons must also be reminded to not exceed the capacity of a wound to degrade and resorb such biomaterials. The concept of the biomaterial wound load becomes important when planning tissue engineered constructs. Wounds that are superficial without thick soft tissue cover may become dehiscent over such biomaterials as they degrade.

Housing the construct

Once the cells have populated the scaffold, the resulting bioimplant or construct could be transplanted into the patient to restore the defect (Figure 2.7). This *ex vivo* derived reconstruction has one major obstacle. The vitality of the bioimplant is entirely dependent upon the vascularity of the recipient bed. Using granules rather than a block scaffold may help the surface area distribution of the bioimplant, but the construct is still totally dependent on the vascularity of its recipient bed. To this end, growth factors such as vascular endothelial growth factor (VEGF) might one day be used to stimulate angiogenesis (Marx *et al.*, 1998) to help vascularize the construct more rapidly after the time of construct implantation. Currently, implantation into an ectopic muscle pouch and then later transplantation of the construct with microsurgical vessel anastomosis is one way to provide immediate perfusion (Mesimäki *et al.*, 2009). This protocol is called *ectopic ossification*. In the future, tissue engineering paradigms might eliminate the need for complex microsurgical repair, greatly shortening the operative procedure for the patient with the goal of reducing the morbidity of reconstruction. This could occur if the construct is implanted directly into a recipient bed with sufficient vascularity and no history of radiation therapy (Figure 2.6d). Such protocols are termed *in situ ossification* and are applied clinical techniques in use today (Sándor *et al.*, 2013; Wolff *et al.*, 2013; Sándor *et al.*, 2014).

Current therapy in the cranio-maxillofacial skeleton

Cell therapy for large bone defects has become a clinical reality (Mesimäki *et al.*, 2009; Thesleff *et al.*, 2011; Sándor *et al.*,

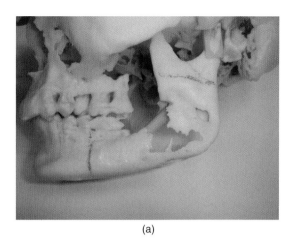

(a)

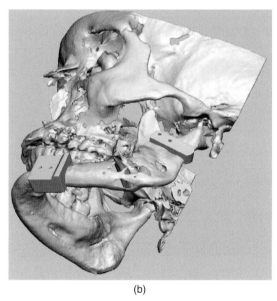

(b)

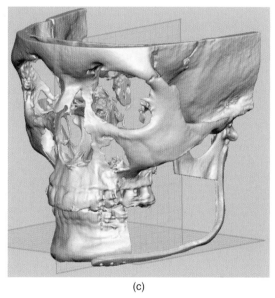

(c)

Figure 2.18 (a) Stereolithic skull model derived from DICOM then STL data files from a CT scan showing a large ameloblastoma lesion of the left body and ramus of the mandible. (b)Virtual preoperative planning using Romexis software with computer generated image of patient showing large ameloblastoma with resection jigs in blue color. Source: Wolff 2013. Permission granted to reproduce figure by *Annals of Maxillofacial Surgery.* (c) Virtual preoperative planning using Romexis software with computer generated image of patient showing large ameloblastoma with resection completed and custom designed reconstruction plate at left ramus and body of mandible. Source: Wolff 2013. Permission granted to reproduce figure by *Annals of Maxillofacial Surgery.* (d) Left ramus and body of mandible exposed, bulging laterally due to the tumor beneath. The resection lines have been scribed. Source: Wolff 2013. Permission granted to reproduce figure by *Annals of Maxillofacial Surgery.* (e) Resections complete and the mandulectomy segment is lifted laterally and superiorly out of the reconstruction plate without removing it. This is a great advantage as the residual mandibular proximal and distal segment retain their orientation relative to each other assuring a good postoperative occlusion. Source: Wolff 2013. Permission granted to reproduce figure by *Annals of Maxillofacial Surgery.* (f) Granules of ASC seeded β-TCP scaffold, RegeOS™ (BioMediTech, Tampere, Finland) are picked up using a cut tuberculin syringe which is useful in inserting the graft material under the titanium hardware. (g) ASC seeded β-TCP granules, RegeOS™ (BioMediTech, Tampere), Finland being inserted beneath a titanium containment mesh restoring the mandibulectomy defect. Permission granted to reproduce figure by *Annals of Maxillofacial Surgery.* (h) Cone beam CT scan showing healed mandibular reconstruction. (i) Cone beam CT scan showing successfully restored and loaded dental implant in regenerated bone.

2013; Wolff *et al.,* 2013; Sándor *et al.,* 2014). Autogenous adipose-derived stem cells (ASCs) are harvested from the subcutaneous fat from the anterior abdominal wall of a patient with a bony defect, due to an ameloblastoma of the mandible for example. Ameloblastoma provides a good model for mandibular reconstruction as it requires a mandibular resection for its treatment. Moreover the resulting wound is larger than critical size. These tumors do not require radiation treatment so that the vascular bed is unaltered, lowering the risk of wound healing complications.

The ASCs are transported to a cell culturing laboratory and separated from surrounding tissue (Figures 2.10 and 2.11)

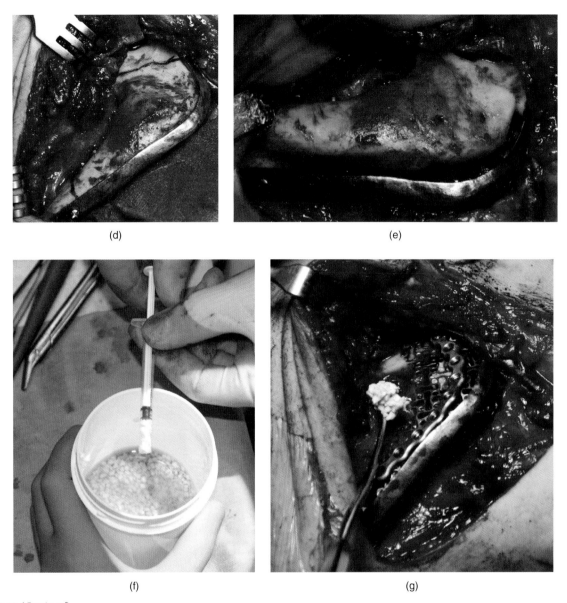

(d)

(e)

(f)

(g)

Figure 2.18 (*Continued*)

(Sándor *et al.*, 2013). The adipose tissue is digested and the ASCs are isolated. The expansion of hASCs occurs in culture conditions ensuring proliferation of hASCs without cell differentiation (in 37 °C, humidified atmosphere, 5% CO2) for 2–5 weeks (Figures 2.12 to 2.15) with appropriate Good Manufacturing Practice (GMP) quality assurance protocols in place which are acceptable to the responsible regulatory agencies. Then the granules of β-TCP are pre-incubated in the culture medium. The β-TCP granules are seeded with the expanded ASCs and BMP-2 has been used in the culture solution. The seeded alloplast and BMP-2 combination is packaged then transported from the laboratory to the operating room from 3 to 5 weeks after the fat harvesting was performed (Figures 2.16 and 2.17). The ASC

seeded β-TCP, RegeOS™, is placed into a titanium mesh cage once the resection is completed and the construct is inserted into the wound (Figures 2.18a to 2.18g). Nine months after placement and with radiographic control, dental implants can be placed into the remodeling construct and the mandibular defect can be rehabilitated with an implant borne prosthesis (Figure 2.18h and 2.18i). The successful placement and masticatory loading of a dental implant is a significant functional test of a living bone regenerate. Biopsy of the regenerated bone is possible at the dental implant insertion site and shows bone formation at the site of the placement of the ASCs seeded β-TCP granule implantation (Figure 2.19).

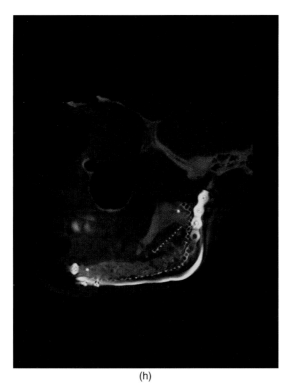

(h)

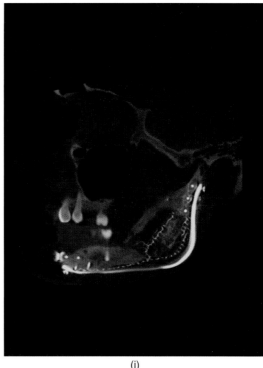

(i)

Figure 2.18 (*Continued*)

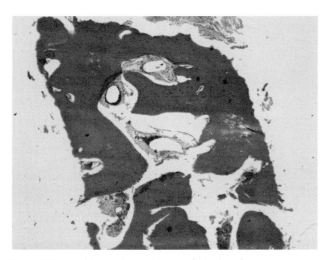

Figure 2.19 Bone biopsy taken at the time of dental implant insertion showing mature bone at regenerated site where dental implant had been placed. Source: Wolff 2013. Permission granted to reproduce figure by *Annals of Maxillofacial Surgery*.

Current therapy concerning cleft lip and palate treatment

Alveolar cleft defects can presently be managed by gingival-periosteoplasty or autogenous bone grafting at the time of maxillary canine or lateral incisor tooth eruption. Autogenous bone from several possible sources remains the gold standard for treating these defects to this day (Figure 2.4).

Behnia *et al.* reported the first use of human mesenchymal stem cells in two patients in a pilot study. Both patients had unilateral cleft lip and palate and were treated with scaffolds of demineralized bone matrix (DBM) and calcium sulfate. The authors followed the defects with computed tomography and reported 34.5% regenerated bone in one case and 25.6% maintenance of bony integrity in the other case (Behnia *et al.*, 2009).

In 2012 the authors reported that they refined their approach in three patients who had a total of four alveolar cleft defects. The authors reported that they had mounted mesenchymal stem cells on biphasic scaffolds with platelet derived growth factor (PDGF) forming the triad of cells, scaffold, and growth factor. Postoperative cleft volumes were measured on CT scans and a mean of 51.3% fill of the bone defect was calculated three months after surgery. While these pilot studies are early reports, involving few patients, the results are encouraging (Behnia *et al.*, 2012). Support for such an approach can be found in the literature where palatal defects in rats have been treated using three-dimensional scaffolds seeded with fat-derived stem cells (Conejero *et al.*, 2006)

Carstens *et al.* reported the reconstruction of a number 7 lateral facial cleft with the expansion of periosteum combined with implantation of a collagen sponge soaked with recombinant human BMP-2 and distraction, which resulted in abundant production of bicortical bone in 12 weeks. This technique was termed distraction-assisted *in situ* osteogenesis or DISO (Carstens *et al.*, 2005).

Another approach is to consider an alternative source of stem cells, as did the group of Bueno *et al.* who sought a new source of stem cells with osteogenic potential using orbicular oris muscle (OOM) fragments, which are routinely discarded during cleft lip cheiloplasty in cleft lip and palate patients. The authors obtained cells from OOM fragments of four unrelated CLP patients. The cells were analyzed with flow cytometry and were positive for five mesenchymal stem cell antigens (CD29, CD90, CD105, SH3, and SH4), while negative for hematopoietic cell markers, CD14, CD34, CD45, and CD117, and for endothelial cell marker, CD31. After induction under appropriate cell culture conditions, these cells were able to undergo chondrogenic, adipogenic, osteogenic, and skeletal muscle cell differentiation, as evidenced by immunohistochemistry. The authors also demonstrated that these cells together with a collagen membrane lead to bone tissue formation in critical-size cranial defects in non-immunocompromised rats. The presence of human DNA in the new bone was confirmed by PCR with human-specific primers and immunohistochemistry with human nuclei antibodies. In conclusion, the authors showed that cells from OOM have phenotypic and behavior characteristics similar to other adult stem cells, both *in vitro* and *in vivo*. There is promise in this approach for bone regeneration and also for possible future muscle regeneration to be used in cleft lip repair (Bueno *et al.*, 2009).

While isolated reports regarding tissue engineering applications in cleft reconstruction exist (Moreau *et al.*, 2007; van Hout *et al.*, 2011), clinical trials and organized reviews are lacking. Janssen *et al.* performed a systematic review of the alveolar cleft literature and found only 16 articles eligible for inclusion. These articles showed a vast heteroegeneity in case selection, data acquisition, and follow-up time. Future studies are desperately needed which are methodologically sound with adequate 3D radiological imaging of both preoperative and postoperative results (Janssen *et al.*, 2014).

Future directions

Other sources of stem cells could be from suction trap aspirates of bone chips harvested during mandibular third molar removal or during osteotomies such as cranioplasty (Lindholm *et al.*, 2003; Khanna-Jain *et al.*, 2010a, b; Lappalainen *et al.*, 2014). This technique would allow stem cell harvesting during routine oral surgical and cranio-maxillofacial procedures (Lappalainen *et al.*, 2014). Third molar removal may also present some other new opportunities. The removed developing third molar follicle may yield follicular cells, cementoblast-like cells, apical papilla, and dental pulp stem cells, which can also be cultured and studied. The receptors of these neural crest affected dental stem cells can be characterized and this is an important first step in the understanding of these cells and their possible future utilization (Khanna-Jain *et al.*, 2010a, b). Further developments in the 3D printing of not only specifically sized scaffolds (Berger *et al.*, 2015) but with the actual 3D printing of scaffolds together with living cells will further perfect the application of tissue engineered constructs.

Conclusions

Surgeons can augment the healing potential of large bone defects by acute and chronic periosteal stretching with distraction osteogenesis, or by using growth factors and stem cells and by augmenting angiogenesis indirectly by the use of hyperbaric oxygen therapy, for example.

While these modalities are of interest, costs, access to the various treatment modalities, and practicality remain as major issues. Future surgeons will likely combine the useful features of stem cell therapy, new biomaterials, and cell signaling molecules to simplify reconstructive measures with the goal of making the reconstruction of bone defects more predictable and less morbid. Clinical successes with allogeneic stem cells (Prasad *et al.*, 2011) make the concept of an off-the-shelf bone regenerative product a future possibility.

References

Avery, C. M. E., Bujtár, P., Simonovics, J., *et al.* (2013) Finite element analysis of bone plates used for prophylactic internal fixation of the radial osteocutaneous donor site using a sheep tibia model. *Med Engineer Phys* **35**:421–1430.

Barr, T., Carmichael, N. M., and Sándor, G. K. (2008) Juvenile idiopathic arthritis: A chronic pediatric musculoskeletal condition with significant dental manifestations. *J Canadian Dental Assoc* **74**:813–821.

Barr, T., McNamara, A. J., Sándor, G. K., *et al.* (2010) Comparison of the osteoinductivity of bioimplants containing rhBMP-2 (Infuse®) and rhBMP-7 (OP-1®). *Oral Surg Oral Med Oral Pathol Oral Radiol Endod* **109**:531–540.

Bauer, S. M., Bauer, R. J., and Velazquez, O.C. (2005) Angiogenesis, vasculogenesis, and induction of healing in chronic wounds. *Vasc Endovascular Surg* **39**:293–306.

Behnia, H., Khojasteh, A., Soleimani, M., *et al.* (2009) Secondary repair of alveolar clefts using human mesenchymal stem cells. *Oral Surg Oral Med Oral Pathol Oral Radiol Endod* **108**:e1–6.

Behnia, H., Khojasteh, A., Soleimani, M., *et al.* (2012) Repair of alveolar cleft defect with mesenchymal stem cells and platelet derived growth factors: A preliminary report. *J Craniomaxillofac Surg* **40**:2–7.

Berger, M., Probst, F., Schwartz, C., *et al.* (2015) A concept for scaffold-based tissue engineering in alveolar cleft osteoplasty. *J Craniomaxillofac Surg* **43**:830–836.

Bourque, W. T., Gross, M., and Hall, B. K. (1992) A reproducible method for producing and quantifying the stages of fracture repair. *Lab Anim Sci* **42**:369–74.

Brown, D. A., Evans, A. W., and Sàndor, G. K. B. (1998) Hyperbaric oxygen therapy in the management of osteoradionecrosis of the mandible. *Adv Otorhinolaryngol* **54**:14–32.

Bueno, D. F., Kerkis, I., Costa, A.M., *et al.* (2009) New source of muscle-derived stem cells with potential for alveolar bone reconstruction in cleft lipand/or palate patients. *Tissue Eng Part A* **15**:427–435.

Burchadt, H. (1983) The biology of bone graft repair. *Clin Orthop* **174**:28–36.

Byrne, A. M., Bouchier-Hayes, D. J., and Harmey, J. H. (2005) Angiogenic and Cell Survival Functions of Vascular Endothelial Growth Factor (VEGF). *J Cell Mol Med* **9**:777–794.

Carmichael, R.P. and Sàndor, G.K. (2008) Use of dental implants in the management of cleft lip and palate. *Oral Maxillofac Clin North Am* **16**:61–82.

Carstens, M. H., Chin, M., Ng, T. and Tom, W. K. (2005) Reconstruction of #7 facial cleft with distraction-assisted in situ osteogenesis (DISO): Role of recombinant human bone morphogenetic protein-2 with Helistat-activated collagen implant. *J Craniofac Surg* **16**:1023–32

Clokie, C. M. and Bell, R.C. (2003) Human transforming growth factor B-1 and its effects on osseointegration. *J Craniofac Surg* **14**:268–277.

Clokie, C. M., Moghadam, H., Jackson, M. T., and Sàndor, G. K. (2002) Closure of critical sized defects with allogenic and alloplastic bone substitutes. *J Craniofac Surg* **13**:111–121.

Clokie, C. M. and Sàndor, G. K. (2008) Reconstruction of 10 major mandibular defects using bioimplants containing BMP-7. *J Canadian Dental Assoc* **74**:67–72.

Clokie, C. M. and Urist, M. R. (2000) Bone morphogenetic protein excipients: Comparative observations on poloxamer. *Plast Reconstr Surg* **105**:628–637.

Conejero, J. A., Lee, J. A., Parrett, B.M., et al. (2006) Repair of palatal bone defects using osteogenically differentiated fat-derived stem cells. *Plast Reconstr Surg* **117**:857–863.

Deckers, M. and Karperien, M. (2000) Expression of vascular endothelial growth factors and their receptors during osteoblast differentiation. *Endocrinology* **141**:1667–1674.

Dragoo, J. L., Choi, J. Y., Lieberman, J. R., et al. (2003) Bone induction by BMP-2 transduced stem cells derived from human fat. *J Orthop Res* **21**:622–629.

Ducy, .P, Zhang, R., Geoffroy, V., et al. (1997) Osf2/Cbfa1: a transcriptional activator of osteoblast differentiation. *Cell* **89**:747–754.

Du Val, M. G., Davidson, S., Ho, A., et al. (2007) Albright's hereditary osteodystrophyt with extensive heterotrophic ossification of the oral and maxillofacial region: How fetuin research may help a seemingly impossible condition. *J Canadian Dental Assoc.* **73**:845–850.

Engsig, M. T., Chen, Q. J., Vu, T. H., et al. (2000) Matrix metalloproteinase 9 and vascular endothelial growth factor are essential for osteoclast recruitment into developing long bones. *J Cell Biol* **151**:879–889.

Ferrara, N., Gerber, H. P., and LeCouter, J. (2003) The biology of VEGF and its receptors. *Nat Med* **9**:669–676.

Fok, T. C. O., Jan, A., Peel, S. A., et al. (2008) Hyperbaric oxygen results in an increase in vascular endothelial growth factor (VEGF) protein expression in rabbit calvarial critical sized defects. *Oral Surg Oral Med Oral Pathol Oral Radiol Endod* **105**:417–422.

Gimble, J. M., Zvonic, S., Floyd, Z. E., et al. (2006) Playing with bone and fat. *J Cell Biochem* **98**:251–266.

Glowacki, J. (1998) Angiogenesis in fracture repair. *Clin Orthop Relat Res* **355**(Suppl 1998):S82 –89.

Grinnemo, K. H., Syven, C., Hovatta, O., et al. (2008) Immunogenicity of human embryonic stem cells. *Cell Tissue Res* **331**:67–68.

Haimi, S., Gorianc, G., Moimas, L., et al. (2009) Characterization of zinc-releasing three dimensional bioactive glass scaffolds and their effect on adipose stem cell proliferation and osteogenic differentiation. *Acta Biomaterialia.* **5**:3122–3131.

Hare, J. M, Traverse, J. H., Henry, T. D., et al. (2009) A randomized, double-blind, placebo-controlled, dose-escalation study of intravenous adult human mesenchymal stem cells (prochymal) after acute myocardial infarction. *J Am Coll Cardiol* **54**:2277–2286.

Hu, Z. M., Peel, S. A., Ho, S. K., et al. (2005) Role of bovine bone morphogenetic proteins in bone matrix protein and osteoblast-related gene expression during rat bone marrow stromal cell differentiation. *J Craniofac Surg* **16**:1006–1014.

Hu, Z., Peel, S., Ho, S. K., et al. (2009a) Comparison of platelet-rich plasma, bovine BMP, and rhBMP-4 on bone matrix protein expression in vitro. *Growth Factors* **27**:280–289.

Hu, Z., Peel, S., Ho, S. K., et al. (2009b). Platelet-rich plasma induces Mrna expression of VEGF and PDGF in rat bone marrow stromal cell differentiation. *Oral Surg Oral Med Oral Pathol Oral Radiol Endod* **107**:43–48.

Hu, Z., Peel, S. A., Lindholm, T. C., et al. (2011) Osteoinductivity of partially purified bovine, ostrich and emu bone morphogenetic proteins in vitro. *J Biomed Mater Res A* **98**:473–477.

Jan, A., Sàndor, G. K. B., Iera, D., et al. (2006) Hyperbaric oxygen results in an increase in rabbit calvarial critical-sized defects. *Oral Surg Oral Med Oral Pathol Oral Radiol Endod* **101**:144–149.

Jan, A., Sàndor, G. K. B., Brkovic, B. M.B., et al. (2009) Effects of hyperbaric oxygen on grafted and non-grafted on calvarial critical-sized defects. *Oral Surg Oral Med Oral Pathol Oral Radiol Endod* **107**:157–163.

Jan, A., Sàndor, G. K. B., Brkovic, B. M.B., et al. (2010) Effects of hyperbaric oxygen on demineralized bone matrix and biphasic calcium phosphate bone substitutes. *Oral Surg Oral Med Oral Pathol Oral Radiol Endodont* **109**:60–67.

Janssen, N. G., Weijs, W. L., Koole, R., et al. (2014) Tissue engineering strategies for alveolar cleft reconstruction: a systematic review of the literature. *Clin Oral Investig* **18**:219–226.

Kebriaei, P., Isola, L., Bahceci, E., et al. (2009) Adult human mesenchymal stem cells added to corticosteroid therapy for the treatment of acute graft-versus-host disease. *Biol Blood Marrow Transplant* **15**:804–811.

Khanna-Jain, R., Agata, H., Vuorinen, A., et al. (2010a) Osteogenic differentiation of human periodontal ligament cells induced by osteogenic supplements with or without bone morphogenetic proteins 2 or 6. *Growth Factors* **28**:437–446.

Khanna-Jain, R., Vuorinen, A., Sàndor, G. K., et al. (2010b) Vitamin D_3 metabolites induce osteogenic differentiation in human dental pulp and human dental follicle cells. *J Steroid Biochem Molec Biol.* **122**:133–141.

Khanna-Jain, R., Mannerström, B., Vuorinen, A., et al. (2012a) Growth and differentiation of human dental pulp stem cells maintained in fetal bovine serum, human serum and serum-free/xeno-free culture media. *Stem Cell Res Ther* **2**:126.

Khanna-Jain, R., Mannerström, B., Vuorinen, A., et al. (2012b) Osteogenic differentiation of human dental pulp stem cells on β-TCP / Poly L-lactic acid-caprolactone three dimensional scaffolds. *J Tissue Engineering* doi:10.1177/2041731412467998.

Kim, J. B., Leucht, P., Lam, K., et al. (2007) Bone regeneration is regulated by wnt signaling. *J Bone Miner Res* **22**:1913–1923.

Kyllönen, L., Haimi, S., Mannerström, B., et al. (2013a) Effects of different serum concentrations on osteogenic differentiation of human adipose stem cells in vitro. *Stem Cell Res Ther* **4**:17.

Kyllönen, L., Haimi, S., Säkkinen, J., et al. (2013b) Exogenously added BMP-6, BMP-7 and VEGF may not enhance the osteogenic differentiation of human adipose stem cells. *Growth Factors* doi: 10.3109/08977194. 2013.817404.

Lappalainen, O. P., Korpi, R., Haapea, M., Korpi, J., et al. (2014) Healing of rabbit calvarial critical-size defects using autogenous bone grafts and fibrin glue. *Childs Nervous System* **31**:581–587.

Larmas, M. and Sàndor, G. K. (2013) Solid nomenclature. The bedrock of science: Similarities and dissimilarities between phenomena and cells of tooth and bone ontogeny. *The Anatomical Record (Hoboken).* **296**:564–567.

Langer, R. and Vacanti, J. P. (1993) Tissue engineering. *Science* **260**:920–926.

Leucht, P., Kim, J. B., Helms, J. A. (2008) Beta-catenin-dependent Wnt signaling in mandibular bone regeneration. *J Bone Joint Surg Am.* **90**: Suppl 1:3–8.

Lindholm, T. C., Peel, S. A. F., Clokie, C. M. L., and Sàndor, G. K. (2003) Cortical bone grafts used to culture bone cells to be used for increasing efficacy of bone morphogenetic proteins in tissue engineered bone substitutes. *J Oral Maxillofac Surg* **61**:Suppl 1:74.

Mannon, P. J. (2011) Remestemcel-L: human mesenchymal stem cells as an emerging therapy for Crohn's disease. *Expert Opin Biol Ther* **11**:1249–1256.

Marx, R., Carlson. E., Eichstaedt. R. *et al.* (1998) Platelet Rich Plasma Growth Factor Enhancement for Bone Grafts. *Oral Surg Oral Med Oral Pathol Oral Radiol Endod* **85**:638–646.

Mesimäki, K., Lindroos, B., Törnwall, J., *et al.* (2009) Novel maxillary reconstruction with ectopic bone formation by GMP adipose stem cells. *Int J Oral Maxillofac Surg* **38**:201–209.

Midy, V. and Plouet, J. (1994) Vasculotropin/vascular endothelial growth factor induces differentiation in cultured osteoblasts. *Biochem Biophys Res Commun* **199**:380–386.

Moghadam, H. G, Urist, M. R., Sàndor, G. K., and Clokie, C. M. (2001) Successful mandibular reconstruction using a BMP bioimplant. *J Craniofacial Surg* **12**:119–127.

Moghadam, H. G., Sàndor, G. K., Holmes, H. I., and Clokie, C. M. (2004) Histomorphometric evaluation of bone regeneration using allogeneic and alloplastic bone substitutes. *J Oral Maxillofac Surg* **62**:202–213.

Moreau, J. L., Caccamese, J. F., Coletti, D. P., Sauk, J. J., *et al.* (2007) Tissue engineering solutions for cleft palates. *J Oral Maxillofac Surg* **65**:2503–2511.

Niida, S., Kaku, M., Amano, H., *et al.* (1999) Vascular endothelial growth factor can substitute for macrophage colony-stimulating factor in the support of osteoclastic bone resorption. *J Exp Med* **190**:293–298.

Panfilov, I. A., de Jong, R., Takashima, S., and Duckers, H. J. (2013) Clinical study using adipose-derived mesenchymal-like stem cells in acute myocardial infarction and heart failure. *Methods Mol Biol.* **1036**:207–212.

Peltoniemi, H. H., Salmi, A., Miettinen, S., *et al.* (2013) Stem cell enrichment does not warrant a higher graft survival in lipofilling of the breast: A prospective comparative study. *J Plast Reconstr Aesthet Surg* EPUB Jul 8.

Prasad, V. K., Lucas, K. G., Kleiner, G. I., *et al.* (2011) Efficacy and safety of ex vivo cultured adult human mesenchymal stem cells (Prochymal™) in pediatric patients with severe refractory acute graft-versus-host disease in a compassionate use study. *Biol Blood Marrow Transplant* **17**:534–541.

Sàndor, G. K. and Carmichael, R. P. (2008) Rehabilitation of Trauma Using Dental Implants. *Oral Maxillofac Clin North Am* **16**:83–105.

Sàndor, G. K., Carmichael, R. P., and Binahmed, A. (2008) Reconstruction of ablative defects using dental implants. *Oral Maxillofac Clin North Am* **16**:107–123.

Sàndor, G. K., Carmichael, R. P., and Brkovic, B. M. (2010) Dental implants placed into alveolar clefts reconstructed with bone grafts and tongue flaps. *Oral Surg Oral Med Oral Pathol Oral Radiol Endod* **109**:e1–e7.

Sàndor, G. K., Lam, D. K., Ylikontiola, L. P., *et al.* (2011) Autogenous bone harvesting techniques in oral and maxillofacial surgery. In: *Oral and Maxillofacial Surgery* (eds Kahnberg K .E., Anderson, L., Pogrel, A.) pp. 383–403. Oxford : Blackwell Munksgaard.

Sàndor, G. K. and Suuronen, R. (2008) Combining adipose-derived stem cells, resorbable scaffolds and growth factors: An overview of tissue engineering. *J Canadian Dental Assoc* **74**:167–170.

Sàndor, G. K., Carmichael, R. P., Ylikontiola, L. P., *et al.* (2012) Healing of large dentofacial defects. *Endodontic Top* **25**:63–94.

Sàndor, G. K., Tuovinen, V.J., Wolff, J., *et al.* (2013) Adipose stem cell (ASC) tissue engineered construct used to treat large anterior mandibular defect: A case report and review of the clinical application of GMP-level ASCs for bone regeneration. *J Oral Maxillofac Surg* **71**:938–950.

Sàndor, G. K. (2013) Tissue engineering: Propagating the wave of change. *Ann Maxillofac Surg* **3**:1–2.

Sàndor, G. K., Numminen, J., Wolff, J., *et al.* (2014) Adipose stem cells used to reconstruct 13 cases with cranio-maxillofacial hard-tissue defects. *STEM CELLS Trans Med* **3**:530–540.

Schilephake, H. (2002) Bone growth factors in maxillofacial skeletal reconstruction. *Int J Oral Maxillofac Surg* **31**:469– 484.

Schmitt, J. M., Hwang, K., Winn, S. R., and Hollinger, J. O. (1999) Bone morphogenetic proteins: an update on basic biology and clinical relevance. *J Orthop Res* **17**:269–278.

Sheikh, A. Y., Gibson, J. J., Rollins, M. D., *et al.* (2000) Effect of hyperoxia on vascular endothelial growth factor levels in a wound model. *Arch Surg* **135**:1293–1297.

Street, J., Winter, D., Wang, J. H., *et al.* (2000) Is human fracture hematoma inherently angiogenic? *Clin Orthop Relat Res* **378**:224–237.

Suuronen, R. and Asikainen A. (2004) Biodegradable materials as tools to fasten bone in face and jaw surgery. *Duodecim* **120**:2002–2007.

Thesleff, T., Lehtimäki, K., Niskakangas, T., *et al.* (2011) Cranioplasty with adipose-derived stem cells and biomaterial: a novel method for cranial reconstruction. *Neurosurgery* **68**:1535–1540.

Tirkkonen, L., Halonen, H., Hyttinen, J., *et al.* (2011) The effects of vibration loading on adipose stem cell number, viability and differentiation towards bone-forming cells. *J Royal Society Interface* **8**: 1736–1774.

Urist, M. R., DeLange, R. J., and Finerman, G. A. (1983) Bone cell differentiation and growth factors. *Science.* **220**(4598):680–686.

van Hout, W. M., Mink van der Molen, A. B., Breugem, C. C., Koole, R., *et al.* (2011) Reconstruction of the alveolar cleft: can growth-factor aided tissue engineering replace autologous bone grafting? A literature review and systematic review of results obtained with bone morphogenetic protein-2. *Clin Oral Investig* **15**:297–303.

Warnke, P. H. and Coren A. J. (2003) First experiences with recombinant human bone morphogenetic protein 7 (osteogenic protein 1) in a human case in maxillofacial surgery. *Plast Reconstr Surg* **111**:2471–2472.

Waselau, M., Patrikoski, M., Juntunen, M., *et al.* (2012) Effects of bioactive glass S53P4 or beta tricalcium phosphate and Bone Morphogenetic Proteins 2 and BMP-7 on osteogenic differentiation of human adipose stem cells. *J Tissue Engineering* **3**:2041731 412467789

Wolff, J., Sàndor, G. K., Miettinen, A., *et al.* (2013) GMP-level adipose stem cells combined with computer-aided manufacturing to reconstruct mandibular ameloblastoma resection defects: Experience with 3 cases. *Ann Maxillofac Surg* **3**:114–125.

Wozney, J. M., Lynch, S. E., Genco, R. J., and Marx, R. E. (1999) *Biology and clinical application of rhBMP-2: Tissue Engineering: Applications for Maxillofacial Surgery and Periodontics.* Chicago, IL: Quintessence, pp. 103–23.

Yeh, L. C. and Lee, J. C. (1999) Osteogenic Protein-1 increases gene expression of vascular endothelial growth factor in primary cultures of fetal rat calvaria cells. *Mol Cell Endocrinol* **153**:113–124.

Zheng, G. P., Ge, M. H., Shu, Q., *et al.* (2013) Mesenchymal stem cells in the treatment of pediatric diseases. *World J Pediatr* **9**:197–211.

CHAPTER 3

The nasolabial region: a revision of the vascular anatomy

Ricardo D. Bennun

Asociacion PIEL, Maimonides University and National University of Buenos Aires, Argentina

Introduction

Anatomy when pertinent to the surgery becomes vital and exciting, and will be called on to influence procedure design (Cloquet, 1821; Debierre, 1890; Arcieri, 1945; Berand, 1982). A comparison of the anatomy of cleft deformity and that which is normal in reference to muscles, blood supply, and specific labial and nasal peculiarities merits our attention and should influence directly any plan for cleft lip surgery.

The anatomy of the cleft deformity reflects not only the embryological failure but the ultimate results of growth and development in the absence of intact dynamic labial and palatal musculature, as well of the lack of structural support of the bony arch; in fact, growth and development exaggerate the asymmetry and with it the difficulty of correction (Delaire, 1977; Pensler, 1985; Viale-Gonzalez, 1970). The nasal septum is a key factor in the height and antero-posterior dimensions of the face (Latham, 1969).

The study of human vascular anatomy employing injectable plastic materials was first described by Schiefferdecker in 1882. Several authors have reported studies of the anatomy of the nasolabial region since then (Salmon, 1936; Harvey, 1975; Manchot, 1889).

In 1952, Conway *et al.* used an arteriographic technique to show the superficial blood supply of the head and neck. They noted a single artery that ran parallel to the superior labial artery located at the nasal base. This artery joined the one on the other side, forming a single columellar artery.

The normal supply

Arterial blood supply to the external nose is achieved by branches of the facial artery, as well as the ophthalmic artery. At the alar base, the facial artery divides into the labial, alar, and angular arteries. The superior labial artery supplies the upper lip and columella. The superior and inferior alar arteries run along the caudal and cephalic margin of the lower lateral cartilage. These supply the lobule. The angular artery runs upward along the lateral nasal wall and supplies the dorsum. It communicates with the dorsal nasal branch of the ophthalmic artery close to the medial orbital angle. All these larger vessels run laterally along the cartilaginous and bony framework and, working in close proximity with the perichondrium and periosteum, they need not necessarily be damaged (Cormack, 1986) (Figure 3.1).

The internal nose receives blood from branches of the ophthalmic artery and from branches of the internal maxillary artery. The antero-superior part of the septum and lateral nasal wall is supplied by the ethmoidal arteries, whereas the postero-inferior part receives blood from the sphenopalatine and descending palatine arteries. The greater palatine artery serves the antero-inferior portion of the nose, running through the incisive canal. It communicates with branches of the sphenopalatine artery. The network of vessels on the anterior septum, just posterior to the vestibular skin, contributes to Kiesselbach's plexus. This area is the most common site for epistaxis (Figure 3.2).

Cleft Lip and Palate Management: A Comprehensive Atlas, First Edition. Edited by Ricardo D. Bennun, Julia F. Harfin, George K. B. Sándor, and David Genecov.
© 2016 John Wiley & Sons, Inc. Published 2016 by John Wiley & Sons, Inc.

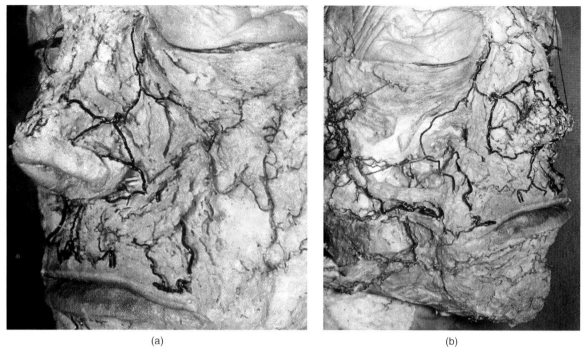

(a)   (b)

Figure 3.1 (a, b) Normal blood supply of the lip and nose region in a fresh adult specimen injected with blue buthaclore colored latex.

Material and methods

We studied 17 fresh cadavers preserved by refrigeration at −5 °C. Our sample included 13 adults (8 males and 5 females), and 4 term and pre-term fetuses. One of the fetuses had bilateral cleft lip and multiple malformations such as Fallot tetralogy, microcephaly, and genital alterations (Figure 3.3).

These specimens were injected with buthaclore colored latex following Cozzi's technique (1984) introducing a catheter in the troncular vessels, at the aortic arc level, using moderate manual pressure with a 20-cc syringe in order to fill up the smaller capillaries of the face, which we controlled by transparence in the oral mucosa. In two cases, the venous system was also filled, with different colored latex. Dissections were performed under 2.5 × magnification.

Intrasurgical findings, in 32 patients with protruded bilateral cleft lip and facial clefts who arrived late to the first consultation, were also included. These patients, without any pre-surgical treatment, were operated on, utilizing a prolabial island flap in a one-stage lip and nose reconstruction procedure (Figure 3.4).

Results

Normal specimens
The lateral nasal (alar) artery, a branch of the angular artery, entered the soft tissues of the nose near the inferior lateral

attachment of the ala nasi. Almost immediately, this vessel divided into two branches which ran along the superior and inferior borders of the alar cartilage, rejoining over the genu forming an arch with multiple anastomoses. Both alar arterial arches joined at the nasal tip, and from this anastomotic union paired collumelar arteries are born. These arteries meet the anastomotic arch of the upper lip, which is formed by the paired basal nasal arteries and superior labial arteries.

The arch at the upper lip has multiple anastomoses. Although the number of branches is variable, we usually found two in the prolabium to be fairly constant, one being deep and the other superficial following the columellar artery (Figure 3.5).

An interesting finding was the absence of the external maxillary or facial artery on one side in a normal fetus specimen. In this case, the circulation of this part of the face was assured by a contralateral external maxillary artery with the same distribution of accessory arteries (Figure 3.6).

Bilateral complete cleft lips specimens
The superior labial artery and the basal nasal artery followed the abnormal muscle insertions along the cleft margin and alar base, and contributed to the lateral nasal artery. This divided into two branches running along the alar cartilages, surrounding them superiorly and inferiorly (Figure 3.7).

The alar arcades met on the opposite side to form paired columellar arteries. These became the prolabial arteries at the columellar–labial junction (Figures 3.8 and 3.9).

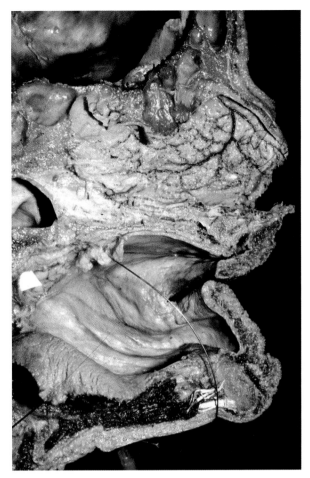

Figure 3.2 Sagittal cut of a normal fresh adult specimen injected with red buthaclore colored latex showing septal and palatal vascular distribution.

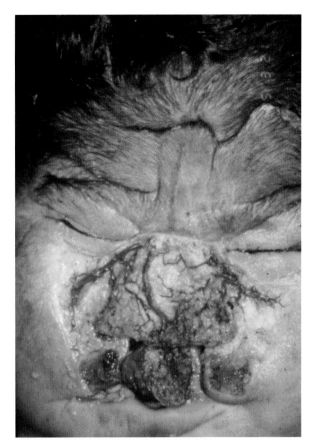

Figure 3.3 The facial vascular distribution in a fetus, with bilateral complete cleft lip.

The anterior palatine artery and the septal arteries were small terminal branches that ensured premaxillary nutrition, but were relatively unimportant to the prolabial blood supply. Thus, in the bilateral complete cleft lip anomaly, major blood supply to the prolabium arises from the nasal columellar prolabial arteries.

In reference to the veins, in bilateral complete cleft lip we found at least two vessels, the most important one being located quite superficially, and with preference on the left side.

In our intrasurgical observations, we have found that there were two anatomical variants at the prolabium vascular distribution.

- In 23 cases (70%), the anastomotic arch of the left alar cartilage continued with a superficial vessel, and the right arch gave a deep branch.
- In 9 cases (30%), both arches made a fusion to give a unique and important artery with a superficial branch to the skin.

The palatine and the septal arteries entered the lip as small terminal branches of relative importance for prolabial blood supply.

Thus, in bilateral cleft cases, the main arterial supply comes from the nasal columellar arteries (superficial).

Discussion

A description of an asymmetrical blood supply between the right facial artery and the left facial artery, as well as their committing veins, was published by King (1954). Cronin, in 1958, proposed lengthening the columella by using skin from the nasal floor and alae.

A comparative arteriographic study between normal and cleft fetuses showed that the philtrum and premaxillary regions in bilateral cleft lips receive their main blood supply from the posterior septal artery and, to a lesser extent, from the lateral nasal artery together with terminal branches of the anterior ethmoidal artery, passing through the columella (Slaughter, 1960). Based on these studies, he concluded that incision and undermining along the border of the bilateral cleft might compromise philtral blood supply. This led him to suggest a two-stage closure of the bilateral defect.

Corso, in 1961, showed in his work on fresh cadavers the advantages of working in three dimensions instead of the bidimensional view an arteriographic study provides.

In 1967, Millard was the first to propose a one-stage bilateral complete cleft lip repair using a "primary" forked flap technique.

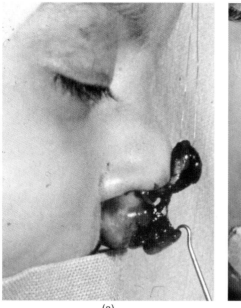 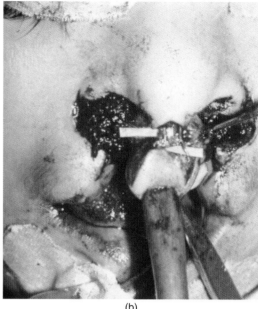

(a)   (b)

Figure 3.4 (a, b) Intraoperative pictures showing both variants of prolabial irrigation.

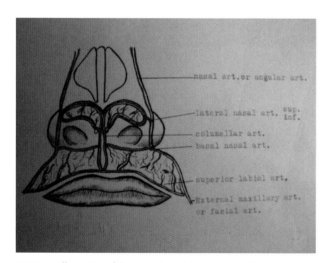

Figure 3.5 Illustration of the normal nasolabial vascular distribution.

He abandoned this technique due to frequent circulatory problems, favoring the stage lip and nose correction.

In 1968, Fara discovered deficient arterial vessels using arteriographic studies in one bilateral incomplete and six bilateral complete clefted mature stillborns. He found deficient arterial vessels on the cleft sides of the philtrum but always a rich vascular network from the septal and columellar arteries. In the lateral elements, he found the arteries along the edges of the cleft turning upward parallel to the muscle bundles. On the lateral side, he noted vessels formed more dense networks than on the philtral side.

Our research on fresh injected specimens showed that the primary blood supply for the premaxilla and prolabium comes from the external maxillary or angular arteries and accessory branches. This allowed us to consider the nasal columellar prolabial region as a single circulatory unit, which permits one-stage correction of a bilateral cleft lip and nose using an island flap (Bennun & Dogliotti, 1986).

Attempts of correction of bilateral complete cleft lip, by Millard 1971, in the same way resulted in prolabial arterial insufficiency. In an effort to avoid this problem, the bilateral lip is traditionally corrected in two stages.

On the other hand, McComb from 1975 continued using the primary nasal construction principle for 15 years. He changed the sequence of repair, first doing the nasal construction and then the lip closure 6 weeks later, always in two stages (McComb, 1986).

More recently, he changed his strategy again, performing primary nasal correction and bilateral lip adhesions followed by a definitive bilateral lip repair a month later (McComb, 1990).

McComb concluded that nasal tip dissection jeopardizes the blood supply to the prolabium and he performed bilateral cleft repair in two stages, leaving the prolabium attached to the premaxilla, while the nose is repaired during the first stage.

Mulliken prefers a single stage repair of lip and nose (1985, 1992).

Reinisch and Sloan (1990) noted that thinning of the philtral flap with the placement of a central dermal suture in an attempt to create a philtral dimple seldom works and jeopardizes the blood supply.

Following Slaughter and Fara's anatomical description, Cutting and Grayson (1983) described a winding prolabial flap, in which they carefully dissect the outer prolabial mucosa, leaving

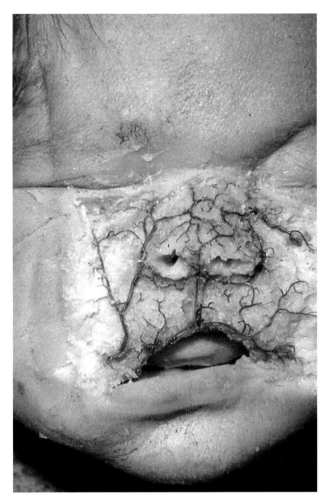

Figure 3.6 The facial artery on one side of the face of a normal fetus is absent. However, the anastomotic vascular arch looks totally normal.

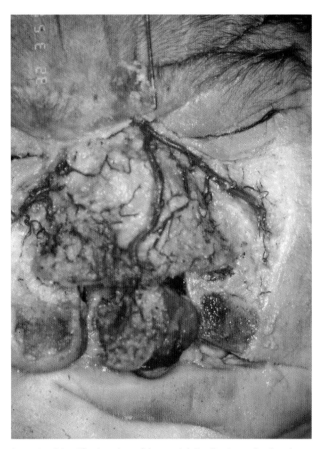

Figure 3.8 Magnification view of the arterial distribution at the dorsal nose area.

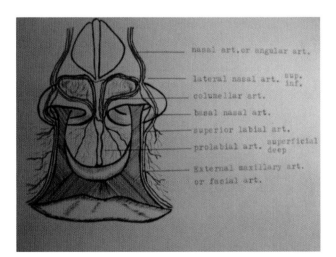

Figure 3.7 Illustration of the altered nasolabial vascular distribution, in the presence of bilateral complete cleft lip.

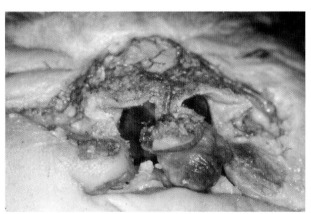

Figure 3.9 Inferior view showing the prolabial artery arriving at the prolabium.

an intact pedicle, thus allowing a subdermal "back cut" between the labial and columellar segments of the prolabium.

In our surgical observations using one-stage correction of bilateral complete cleft lip and employing an island pro labialflap (32 cases), we found two types of prolabial vascular distribution and we had no prolabial necrosis.

Conclusions

We conclude that skin flaps can be designed in different ways, but the key will always be an exact knowledge of the vascular distribution and careful dissection in order to preserve the correct vessels.

We confirm the presence of a bilateral nasal basal artery in 100% of our dissections.

The facial artery was absent on one side of the face in one normal stillborn case.

The superficial anastomosis between nose and lip, in the presence of bilateral cleft lip anomaly, is more important than the deep anastomosis mentioned in the literature.

We believe the prolabial island flap is a valid option for the surgeon, in order to solve difficult bilateral cases with protruded premaxilla and without presurgical treatment, for adult patients who arrive late to the first consultation, or eventually to solve bilateral cleft lip in medial clefts.

References

Arcieri, J. P. (1945) *The Circulation of the Blood and Andrea Casalpino of Arezzo*. New York: S.F. Vanni.

Bennun, R. D., Dogliotti, P. L. (1986) Anatomical bases for one stage repair of bilateral cleft lip. 8th Congress European Association for Maxillo-Facial Surgery, Abstracts: p. 240.

Berand, B. J. (1982) *Atlas complet d'anatomie chirurgicale topographique. 1er partie comprendant les regions de la tete et du cou*. Paris: G. Bailhiere.

Cloquet, J. (1821) *Anatomie de l'homme: Description et figures litographies de toutes les parties de corp humain* Vol. **4**, Paris: C de Lastegrie.

Conway, H., Stark, R. B., and Kavanaugh, J. D. (1952) Variations of the temporal flap. *Plast Reconstr Surg* **9**(5):410–423.

Cormack, G. C., Lamberti, B. G. H. (1986) *The Arterial Anatomy of Skin Flaps*. Edinburgh: Churchill-Livingstone.

Corso, P. F. (1961) Variations of the arterial, venous and capillary circulation of the soft tissues of the head by decades as demonstrated by the methyl methacrylate injection technique, and their application to the construction of flaps and pedicles. *Probl Sovrem Neirokhirurgii* **27**:160–184.

Cozzi, EP: Personal communication, 1984.

Cronin, T. D. (1958) Lengthening columella by use of skin from nasal floor and alae. *Plast Reconstr Surg Transplant Bull* **21**(6):417–426.

Cutting, J. F., Grayson, B. (1993) The prolabial unwinding flap method for one stage repair of bilateral cleft lip, nose and alveolus. *Plast Reconstr Surg* **91**(1):37–47.

Delaire, J., Fève, J. R., Chateau, J.P., *et al.* (1977) Anatomy and physiology of the muscles and median frenulum of the upper lip. Initial results of selective electromyography. *Rev Stomatol Chir Maxillofac* **78**(2):93–103.

Debierre, C. H. (1890) *Traite elementaire d'anatomie de l'homme*. Tome premier. Paris: Felix Alcon.

Fara, M. (1968) Anatomy and arteriography in cleft lip in stillborn children. *Plast Reconstr Surg* **42**:29–36.

Harvey, W. (1975) Classic pages in obstetrics and gynecology. Exercitatio anatomica de motu cordis et sanguinis in animalibus. *Am J Obstet Gynecol* **121**(7):1007.

King, T. S. (1954) The anatomy of hare lip in man. *J Anat* **87**:447.

Latham, R. A. (1969) The septo-premaxillary ligament and maxillary development. *J Anat* **104**(3):584–586.

Manchot, C. (1889) *Die hautarterien des Menschlichen Korpus*. Leipzig: F.C.W. Vogel. (Reprinted as: Manchot, C. (1983) *The Cutaneous Arteries of the Human Body*, New York, NY: Springer.)

McComb, H. (1975) Primary repair of the bilateral cleft lip nose. *Brit J Plast Surg* **28**(4):262–267.

McComb, H. (1986) Primary repair of the bilateral cleft lip nose. *Plast Reconstr Surg* **77**(5):701–716.

McComb, H. (1990) Primary repair of the bilateral cleft lip nose. A 15 year review and a new treatment plan. *Plast Reconstr Surg* **86**(5):882–889; discussion 890–893.

Millard, D. R. (1967) Bilateral cleft lip and a primary forked flap: A preliminary report. *Plast Reconstr Surg* **39**(1):59–65.

Millard, D. R. (1971) Closure of bilateral cleft lip and elongation of columella by two operations in infancy. *Plast Reconstr Surg* **47**(4):324–331.

Mulliken, J. B. (1985) Principles and techniques of bilateral complete cleft lip repair. *Plast Reconstr Surg* **75**(4):477–487.

Mulliken, J. B. (1992) Correction of the cleft lip nasal deformity: evolution of a surgical concept. *Cleft Palate-Craniofac J* **29**: 540–545.

Pensler, J. M., Ward, J. W. and Parry, S. W. (1985) The superficial musculo-aponeurotic system in the upper lip: an anatomic study in cadavers. *Plast Reconstr Surg* **75**(4):488–94.

Reinisch, J.F. and Sloan, G. M. (1990) Complications of cleft lip repair. In Bardach, J. and Morris, H. (Eds) *Multidisciplinary Management of Cleft Lip and Palate*. Philadelphia: Saunders.

Salmon, M. (1936) *Arteres et muscles de la tete et du cou*. Paris: Masson.

Schiefferdecker, P. (1882) A concentrate solution of celloidin formula. *Arch Anat. Physiol.*

Slaughter, W. B, Henry, J. W., Berger, J. C. (1960) Changes in blood vessel patterns in bilateral cleft lip. *Plast Reconstr Surg Transplant Bull* **26**:166–179.

Viale-Gonzalez, M. and Ortiz-Monasterio, F. (1970) Observations on growth of the columella and pro labium in the bilateral cleft lip. *Plast Reconstr Surg* **46**(2):140–144.

CHAPTER 4

Epidemiological data about nonsyndromic oral clefts in Argentina

Ricardo D. Bennun

Asociacion PIEL, Maimonides University and National University of Buenos Aires, Argentina

Introduction

At a first glance oral clefts (OC) seem an ideal group for congenital malformations study. They are among the most common congenital malformations and, compared to most other anomalies, easily diagnosed and described. Despite these characteristics the statistical power of most etiological studies is low, particularly because most studies subdivide OCs into cleft lip with or without cleft palate and isolated cleft palate, and furthermore into syndromic and nonsyndromic cases. For that reason, emerging international collaborative efforts are essential to obtain reasonable statistical power in analyses of the subgroups.

Most countries have undergone dramatic changes over the last century in terms of living conditions, work environment, health care, and lifestyle. Therefore, it is of considerable interest to test whether the frequency of OCs is associated with these changes.

The standard epidemiological characteristics of OC are important both for scientific purposes and for public health planning. These data are usually obtained through population-based clinical records, cleft treatment centers, surveillance systems, or birth certificates. The completeness of such files greatly depends on the practice and organization of the country providing them.

An essential problem of all studies is that they use only cases with OC who have survived at least two trimesters. Hence, it is not possible to distinguish factors that increase the risk of OC in fetuses and factors that enhance the survival chances of OC fetuses. However, prevalence measures of OCs are the basis of epidemiology research in this subject; therefore, high-quality methods of collecting prevalence data are essential. For assessing environmental risk factors, the case-control study uses cases ascertained shortly after birth from a well-defined population and has four or five controls for each case.

This research had the aim of collecting a representative sample of nonsyndromic OC patients coming from a population of affected infants, treated by the same interdisciplinary team, with the objective of being instrumental in identifying primary prevention strategies and preparing a national program to play a key role in the evaluation of their effectiveness.

Method

The Cleft Lip/Palate Program in Argentina, was inaugurated in 1985. The first intention was multidisciplinary work in a public hospital. With the aim of increasing treatment results and data collection, a protocol and a complete data record – including risk factors – were implemented through a national consensus of participating teams.

Population covered

Argentina registered in 2013 a population of 41 446 246 inhabitants. Females are in the majority with 51.06% of the total. Population density is low, with 15 inhabitants by km^2. PIB per capita is 19,765 dollars, the highest in South America. Argentina has 750 000 new lives born per year, and according to RENAC (National Registry of Congenital Anomalies of Argentina) the prevalence for cleft lip/palate is 10 000:12 (Groisman *et al.*, 2013a, b).

Case definition

The population under study was a group of 2937 patients. We added 1129 new patients in reference to our previous research (Bennun, 2001). The inclusion criteria included all live-born infants affected with nonsyndromic oral clefts, without

Cleft Lip and Palate Management: A Comprehensive Atlas, First Edition. Edited by Ricardo D. Bennun, Julia F. Harfin, George K. B. Sándor, and David Genecov.
© 2016 John Wiley & Sons, Inc. Published 2016 by John Wiley & Sons, Inc.

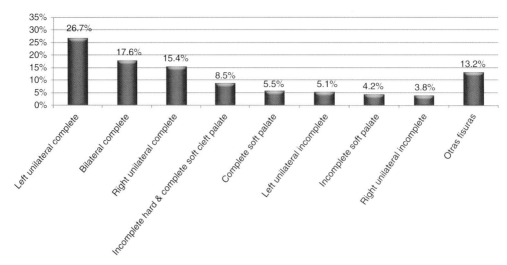

Figure 4.1 Cleft distribution.

distinction of age or sex. All these patients were assisted by the same interdisciplinary team, in three different national reference centers, during the period between July 1990 and August 2012.

The patient medical record included:
- General patient information.
- Parent's information.
- Family history (including complication during pregnancy and birth, genetics and environmental factors).
- Risk factors (as cigarette smoking, alcohol consumption, medications and illnesses, and socioeconomic status).
- Diagnosis description of cleft.
- Associated malformations.

The present study is a description of case research, where the percentage distribution of registers was estimated, preparing uni- and bivariate tables for the analysis of different relationships between the three subgroups of oral clefts mentioned in the literature: Cleft Lip (CL), Cleft Lip and Palate (CL/P) and isolated Clef Palate (CP). For data charge and statistical analysis we used Microsoft Access, version 2010.

Results

- We found 45 variations of cleft presentation, considering their anatomical distribution and side. Unilateral complete cleft lips were the most frequent (42.1%), followed by bilateral complete cleft lips (17.6%) (Figure 4.1).
- The primary and secondary palate were affected in 61.8% of cases, isolated secondary palate in 19.5%; the primary palate only compromised 14.8%, and primary and secondary palate affection without connection was encountered in 3.9% of the total. The left side was prevalent in unilateral clefts (31.8%) (Figure 4.2).
- The general sex distribution of this series showed 55% of males and 45% of females affected. Considering only the

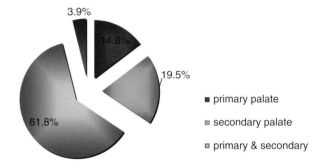

Figure 4.2 Types of cleft.

three more frequent forms with cleft lip/palate the relation increased to 58 : 42%, however an inverted proportion of 42 : 58% was found when checking isolated cleft palate (Figure 4.3).
- Associated congenital malformations were present in 13.9% of the cases, and the severity of cleft influence was confirmed (Figures 4.4 and 4.5).
- 44% of fathers and 31% of mothers were older than 34 years old, considering both parents the average represented 26% (Figure 4.6).
- A first or a second degree of family history was found in an average of 19.6% of the patients (Figure 4.7).
- External environmental risk factors analysis showed no significant evidence; however, when matching maternal cigarette smoking with maternal alcohol intake, an increasing percentage was found.
- The majority of patients (73.6%) were from Buenos Aires. In fact, more than 50% of the total inhabitants of the country live in this province.
- 68.2% of patients were categorized as low income, and 61.3% of this group were unemployed or without health insurance (Figures 4.8 and 4.9).

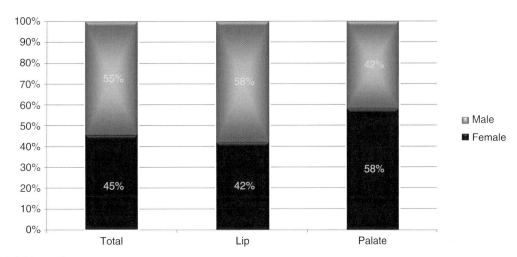

Figure 4.3 Oral cleft by gender.

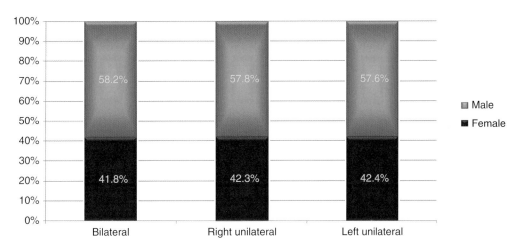

Figure 4.4 Oral lip by gender.

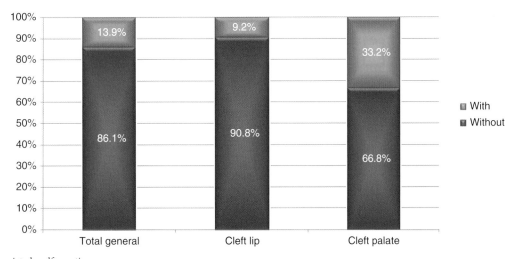

Figure 4.5 Associated malformations.

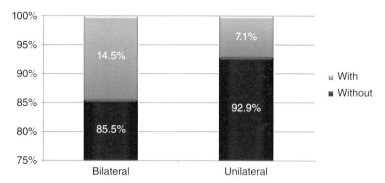

Figure 4.6 Associated malformations according to severity.

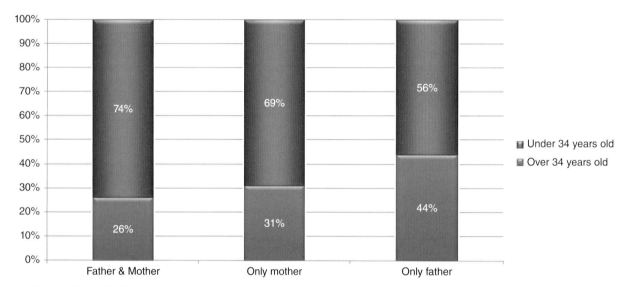

Figure 4.7 Parental age and clefts.

Discussion

Oral clefts have been the subject of many studies that have increased our knowledge of their epidemiology. For instance, studies on the variation in prevalence by race/ethnicity have shown a high rate of oral clefts in Asians, followed by whites and African-Americans (Vanderas, 1987). Etiologic studies have identified possible increases in the risk of oral clefts with a number of factors, including maternal smoking (Khoury *et al.*, 1989; Lieff *et al.*, 1999), alcohol consumption (Shaw *et al.*, 1999; Grewal *et al.*, 2008), and occupational factors (Lorente *et al.*, 2000). Data for these studies have come from population-based surveillance systems for birth defects.

None of the environmental risk factors studied to date stand out as a strong and consistent risk factor for oral clefts. There is a tremendous amount of heterogeneity in the study design and assessment of exposures.

The notion that environmental factors interact with the genoma in the production of diseases emerged around the middle of the nineteenth century, when certain individuals were observed to be more resistant than others to communicable diseases. Almost 100 years passed, however, before epidemiologists interested in genetics and geneticists interested in epidemiology were able to identify environmental and genetic factors involved in the pathologic process.

Descriptive and analytic are the two types of research strategies used by genetic epidemiology. The descriptive strategy, at the population as well as the family level, is based on the study of time, location, and the individual. Analytic studies answer the "why" and "how" question of genetic epidemiology (Wyszynski, 2002).

It is likely that the mystery surrounding the etiology of oral clefts will be unlocked as technology advances and the ability to examine gene–environment interaction increases.

Information provided by this research was useful for creating our present treatment protocol, understanding patient and family requirements, and increasing results and decreasing sequels.

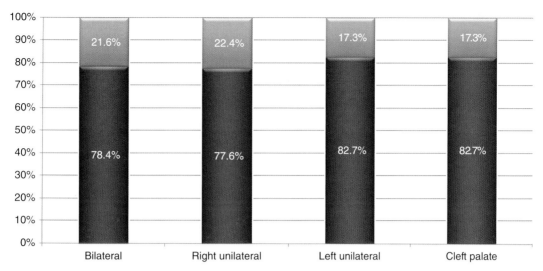

Figure 4.8 Family background of clefts.

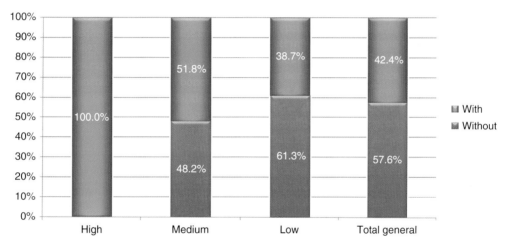

Figure 4.9 Socio economic status/health insurance.

Conclusions

Clinical and epidemiological research studies of defined geographic populations can serve as a means of establishing important data for genetic counseling and as a first step in identifying strategies best suited for identification of causes and the outline of health programs that could lead to the improvement of health public politics concerning the prevention, diagnosis, treatment, and rehabilitation of OCs in any country.

They are additionally likely to play an important role in population-based studies of the long term effects of OCs on children's health and development, and of prognostic and risk factors for developmental and prevent morbidity associated with OC, thereby improving the quality of life of affected children and their families.

Better social and economic conditions of the population are essential to reduce prevalence of congenital malformations. Government programs, although an obligation, are absent in most developing countries. Multidisciplinary teams must be trained to solve a child's problems through observing that they are not only a lip/palate but a human too. Only in this way will we receive loyalty from our patients and avoid treatment rejection and gain totally rehabilitated patients with long term follow-ups.

References

Bennun, R. D. (2001) Epidemiological research in 1808 cases of non syndromic oral cleft in Argentina. Master's Thesis in Epidemiology and Environmental Health Politics. Nat. Univ. of Lanus, Buenos Aires.

Groisman, B., Bidondo, M. P., Barbero, P., *et al.* (2013a) RENAC: National Registry of Congenital Anomalies of Argentina. *Arch Argent Pediatr* **111**(**6**):484–494.

Groisman, B., Bidondo, M. P., Gili, J. A. *et al.* (2013b) Strategies to achieve sustainability and quality in birth defects registries: The experience of the National Registry of Congenital Anomalies of Argentina. *J Registry Manag* **40**(**1**):29–31.

Grewal. J., Carmichael, S. L., Ma, C. *et al.* (2008) Maternal periconceptional smoking and alcohol consumption and risk for select congenital anomalies. *Birth Defects Res A Clin Mol Teratol* **82**(**7**):519–526.

Khoury, M. J., Gomez-Farias, M., and Mulinare, J. (1989) Does maternal cigarette smoking during pregnancy cause cleft lip and palate in offspring? *Am J Dis Child* **143**(**3**):333–337.

Lieff, S., Olshan, A. F., Werler, M., *et al.* (1999) Maternal cigarette smoking during pregnancy and risk of oral clefts in newborns. *Am J Epidemiol* **1**;150(**7**):683–694.

Lorente, C., Cordier, S., Bergeret, A. *et al.* (2000) Maternal occupational risk factors for oral clefts. Occupational Exposure and Congenital Malformation Working Group. *Scand J Work Environ Health* **26**(**2**):137–145.

Shaw, G. M. & Lammer, E. J. (1999) Maternal periconceptional alcohol consumption and risk for orofacial clefts. *J Pediatr* **134**(**3**):298–303.

Vanderas, A. P. (1987) Incidence of cleft lip, cleft palate, and cleft lip and palate among races: a review. *Cleft Palate J* **24**(**3**):216–225.

Wyszynski, D. F. (2002) *Cleft Lip and Palate from Origin to Treatment.* New York, NY: Oxford Univ Press Inc.

CHAPTER 5

International multicenter protocol

Ricardo D. Bennun[1], Suvi P. Tainijoki[2], Leena P. Ylikontiola[3], George K. B. Sándor[4], and Vanesa Casadio[5]

[1] Asociacion PIEL, Maimonides University and National University of Buenos Aires, Argentina
[2] University of Oulu, Finland
[3] Oulu University Hospital, University of Oulu, Finland
[4] Tissue Engineering, University of Oulu, and Institute of Biosciences and Medical Technology, University of Tampere, Finland
[5] Speech Therapists of Asociacion PIEL, Argentina

Introduction

The goal of this chapter is to provide parameters for the care of children with cleft lip and palate, in an interdisciplinary range of expertise including anesthesiology, dentistry, genetics, nursing, plastic surgery, oral and maxillofacial surgery, orthodontics, otolaryngology, pediatrics, psychology, public health, radiology, and speech-language pathology (Bennun & Manassero, 1988; Lee, 1999; Shaw *et al.*, 2001). The objective is to reach a consensus and draft specialty-specific parameters of care based on the literature and/or on the expert opinion of our professional team and to present you with the recommendations of multidisciplinary groups to facilitate exchange across disciplines and provide feedback between the members (Wyszynski *et al.*, 2003 and 2005; Adetayo *et al.*, 2012; Fitzsimons *et al.*, 2013; Piombino *et al.*, 2014).

Early evaluation of a child with cleft lip and palate is imperative and should begin perinatally. Proper timing of interventions is critical. Moreover, coordinated care is necessary because of the complexity of the medical, surgical, and psychosocial factors. While early management may lead to better outcomes (e.g. fewer operations and lower cost) the continuity of care in a team setting is essential because outcomes are measured throughout the child's growth and development (Campbell *et al.*, 2010; Paiva *et al.*, 2014).

To be considered successful the present protocol treatment must be implemented until the age of 6 years, to allow the child to enter a normal school education.

Overview of key treatment by age

(See Figure 5.1.)

Prenatal diagnosis:
- Parent's consultation with the team coordinator.
- Family handling and understanding of diagnosis and treatment needs.
- Indication of main interventions,

Supporting delivery:
- Avoid baby separation from parents, oral tube utilization, and prolonged hospital stay.

Orofacial dysmorphology:
- Participate in the diagnosis and collection of pertinent records.
- Distinguish between syndromic and nonsyndromic.

Oral health:
- Oral examination.
- Dentist should collect an impression to build the oral plate.
- Early presurgical treatment.

Psychosocial support:
- Address barriers to medical and healthcare with family.
- Monitor parent–child issues.
- Referral to parent support groups.

Suction:
- Assess feeding and swallowing with interdisciplinary team.

Cleft Lip and Palate Management: A Comprehensive Atlas, First Edition. Edited by Ricardo D. Bennun, Julia F. Harfin, George K. B. Sándor, and David Genecov.
© 2016 John Wiley & Sons, Inc. Published 2016 by John Wiley & Sons, Inc.

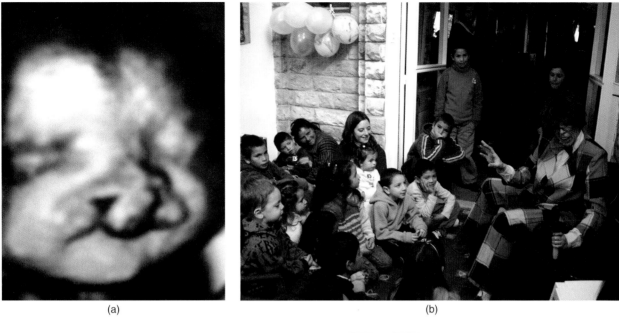

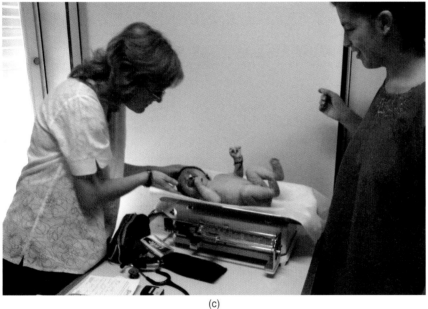

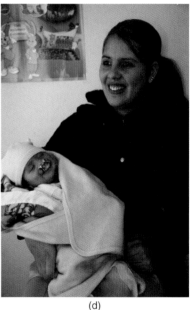

Figure 5.1 (a–l) Different aspects of the interdisciplinary treatment can be observed.

Speech and language support:
- Counsel parents on early stimulation development.
- Assessment of early vocal output and communicative behavior.

General pediatric health:
- Pediatric care provider screening and presurgical evaluation.

ENT health:
- Physical assessment of oral and pharyngeal structures.
- Middle ear status diagnosis.

Surgical reconstruction:
- Lip and nose primary reconstruction from 2 to 6 months.

Anesthesiology:
- The airway skills of an experienced pediatric anesthesiologist are required to provide clinical care during operative procedures in order to maximize success and minimize risk.
- The use of local and regional anesthesia with epinephrine as a complement is useful in reducing bleeding, pain, and general anesthesia dose, and to allow ambulatory care surgeries.

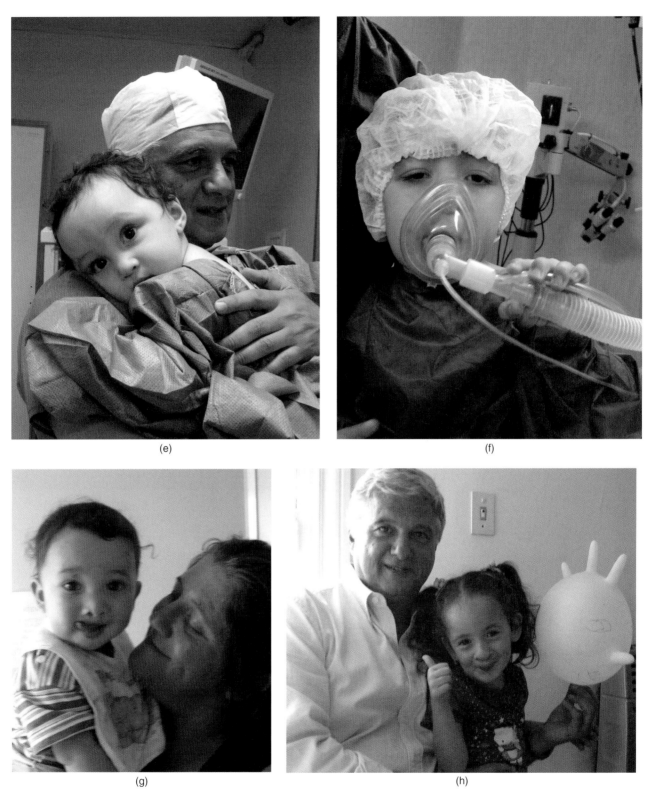

(e)

(f)

(g)

(h)

Figure 5.1 (*Continued*)

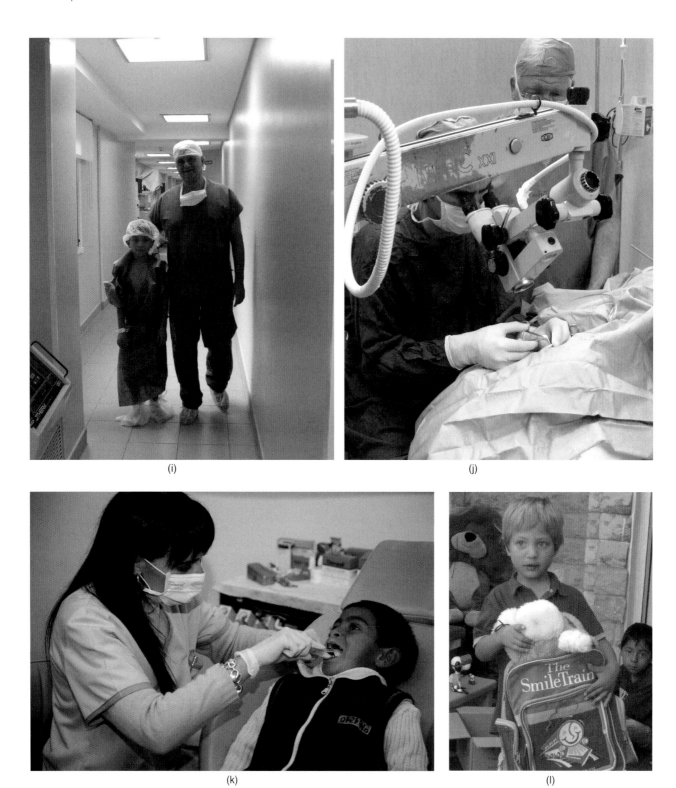

(i)

(j)

(k)

(l)

Figure 5.1 (*Continued*)

Oral health:
- Nasal component removing and oral plate adaptation.
- Caries prevention anticipatory guidance.

ENT health:
- Follow-up for patients with recurrent infections, hearing loss, Eustachian tube dysfunction, miringotomy tube indication.

General pediatric health:
- Pediatric care provider screening and presurgical evaluation.

Surgical reconstruction:
- Complete cleft palate closure from 8 to 14 months.
- Miringotomy tube insertion.

Complete diagnostic assessment (2 years):
- Address barriers to medicine and healthcare within family.
- Speech and language development.
- Facial growth and development.
- Scars and aesthetic evaluation.

Complete sequels detection (4–6 years):
- Annual pediatric care provider screening.
- Monitor dental development and malocclusion.
- Assess Eustachian tube dysfunction, recurrent infections, sleep apnea, airway issues.
- Monitor school achievement, screen for precursors of learning disability, and assess emotional and behavioral functioning.
- Evaluation of language comprehension and competence, and phonologic and phonetic development.

Complete sequels treatment (6–12 years):
- After permanent teeth eruption orthodontics treatment must be implemented.
- The interdisciplinary team must be ready to solve any dysfunctional condition.

Observations on feeding an infant with cleft lip and palate: the Oulu perspective

Suvi P. Tainijoki, Leena P. Ylikontiola, George K. Sándor

All babies can be fed and will eventually learn to eat. It is exceedingly rare to have cleft infants who require nasal feeding tubes or gastrostomies, although they can be necessary in severe cases when infants tire and are at risk of respiratory distress. The goal of the feeding expert of the cleft team is to find an individualized feeding method that is suitable for both the baby and the mother. The objective is to establish a feeding technique in the most natural way to promote bonding between the infant and the mother. Breast milk is always advocated, even if the delivery method of the breast milk may vary from patient to patient.

The size and structure of the cleft often affects whether or not the child succeeds at breast feeding and does not fatigue. Infants with lip clefts may succeed with breast feeding if the

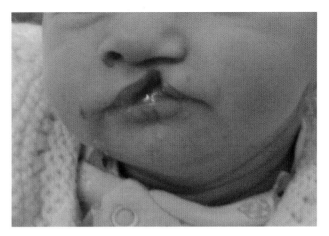

Figure 5.2 Incomplete cleft lip infant who could successfully breast and bottle feed.

lip cleft opening is small and does not involve the hard palate (Figure 5.2). The same is true for small clefts of the soft palate. In comparison, breast feeding successes with palatal clefts involving the hard palate are not impossible, but are rare. Clefts of the hard palate provide an open access from the mouth to the nasal cavity. As a result, the mouth is unable to generate the suction or the vacuum required for feeding. In hard palate cleft palate patients, breast milk can be delivered by pumping example, and then placing the breast pump acquired milk into a feeding bottle for delivery to the baby. Both electrical and manual breast pumps are possible and encouraged.

Bottle feeding with breast milk can be tried first with a normal nipple (Figure 5.3) or if necessary with a flat anatomical nipple. If the opening in the nipple is too small, then the nipple hole is made by cutting with sharp scissors with the incision having the shape of a cross (+). However, the hole should be kept small enough such that the flow of milk is not too profuse while feeding the baby.

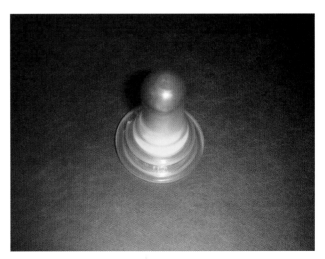

Figure 5.3 Normal nipple used most often in the Oulu University Hospital.

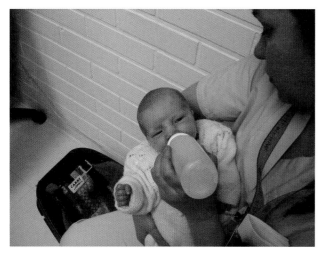

Figure 5.4 The patient is feeding from a bottle in a semi-vertical position.

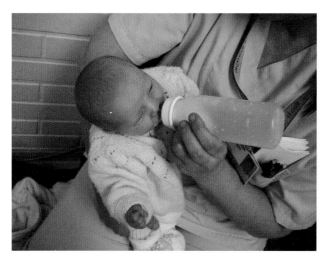

Figure 5.5 Near the end of feeding, the infant assumes a more vertical position to prevent the swallowing of air.

Special feeding bottles, for example the Pigeon feeding bottle, are provided with a valve so there is no negative pressure in the bottle, and this facilitates the ease of the baby's feeding. Milk should run at the child's own speed, albeit low suction power is better. The child sucks between the rests because the milk does not run-off too profusely.

The feeding process works best in a peaceful place with the mother holding the child in her lap, in an almost vertical position (Figure 5.4). When arms are upright, the feeding child does not swallow so much air, and can feed successfully (Figure 5.5). While still eating, near the end of feeding it is good to raise the head of the child on the mother's shoulder to allow the child to "burp" and allow swallowed air to escape.

Early on, the baby eats and sleeps at its own pace. For cleft babies, eating is often slow, with the baby eating only small amounts each time. The intervals between eating are usually short, being 2–3 hours in the beginning. This, however, is only

a guide. The mother should try to adopt the baby's own rhythm as soon as possible.

During the initial feedings it is a good idea to monitor the baby's eating, for example by recording the quantities of milk ingested and the meal times. This will document the amount of milk ingested each day. In Finland, the baby's growth and development are monitored on a weekly basis for weight and the cleft nurse calls at the baby's home to speak with the mother as necessary at the beginning. If necessary, the mother can also contact the cleft nurse whenever she may have questions.

Nasal suctioning

Despite all efforts and precautions, cleft infants have a tendency to regurgitate milk into their noses. While this is not dangerous, it causes extra mucosal secretions and wheezing in the respiratory tract. This can be ameliorated by suctioning secretions from the nose, using a nasal suction, for example. These nasal suctions are available in Finnish pharmacies.

Sleeping position

The child's sleeping position is best with a bit of a head elevation. This facilitates the removal of air from the stomach and prevents the milk, which is so irritating to the baby's nose, from rising into the nasal cavity. Those infants with a small retrusive mandible particularly should sleep lying on their side. Their sleeping position should be alternated from side to side.

Pacifiers

Having a cleft is not in itself a barrier to the use of soothers or pacifiers, but its use is limited due to poor suction power. Soothers can be held in the child's mouth and the child calms down from crying when receiving the pacifier and becomes more content (Figure 5.6). In our practice, dynamic nasoalveolar (NAM) molding devices also work as pacifiers and have replaced pacifiers in cases treated with dynamic NAM (Figure 5.7).

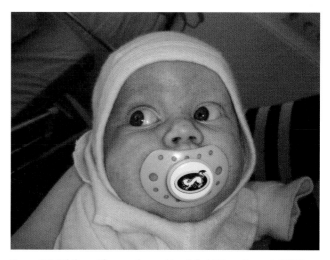

Figure 5.6 While pacifiers can be used by cleft children, dynamic NAM devices have replaced pacifiers in our unit in those patients being managed with dynamic NAM.

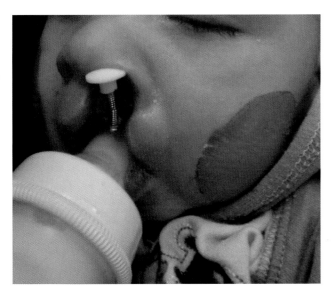

Figure 5.7 Infant feeding while wearing a dynamic NAM device who has never even used a pacifier.

Detailed speech therapist work

Vanesa Casadio

Introduction

The objective of this presentation is to detail the different stages in the speech therapy treatment for recovery of children with oral clefts that we do at Asociacion PIEL (Figure 5.8).

The speech therapist begins work before the lip and palate reparation, this will be from the first day of life, giving the mother the first indications on how to feed the baby. The speech therapist will also have to take full account of the different areas to stimulate, according to the different stages in the development and growth of the child.

Family collaboration will be essential during these stages in order for the baby to have a favorable treatment and evolution, without maturation delays.

Our work is aimed at the functional part of the process through early stimulation, having in mind the objectives of improving the respiratory, swallowing and chewing functions, and speech articulation, to gain better comprehensibility during communication. The speech therapist has to work in a team, together with the maxillofacial surgeon, the pediatric dentist, the ear, nose and throat specialist, and the pediatrician, to coordinate their actions.

Stage 1. From birth to cheiloplasty

Objective of the treatment: Promote maternal nutrition. General stimulation in the stomatognathic system.
- ° Early stimulation.
- ° Avoid tube feeding.
- ° Suction stimulation.
- ° Use of pacifier.
- ° Use of baby bottle, nipple selection.

- ° Feeding patterns.
- ° Strengthening bond between mother and child.
- ° Hearing screening.

Stage 2. Until palatoplasty

Objective of the treatment: General stimulation in the communication area and speech. Assistance every 1, 2, or 3 months, according to the needs of each particular case.
- ° Early stimulation.
- ° Dietary change, determined by the child maturation.
- ° Stimulation through vocal games. Vowel phonemes and consonant phonemes from 6 months and so on.
- ° Motor control.
- ° Hearing screening.

Stage 3. From palatoplasty until year 4

Objective of the treatment: Improve speech and comprehensive–expressive language development through systemized treatment.
- ° Guidelines.
- ° Stimulation of the velar mucous.
- ° Stimulation of the speech by onomatopoeia sounds.
- ° Comprehensive–expressive language.
- ° Gestural and facial mime.
- ° Nasal permeability.
- ° Hearing screening.

From 24 months and onward

- ° Control in the process of language development.
- ° Control in dietary change.
- ° Systematized treatment using games.
- ° Assist in the speech development in the different linguistic aspects: phonological, grammatical, and semantic.
- ° Respiratory control.
- ° Body posture control.
- ° Velo palatine exercises.
- ° Articulations of the occlusal–fricative phonemes.
- ° Labial, lingual, velar, and mandibular praxis.
- ° Auditory discrimination.

Stage 4. From year 4 till year 6

Objective of the treatment: Improve articulation: manner and place. Resonance. Audition.
- ° Evaluation of the velo pharyngeal competence. Rinofibroscopy.
- ° Evaluation of articulations.
- ° Hearing screening through the audiological procedure: oeas, acoustic impedance, audiometry, and tone and speech testing.
- ° Systematized diagnosis and treatment.

Feeding

Feeding is stimulation, because the supporting points used by the tongue to suck and swallow are also the ones that prepare the support points for speech and later language development.

Stage 1. from birth to cheiloplasty

Objective: To retire the SNG if there is one. Mother–child

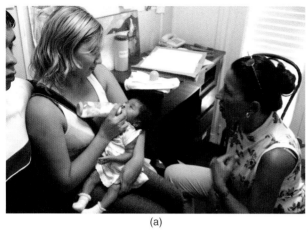
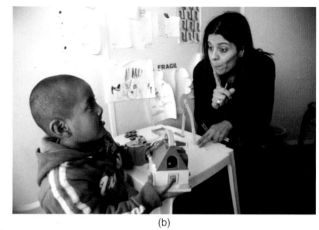

(a)   (b)

Figure 5.8 (a, b) Early stimulation and speech pathology rehabilitation sessions.

bonding. Losing fear when feeding the baby. Assimilation and weight gain.
° Guidelines:
° Breast feeding.
° Baby bottle.
° Pacifier.
° Posture.
° Feeding time.
° Symmetry.

Stage 2. from 3 to 6 months
Objective: Supervision and monitoring the baby's weight. Supervision and monitoring of the oral–facial musculature functions.
° Suction.
° Breathing.
° Audition.
° Breast feeding.
° Baby bottle.
° Pacifier.

Stage 3. from 6 months until 24 months
Objective: Give proprioceptive stimulation with temperature and textures through dietary change. Lingual stimulation and muscular peri and intraoral stimulation.
° Incorporation of semi-solids and solids.
° From 6 months, pediatricians generally recommend the introduction of mushy foods (such as porridge).
° Utensil: flat spoon.
° Gradually add solid elements to improve chewing and the formation of the alimentary bolus in swallowing stages.
° Liquid incorporation: water, drinking it with a straw, then with a baby cup and later with a cup.

Useful advice:
° Follow the pediatrician's instructions, do not prolong the mushy food stage.

° Follow the recommended period for using a baby bottle – it is until 18–24 months of age.
° While feeding, place the child in front of you/of the mother, and make sure there is no choking.
° Chewing is necessary for jaw growth and good teething.
° Soda and other sugared drinks and candies are NOT indicated for children.
° Use a baby bottle only for milk.
° Juices, water, and infusions have to be drunk from a glass or a cup.

Hygiene:
° After the feeding with milk or mushy food, offer the child water. This will contribute to mouth and nose hygiene.
° After every food intake, brush their teeth.
° Keep the nose clean of mucus by inhaling vapors, using a physiological solution.
° Clean the plaque off after every meal.

Early speech stimulation

- Vocalization > First words > easy phrases.
- Talking with the baby (sounds).
- Anticipate actions with the baby and for the baby. (Example: "Let's go to the water" to bathe him.)
- The more difficult letters for a child with cleft lip and cleft palate are P, T, K, and later R.
- Many children don't move their lips and tongue to talk. Therefore, we have to play with noises, massage the lips and palate, and play making movements with the tongue and the lips.
- Later (8–10 months) put yourself in front of the child for him/her to see you, touch you, and hear every sound and where is it placed. This must continue for a protracted period of time.
- Then, play with the sounds of vehicles, animals, and musical instruments.
- Play by blowing air.

- Play by making gargles.
- Play with words (short words).
- Play with a ball (throw the ball, pronouncing the words "Pa – Sha – Ja, etc.).

Useful advice:
- Place yourself in front of the child for him/her to see where every sound goes.
- Use the mirror.
- Don't correct him/her when he/she talks.
- Don't ask the names of the objects all the time.
- Talk slowly (to give him/her time to place his/her tongue).
- Work (or play) every day a little bit to stimulate speech and vocabulary.
- Brothers or sisters and grandparents are also good stimulators.

Motor development

General motor development (gross motor development).
Manual motor development (fine motor development).
- Give the child the possibility of being on the floor, lying face down, and also on his or her back.
- The baby at 4 or 5 months begins to roll back, at 6 months he/she will sit down, at 8 months crawl, and at 12 months begin walking (toddler).
- Encourage the child to develop his/her physical skills that contribute to general maturation.
- It is also important that while growing up the child can use his/her hands to manipulate objects for himself/herself (fine motor development: use dough, screw, attach, etc).

Useful advice:
- Encourage his/her independence (e.g., sleeping alone, use a comforter of his/her choice).
- Do not use a walker – it is better to use a playpen if you need to keep the child safe.

References

Adetayo, O., Ford, R., and Martin, M. (2012) Africa has unique and urgent barriers to cleft care: Lessons from practitioners at the Pan-African Congress on Cleft Lip and Palate. *Pan Afr Med J* **12**:15.

Bennun, R. D. and Manassero, G. M. (1988) Tratamiento primario de la fisura labio alveolo palatina. *Revista del Hospital de Niños "R. Gutierrez"* **30**:97–100.

Campbell, A., Costello, B. J., and Ruiz R. L. (2010) Cleft lip and palate surgery: An update of clinical outcomes for primary repair. *Oral Maxillofac Surg Clin North Am* **22**(**1**):43–58.

Fitzsimons, K. J., Copley, L. P., Deacon, S. A., *et al.* (2013) Hospital care of children with a cleft in England. *Arch Dis Child.* **98**(**12**):970–974.

Lee, S. T. (1999) New treatment and research strategies for the improvement of care of cleft lip and palate patients in the new millennium. *Ann Acad Med Singapore* **28**(**5**):760–767.

Paiva, T. S., Andre, M., Paiva, W.S., *et al.* (2014) Aesthetic evaluation of the nasolabial region in children with unilateral cleft lip and palate comparing expert versus nonexperience health professionals. *Biomed Res Int* **2014**:460106.

Piombino, P., Ruggiero, F., Dell'Aversana Orabona, G., *et al.* (2014) Development and validation of the quality-of-life adolescent cleft questionnaire in patients with cleft lip and palate. *J Craniofac Surg* **25**(**5**):1757–1761. doi: 10.1097/SCS.0000000000001033.

Shaw, W. C., Semb, G., Nelson, P., *et al.* (2001) The Eurocleft project 1996–2000: Overview. *J Craniomaxillofac Surg* **29**(**3**):131–140; discussion 141–142.

Wyszynski, D. F., Perandones, C., and Bennun, R. D. (2003) Attitudes toward prenatal diagnosis, termination of pregnancy, and reproduction by parents of children with nonsyndromic oral clefts in Argentina. *Prenat Diagn* **23**(**9**):722–727.

Wyszynski, D. F., Perandones, C., Yannibelli, P. *et al.* (2005) Family environment of individuals with oral clefts, in Argentina. *Cleft Palate Craniofac J* **42**(**2**):185–191.

PART 2

Present primary surgical reconstruction

Dynamic presurgical nasoalveolar remodeling in unilateral and bilateral complete cleft: the DPNR technique

Ricardo D. Bennun[1] and Analia C. Langsam[2]
[1] Asociacion PIEL, Maimonides University and National University of Buenos Aires, Argentina
[2] Pediatric Dentist Asociacion PIEL, Argentina

Introduction

In a normal baby with intact lips and palate, the muscles of the lip, cheek, and pharynx use their usual sphincter-like action against the developing maxillary and mandibular arches. The compressive external muscular forces neutralize the expansion forces of the tongue. The neonatal arch form changes as these forces modify with growth and maturation; yet the opposing muscles always maintain a precise and dynamic balance with each other. When this muscular balance is upset, the arch form and teeth relationship is altered.

Understanding the cleft anatomy

A cleft of the lip and palate is the result of the fusion failure of lip elements and palatal segments, within the first eight weeks of fetal life. The loss of muscular continuity of the orbicularis oris buccinator-superior constrictor ring in complete unilateral and bilateral clefts changes the normal muscular force diagram.

Because clefts differ in their location and magnitude, lip and palate clefts can vary in the degree of geometric distortion, as well as in the size and shape of the cleft palatal segments. The muscular forces that act on the bony platform of the palate and pharynx begin very early in intrauterine life; therefore, the palatal and facial configuration at birth has been formed over the major portion of the infant's existence prior to birth.

The cleft lip and palate deformities are complex, with the involvement of not only the palate and lip but also the nose. The shape of the nose is affected in all three planes of space (Figure 6.1).

Unilateral complete cleft lip and palate

The deformity appears as distortion, displacement, and probably tissue deficiency of nasal and maxillary structures. The maxilla is widely "open" at the level of the pyriform aperture.

Medially, the premaxilla is pulled toward the normal side, together with the nasal septum, columella, and nasal spine. The medial alveolar bone is also rotated superiorly. The tongue, being elevated in the cleft, can also play a role in widening the defect.

Laterally, the maxilla and base of the nostril are pulled away from the midline, and the lower lateral cartilage is displaced inferiorly. The maxilla is also often displaced superiorly and a certain degree of lateral retrusion can be observed.

The lower turbinate can sometimes be interposed between the edges of the cleft maxilla. The orbicularis oris, instead of having a normal insertion in the medial lip element, is attached laterally, exerting lateral and superior traction on the base of the nostril and the pyriform aperture.

It is very interesting to observe the contraction of the orbicularis on an unrepaired cleft and see the widening of the nostril as the patient smiles. It makes it easier to understand how the abnormal muscular insertions have to be completely released from the nose and maxilla before muscular repair can be effectively achieved.

The nasal tip has specific distortions, a displacement down the crus medialis produces a shorter collumellar side and deficient projection of the nasal tip, the shift alar cartilages produce a bifid nasal tip, and the union between the crus medialis and the lateral crus become more released. An increased nasal base makes the alar cartilage collapse (Figure 6.2).

Cleft Lip and Palate Management: A Comprehensive Atlas, First Edition. Edited by Ricardo D. Bennun, Julia F. Harfin, George K. B. Sándor, and David Genecov.
© 2016 John Wiley & Sons, Inc. Published 2016 by John Wiley & Sons, Inc.

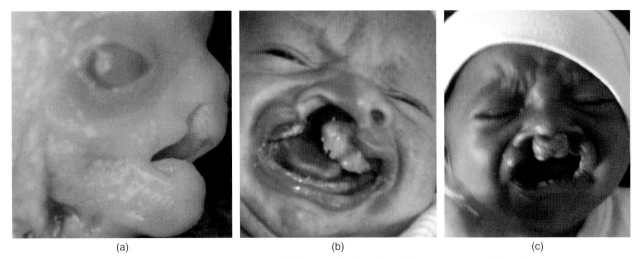

Figure 6.1 (a) Unilateral complete cleft lip and palate in a 12-week old fetus. (b, c) Unilateral and bilateral complete cleft lip and palate in two newborns showing distortion produced during intrauterine life.

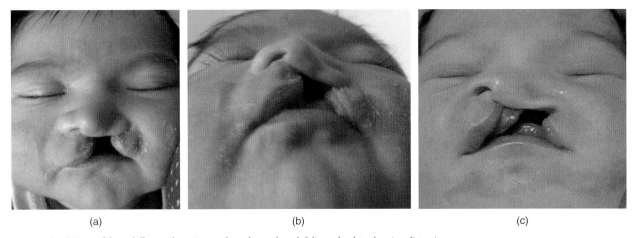

Figure 6.2 (a–c) View of three different planes in a unilateral complete cleft lip and palate showing distortions.

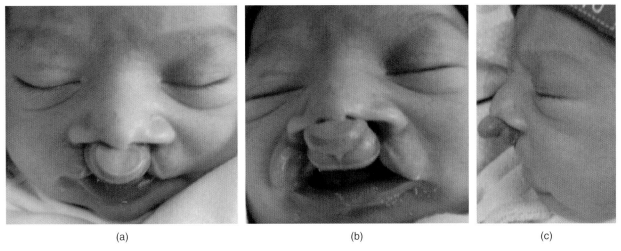

Figure 6.3 (a–c) View of three different planes in a bilateral complete cleft lip and palate showing distortions.

Bilateral complete cleft lip and palate

Bilateral cleft lip and palate are typically characterized by shortened columella, the premaxilla remaining suspended from the tip of the nasal septum with alveolar segments remaining behind and with stretched alar cartilages over the cleft. The premaxilla may be small or large, symmetrical or asymmetrical (Figure 6.3).

Concepts and nomenclature

The general concepts concerning remodeling have been organized by Frost (1993). Based on Frost and Schonau's proposals (2000), researchers have shown that bone and tissue remodeling includes cellular activities and biomechanical events that restore form to damaged or distorted tissues.

Remodeling can be confused with molding. This process can be viewed as the procedures that shape maturing tissues (Grayson et al., 1993). Remodeling is a fundamental part of the growth process and calls for sequential changes in the shape and size of each region (Enlow, 1982).

Developmental insufficiency can lead to bone and soft tissue deficits. Utilization of the regenerative capacity of bone and soft tissues has produced a diverse spectrum of modalities to correct these deficits: including autogenous grafts, allogenic bank bone and cartilage, synthetic materials, recombinant therapeutics (e.g., growth factors), and mechanical devices (such as nasal stents).

An increasing number of biological factors associated with bone and cartilage homeostasis and regeneration are being identified. Attempts have been made to organize these factors into categories or classes, such as hormones, prostaglandins, cytokines, and growth factors (Hollinger & Wong, 1996).

In general, growth factors and cytokines are mediators of normal cellular growth, embryogenesis, wound repair, and oncogenesis (Herndon et al., 1993). In addition, a specific growth factor or cytokine may have either an inhibitory or stimulatory effect, or it may be both dependent on the cellular interaction and gradients of local factors (Robinson, 1993). For the purpose of this chapter, cytokines will be considered regulators for growth and differentiation of cells of the immune and hematopoietic systems.

Background

In the treatment of cleft lip nasal deformity, correction of the nose continues to be the greatest challenge. In patients with unilateral cleft lip/palate, the nasolabial defect influences the physical appearance of the child. Hence it is recommended to perform nasal remodeling prior to primary lip repair. Considering that the nose is an important component of facial esthetics, correction of the nasal symmetry and nasolabial fold is an important objective.

Clefting is due to disturbance of embryogenesis, and the proper closure of all involved structures should be achieved as soon as possible to favor normal growth of the face (Millard, 1896). Several approaches have been used in order to reduce nasal asymmetry early in life using surgery alone or in conjunction with other approaches.

Auricular cartilage can be remodeled with permanent results if treatment is started within six weeks of life (Matsuo et al., 1984). During this period, there are high levels of maternal estrogen in the fetal circulation which generates an increase in hyaluronic acid in blood. Hyaluronic acid (HA) modifies cartilage, ligament, and connective tissue elasticity by breaking down the intercellular matrix (Hardingham & Muir, 1972; Kenny, 1973).

Levels of estrogen start dropping at six weeks of age. It is based on this principle that the concept of nasoalveolar remodeling works (Shetty et al., 2012).

Repair of early gestation fetal skin occurs in the absence of acute inflammation, without excessive fibroblast infiltration, and without massive collagen deposition. The healed wound resembles normal skin and, hence, reflects a regenerative-like process (West & Kumar, 1989; Thomas et al., 1998).

Fetal skin repair occurs in the presence of abundant HA throughout the repair process (weeks), whereas in adults skin repair HA levels peak at two to four days and then fall rapidly (Chen et al., 1989). The results demonstrate that HA affects the cellular and matrix events in fetal healing and suggest that HA plays an important role in the process of fetal regeneration (Adzick et al., 1985; Chen et al., 1989; Adzick & Lorenz, 1994).

It is also suggested that nasolaveolar remodeling stimulates immature nasal chondroblasts, producing an interstitial expansion that is associated with an improvement in the nasal morphology (Hamrick, 1999).

Presurgical infant orthopedic

The concept of presurgical maxillary orthopedics describes the use of serial appliances to approximate the alveolar cleft segment (McNeil, 1950). Many changes have taken place in appliance design, from McNeil's concept to the actual concept of dynamic nasoalveolar remodeling (Hotz & Gnoinski, 1976; Murthy et al., 2013).

These appliances can be classified as: active or passive; presurgical or postsurgical; and intra-oral or extra-oral. Active appliances move alveolar cleft segments in a predetermined manner with controlled forces, whereas passive appliances deliver no force but act as a fulcrum upon which forces created by surgical lip closure contour and mold the alveolar segments in a predictable fashion (Berkowitz, 1977).

The use of presurgical rigid nasal stents in newborns with unilateral or bilateral cleft lip and palate was introduced as early as

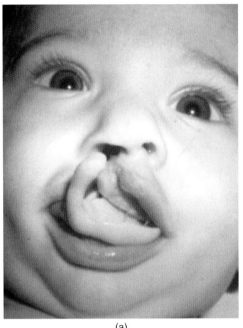
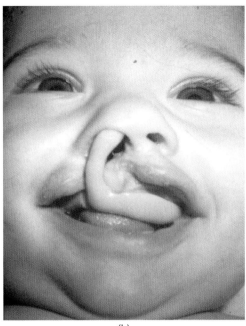

(a)   (b)

Figure 6.4 (a, b) The original nasal stent introduced in 1987.

1987. This protocol, used in a group of 80 patients, was published in Spanish by Dogliotti *et al.* (1991). A six-year follow-up of these patients, in English, is available (Bennun *et al.*, 1999, 2001). At that time the idea was popularized as the nasoalveolar molding (NAM) technique (Grayson *et al.*, 1999) and was adopted by other groups (Figure 6.4).

Dynamic presurgical nasoalveolar remodeling (DPNR technique)

A fundamental principle of reparative medicine, which governs our efforts to regenerate differentiated tissue, is to organize the reparative circumstances to recapitulate selected aspects of embryonic developmental sequence, including attempts to mimic the embryonic microenvironment in which tissue initiation, formation, and expansion take place (Caplan, 2002).

Tissue engineering ought not to focus on whether or not to utilize *in vivo* remodeling approaches, but rather on how to best induce the most desirable remodeling (Greisler, 2002).

DPNR represents a unique form of clinical tissue engineering. Using easily controlled mechanical conditions, an orthopedist is able to guide the position/formation of new tissues and their spatial orientation. This happens without application of any growth factor or other controlling agents.

The principle behind this procedure is the use of the force generated during suction and swallowing. This force can be transmitted by means of a nasal dynamic component to produce remodeling effects on the nasal structures, and also in the lip function by stimulating labial muscle contraction.

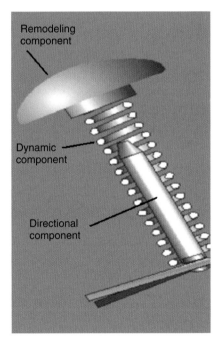

Figure 6.5 The dynamic nasal device introduced in 2002.

This newly designed intraoral appliance consists of two elements:

(1) a perfectly adapted conventional acrylic intraoral plate, and
(2) a dynamic nasal bumper attached to the vestibular flange of the intraoral plate (Bennun *et al.*, 2002; Bennun & Figueroa, 2006) (Figure 6.5).

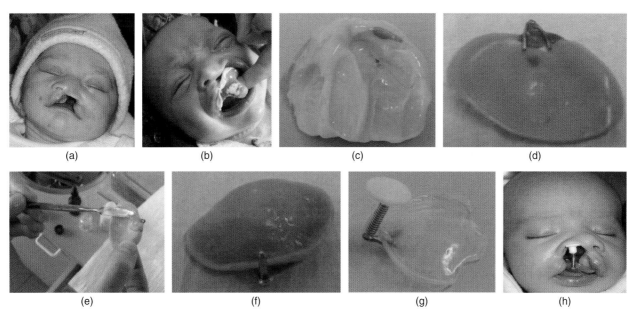

Figure 6.6 (a–h) Step-by-step manufacture process in a newborn patient.

The alignment of the alveolar segments creates a foundation upon which excellent results of lip and primary nasal surgery are dependent in the repair of the cleft lip and palate patient (Bennun & Langsam, 2009).

The purpose of this chapter is to illustrate the step-by-step manufacture and application process of the nasoalveolar remodeling appliance used to direct the growth and repositioning of the alveolar ridge, lips, and nose in the presurgical treatment of cleft lip and palate (Figure 6.6).

Objectives of dynamic presurgical nasoalveolar remodeling (DPNR technique)

- Forces applied on nasal and alveolar processes allow growth, remodeling, and repositioning of the deformed nasal cartilages and maxillary arch.
- Normalizing the cleft side of the columella.
- Removing the intranasal bridge.
- Placement of the lip segments in a more anatomically correct position, facilitating lip repair without scarring.
- DPNR is recommended to produce more favorable bone formation by reducing the size of the cleft in order to decrease the need for secondary alveolar bone grafts.
- Decreasing the cost of treatments and the number of surgical procedures.
- Improving nasal esthetics.

Study population

We implemented our DPNR technique treatment protocol in all patients who had their first consultation within 15 days of life.

We planned a prospective research project where the main nasolabial anthropometric parameters were included.

These parameters were directly verified – by the same person – at the first consultation, immediately before lip and nose repair, and at the time of cleft palate closure, both under general anesthesia; final control was at the age of 6.

The study included patients treated in our hospital from March 2002 to March 2012, and operated on by the same senior surgeon.

The population included 86 patients with unilateral cleft lip and palate (50 males and 36 females), and 48 patients with a bilateral cleft lip and palate (26 males and 22 females).

The control group consisted of 48 healthy 6-year old children (24 males and 24 females).

Statistical analyses were performed using SAS version 9.3 (SAS Institute Inc.).

Step-by-step procedure description

The treatment is initiated at the external border of the alar nose, to obtain muscle and mucosa relaxation, and with a posterior elongation of the nasal muscles causing alar depression. The aim is internal nasal bridge removal.

In a second step, the odonto-pediatrician centralizes the nasal component to ameliorate the alar cartilage breaking down. If this modification is achieved during the first month, the distortion can be eliminated from memory tissues.

In a posterior visit the expert will follow up with centralization of the nasal device, to push up and reposition the crus medialis to achieve a longer collumelar side.

Once all these modifications are accomplished, the specialist will change the directional component for a longer one, with the aim of gaining more nasal tip projection. The nasal device

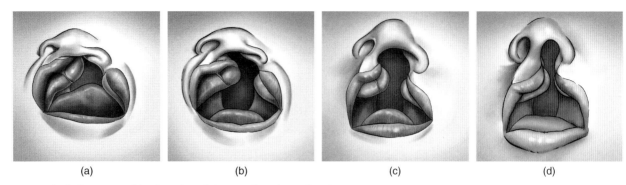

Figure 6.7 (a–d) Illustrations of the chronological changes achieved in unilateral cases.

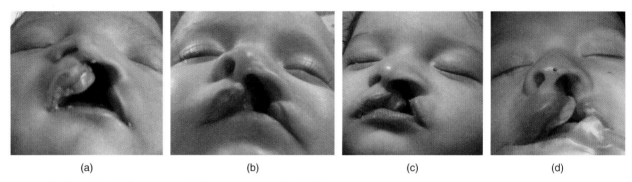

Figure 6.8 (a–d) Initial to final improvement before surgery in a unilateral cleft patient.

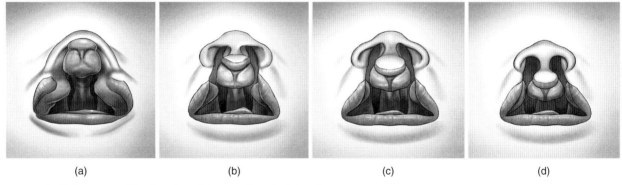

Figure 6.9 (a–d) Illustrations of the chronological changes achieved in bilateral cases.

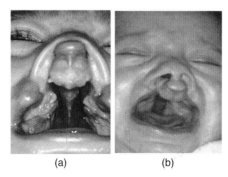

Figure 6.10 (a) Initial and (b) final pictures showing improvement in a bilateral cleft patient.

in this way also produces labial muscle traction and a subsidiary vertical high increase of the lip on both sides of the cleft (Figures 6.7–6.10).

Results

This study revealed that minimal nasal morphology differences remained between the DPNR-treated group and the age-matched, sex-matched, normal control group. However, these differences were significantly less than the discrepancies encountered with the not presurgically treated group of our previous research.

The unilateral series

See Figures 6.11 to 6.17.

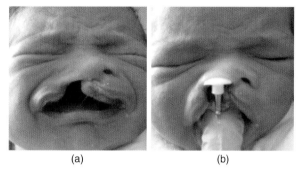

(a)   (b)

Figure 6.11 (a, b) Nasal cartilage can be remodeled with permanent results if treatment is started within 6 weeks of life.

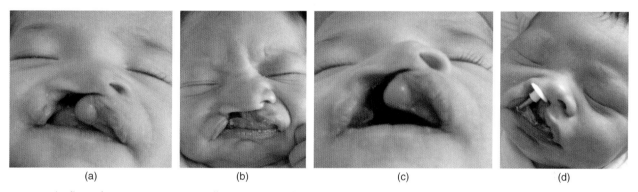

(a)   (b)   (c)   (d)

Figure 6.12 (a–d) Avoiding tongue inter-position allows a passive guided arch correction. Nasal and alveolar modification should be initiated during the first week.

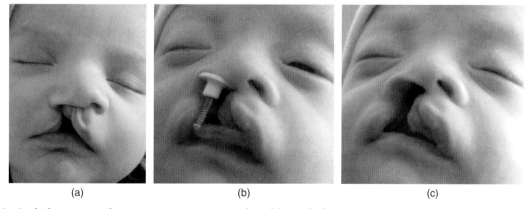

(a)   (b)   (c)

Figure 6.13 (a–c) A high percentage of permanent improvements are achieved during the first month.

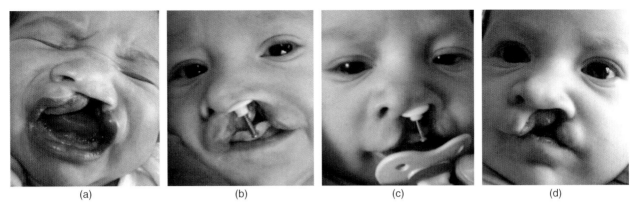

Figure 6.14 (a–d) The nasal device produces labial muscle traction and a subsidiary vertical height increase of the lip on both sides of the cleft.

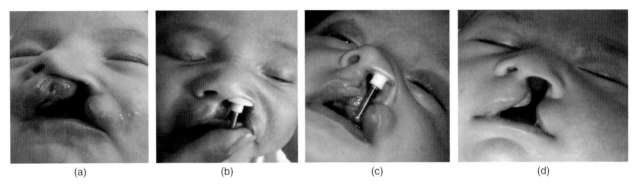

Figure 6.15 (a–d) DPNR is recommended to contribute to a more favorable bone formation by reducing the size of the cleft in order to decrease the need for secondary alveolar bone grafts.

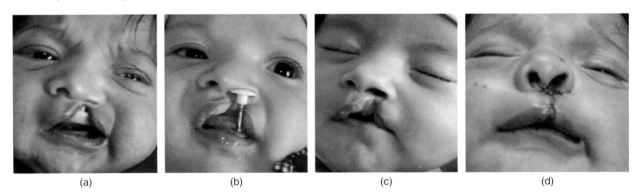

Figure 6.16 (a–d) In the presence of an incomplete cleft lip with or without cleft palate, short term implementation of DPNR can be an option to avoid surgical nose correction.

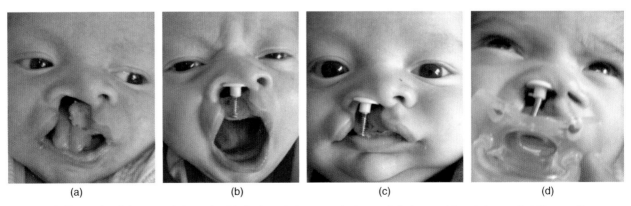

Figure 6.17 (a–h) Introduced changes make it comfortable for the oral plate to stay in the mouth for longer without being expelled. The use of tape or adhesives is not necessary. The intranasal bridge can be totally removed.

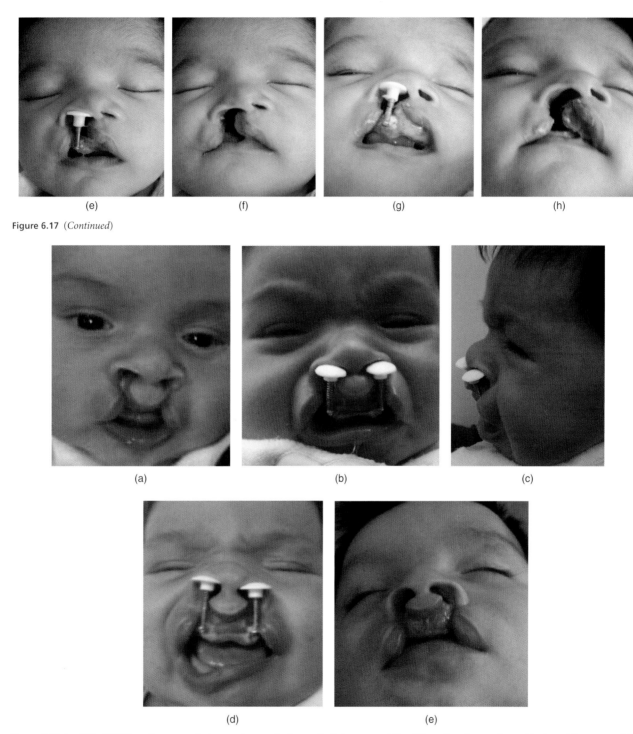

(e)   (f)   (g)   (h)

Figure 6.17 (*Continued*)

(a)   (b)   (c)

(d)   (e)

Figure 6.18 (a–e) The DPNR appliance acts during suction, producing gradual tissue remodeling. Bilateral push up and repositioning of the crus medialis allows the achievement of a longer collumela and more nasal tip projection. Working in this way the device also produces labial muscle traction and a subsidiary vertical height increase of the lip on both sides of the cleft.

The bilateral problem

See Figure 6.18.

Dealing with asymmetry

See Figures 6.19 to 6.21.

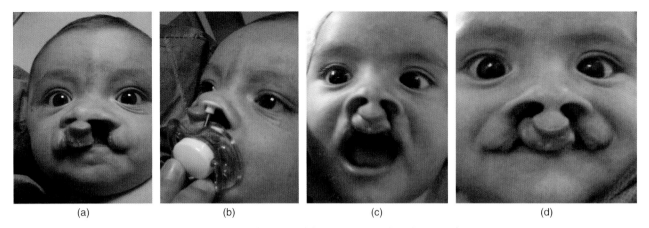

Figure 6.19 (a–d) Asymmetrical cases are an indication. We have treated this patient as a unilateral case to achieve symmetry.

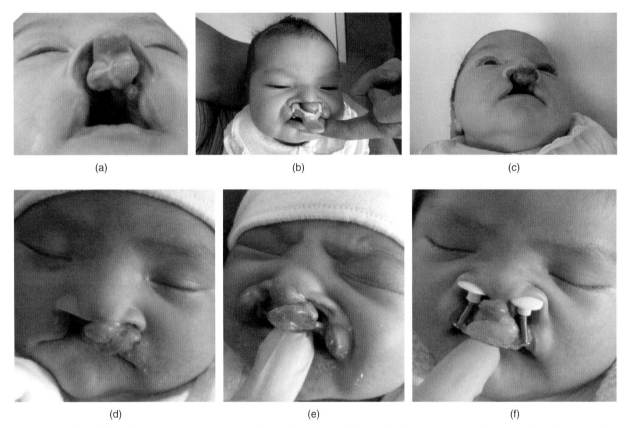

Figure 6.20 (a–i) Centralizing the premaxilla at the moment of impression we can build a modified plate to maintain the premaxilla in the center. After obtaining symmetry we are ready to start nose remodeling.

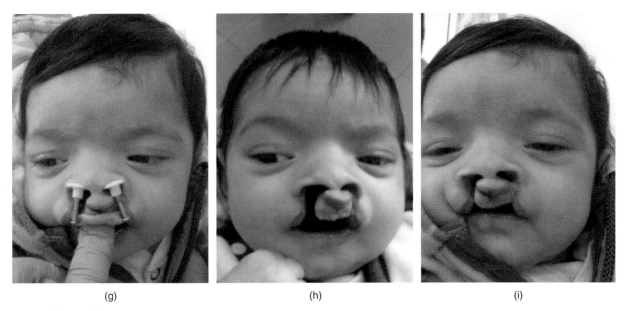

(g)　　　　　　　　　　　(h)　　　　　　　　　　　(i)

Figure 6.20 (*Continued*)

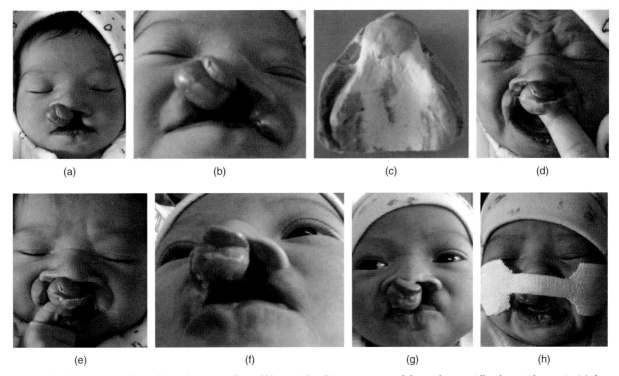

(a)　　　　　　(b)　　　　　　(c)　　　　　　(d)

(e)　　　　　　(f)　　　　　　(g)　　　　　　(h)

Figure 6.21 (a–p) The process of centralizing the premaxilla could be considered instantaneous and the newborn rapidly adapts without pain. (g) shows the premaxilla changes after 48 h. In cases of very protruded premaxilla, after centralization we can use an elastic mask to improve results. Nose remodeling is indicated as soon as possible. (k–m) show the device acting during suction. (o, p) show the frontal and inferior view of the immediate postop result. The possibility of having well-conformed and repositioned alar cartilages with more relaxed nose and labial tissues makes the surgical reconstruction easier.

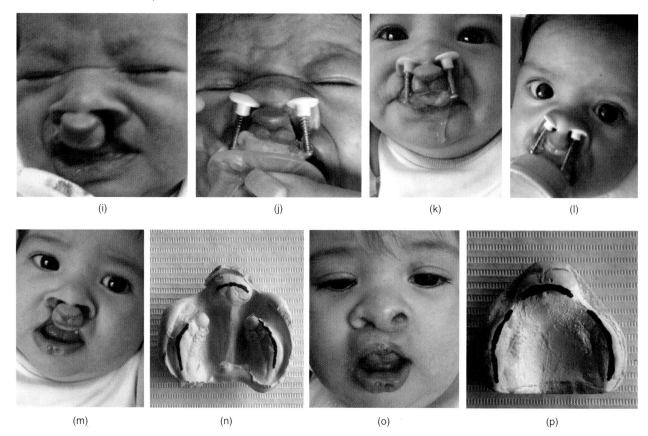

(i)   (j)   (k)   (l)

(m)   (n)   (o)   (p)

Figure 6.21 (*Continued*)

Discussion

Some types of surgery performed on the tip of the nose, such as secondary rhinoplasty on cleft lip and palate (CLP) patients, may have an uncertain end result due to difficulty in maintaining the surgically created status constant over time.

This is precisely the reason behind the multiple proposals and surgical techniques presented by various authors through the years, in order to produce a long-lasting, valid, surgical result. The problem has been approached through implementing varied and creative methods and still remains partially unsolved. Experience has shown that application of a dynamic nasal splint has contributed efficiently to maintaining the surgical results by opposing healing contraction (Cenzi & Guarda, 1996).

Based on a literature review, nasal molding seems to be more beneficial and effective with better long-term results (Matsuo *et al.*, 1991; Singh *et al.*, 2005). However, the effect of alveolar molding needs to be studied further to assess the long-term beneficial effects (Baek & Son, 2006). More favorable results were obtained when gingivoperiosteoplasty was performed along with primary lip repair (Smahel & Müllerová, 1988). Hence it can be concluded that not only the interdisciplinary approach but also a thorough knowledge of the changing concepts of nasoalveolar molding and timing of initiation are essential to improve results (Matsuo *et al.*, 1989; Abbot & Meara, 2012).

Considering the physiopathology of the nasolabial deformity, it is clear how important early prevention of unfavorable factors is. Taking into consideration wound healing concepts we can conclude that premature treating of tissues "without memory" allows avoidance of alar cartilage deformity fixing.

The DPNR technique does not rely on the relatively static force exerted by an orthopedic plate held in place by means of tape or adhesives.

Introduced changes make it more comfortable to keep the oral plate in the mouth longer without being expelled, and also means the use of tape or adhesives is not necessary.

A new, well-adapted nasal component allows better remodeling effects, reducing the time and frequency of visits and avoiding tissue lesions.

The device can be employed in any child and in any type of cleft, and a completed successful treatment results in fewer economic and social costs than any other described procedure.

The possibility of easily modifying the device size and impact direction, allows step-by-step treatment of all the components of nasal distortion, reproducing the described distortion process in an opposing manner.

The possibility of achieving a well-conformed and repositioned alar cartilage with more relaxed nose and labial tissues makes surgical reconstruction easier.

It avoids aggressive surgical dissection and diminishing scars, benefiting normal facial growth and development.

A reduced number of surgical procedures and the shortening of treatments contributes to reduced social and monetary expenses and facilitates normal social insertion of the child at school age.

Conclusions

The DPNR appliance acts via suction, producing gradual tissue remodeling. The device's nasal components are easily adjusted to allow the correction of any distortion of the lip and nose region.

The nasal bumper acts not only on the nasal structures but also on the lip function by stimulating labial muscle contraction. It has been observed that after use of DPNR technique, the length of both cleft sides of the lip improves.

When this protocol is instituted early, it can avoid memory fixation of cartilage and other tissue.

This action over the lip may also help to produce muscular bone on the anterior maxilla, which in turn may be favorable to further approximate the alveolar cleft segments.

The DPNR technique is a worthwhile option to improve cleft nasal deformity and palatal arch conformation previous to surgery, facilitating the reconstructive procedure and improving postop outcomes.

The simplicity of design makes it very useful in any form of unilateral or bilateral cleft presentation.

Although it is not a "magic" solution, presurgical remodeling gives the surgeon the possibility of working with less distorted and more flexible tissues.

This way, repair and closure will be less aggressive – wide cheek dissection will not be necessary – and free of any tension. Fewer scars mean fewer possibilities of maxillary retrusion.

The key to dissection will be the total liberation and normal repositioning of all the mal-inserted nasal and labial structures around the pyriform aperture. Subperiosteal dissection is not necessary.

The muscles once placed in the right position will contribute to complete in a perfect way the palatal arch closure and to prevent oronasal fistulas.

Because of its good results and simplicity, this approach is to be recommended to benefit children in less developed countries, where numerous surgeries are not possible and the percentage of sequels is high. Well-trained pediatric plastic surgeons and dedicated teams still remain an obvious requirement.

References

Abbott, M. M. and Meara, J. G. (2012) Nasoalveolar molding in cleft care: Is it efficacious? *Plast Reconstr Surg* **130**(3):659–666.

Adzick, N., Harrison, M., and Glick, P. (1985) Comparison of fetal, newborn and adult wound healing by histologic, enzyme-histochemical and hudroxyptoline determination. *J Pediatr Surg* **20**:315.

Adzick, N. S. and Lorenz, H. P. (1994) Cells, matrix, growth factors, and the surgeon. The biology of scarless fetal wound repair. *Ann Surg* **220**:10–18.

Baek, S. H. and Son, W. S. (2006) Difference in alveolar molding effect and growth in the cleft segments: 3-dimensional analysis of unilateral cleft lip and palate patients *Oral Surg Oral Med Oral Pathol Oral Radiol Endod* **102**(2):160–168.

Bennun, R. D., Perandones, C., Sepliarsky, V. A., *et al.* (1999) Non-surgical correction of nasal deformity in unilateral complete cleft lip: a 6 years follow-up. *Plast Reconstr Surg* **3**:616–630.

Bennun, R. D., Perandones, C., Sepliarsky, V. A., *et al.* (2001) Non-surgical correction of nasal deformity in unilateral complete cleft lip: a 6 years follow-up. *Year Book of Plast Reconstr and Aesthetic Surg* **1**:16–17.

Bennun, R. D., Zaszczynski, S., and Celnik, R. (2002) Remodelacion naso-labial pre-quirúrgica en fisura labio alveolo palatina: Nuevo diseño del componente nasal. *Rev Arg Ortodon* **66**:16–21.

Bennun, R. D. and Figueroa, A. A. (2006) Dynamic Presurgical Naso Alveolar Remodeling in Patients with unilateral and bilateral cleft lip and palate: Modification to the original technique. *Cleft Palate Craniofac J* **43**:639–648.

Bennun, R. D. and Langsam, A. C. (2009) Long term results after using Dynamic Presurgical Nasoalveolar Remodeling technique in patients with unilateral and bilateral cleft lips and palates. *Craniofac Surg J* **20**(1):670–674.

Berkowitz, S. (1977) Cleft lip and palate research: An updated state of the art. Section III: Orofacial growth and dentistry: A state of the art report on neonatal maxillary orthopedics. *Cleft Palate J* **14**:288–301.

Caplan, A. I. (2002) In vivo remodeling. *Ann NY Acad Sci* **961**:307–308.

Cenzi, R. and Guarda, L. A. (1996) A dynamic nostril splint in the surgery of the nasal tip: technical innovation. *J Cranio Maxillofac Surg* **24**(2):88–91.

Chen, W. Y., Grant, M. E., Schor, A. M., *et al.* (1989) Differences between adult and foetal fibroblasts in the regulation hyaluronate synthesis: correlation with migratory activity. *J Cell Sci* **94**:577.

Dogliotti, P. L., Bennun, R. D., Lozoviz, E., *et al.* (1991) Tratamiento no quirurgico de la deformidad nasal en el paciente fisurado. *Rev Ateneo Argent Odontol* **27**:31–35.

Enlow, D. H. (1982) *Handbook of Facial Growth*. Philadelphia, PA: W.B. Saunders.

Frost, H. M. (1993) Suggested fundamental concepts in skeletal physiology. *Calcif Tissue Int* **52**(1):1–4.

Frost, H. M. and Schonau, E. (2000) The "muscle-bone unit" in children and adolescents: A 2000 overview. *J Pediatr Endocrinol Metabol* **13**(6):571–590.

Grayson, B. H., Cutting, C. and Wood, R. (1993) Preoperative columella lengthening in bilateral cleft lip and palate. *Plast Reconstr Surg* **92**(7):1422–1423.

Grayson, B. H., Santiago, P., Brecht, L. *et al.* (1999) Presurgical naso-alveolar molding in patients with cleft lip and palate. *Cleft Palate Craniofac J* **36**:486–498.

Greisler, H. P. (2002) Regulated in vivo remodeling. *Ann NY Acad Sci* **961**:309–311.

Hamrick, M. W. (1999) A chondral modeling theory revisited. *J Theor Biol* Dec 7;(201)**3**:201–208.

Hardingham, T. E. and Muir, H. (1972) The specific interaction of hyaluronic acid with cartilage proteoglycans. *Biochem Biophys Acta* **279**:401–405.

Herndon, D. N., Nguyen, T. T., and Gilpin, D. A. (1993) Growth factors, local and systemic. *Arch Surg* **128**:1227–1233.

Hollinger, J. O. and Wong, M. E. K. (1996) The integrated processes of hard tissue regeneration with special emphasis on fracture healing. *Oral Surg Oral Med, Oral Path, Oral Radiol* **82**:594–606.

Hozt, M., Gnoinski, W. (1976) Comprehensive care of cleft lip and palate children at Zurich University: A preliminary report. *Am J Orthod* **70**:481–504.

Kenny, F. M., Angsusingha, M., Chen, P. K. *et al.* (1973) Unconjugated estrogens in the perinatal period. *Pediatr Res* **10**:976–981.

Matsuo, K., Hirose, T., and Tomono, T. (1984) Nonsurgical correction of congenital auricular deformities in early neonatal period. *Plast Reconstr Surg* **73**:38–50.

Matsuo, K., Hirose, T., Otagiri, T., *et al.* (1989) Repair of cleft lip with nonsurgical correction of nasal deformity in the early neonatal period. *Plast Reconstr Surg* **83**(**1**):25–31.

Matsuo, K., Hirose, T., Otagiri, T., *et al.* (1991) Preoperative non-surgical over-correction of cleft lip nasal deformity. *Br J Plast Surg* **44**(**1**):5–11.

McNeil, C. K. (1950) Orthodontic procedures in the treatment of congenital cleft palate. *Dent Rec* **70**:126–32.

Millard Jr., D. R. (1986) *Principalization of Plastic Surgery*. Boston, MA: Little Brown.

Murthy, P. S., Deshmukh, S., Bhagyalakshmi, A., *et al.* (2013) Pre surgical nasoalveolar molding: Changing paradigms in early cleft lip and palate rehabilitation. *J Int Oral Health* **5**(**2**):76–86.

Robinson, C. J. (1993) Growth factors: Therapeutic advances in wound healing. *Ann Med* **25**:535–553.

Shetty, V., Vyas, H. J., Sharma, S. M., *et al.* (2012) A Comparison of results using nasoalveolar molding in cleft infants treated within 1month of life versus those treated after this period: development of new protocol. *Int J Oral Maxillofac Surg* **41**(**1**):28–36.

Singh, G. D., Levy-Bercowski, D., and Santiago, P. E. (2005) Three-dimensional nasal changes following nasoalveolar molding in patients with unilateral cleft lip and palate: Geometric morphometrics. *Cleft Palate Craniofac J* **42**(**4**):403–409.

Smahel, Z. and Müllerová, Z. (1988) Effects of primary periosteoplasty on facial growth in unilateral cleft lip and palate: 10-year follow-up. *Cleft Palate J* **25**(**4**):356–361.

Thomas, B. L., Krummel, T. M., Melany, M., *et al.* (1998) Collagen synthesis and type expression by fetal fibroblasts in vitro. *Surg Forum* **39**:642–644.

West, D. C. and Kumar, S. (1989) The effect of hyaluronate and its oligosaccharides on endothelial cell proliferation and monolayer integrity. *Exp Cell Res* **183**:179–196.

CHAPTER 7
Pediatric anesthesia considerations

Luis Moggi[1], Diofre Ponce[1], and María Bevilacqua[2]
[1]Children Hospital of Buenos Aires, Argentina
[2]National Pediatric Hospital of Buenos Aires, Argentina

Introduction

In our experience, optimal cosmetic results for cleft lip repair occur when lip and nose reconstruction is performed between 2–5 months of age. This leads to immediate improvement in suction and decreases the parent's anxiety.

The current general consensus is to close palatal clefts in one procedure at about 6–9 months, at which time the child begins the process of phonation, or voicing (Carreno *et al.*, 2000).

Both procedures – cleft lip repair and cleft palate closure – must be done with extreme caution to prevent maxillary growth alterations.

Sometimes, because of the presence of a cleft lip and palate, the child fails to develop a successful combination of both generating negative intraoral pressure and intraoral muscular movements to suck the nipple. The inability to coordinate feeding and breathing correctly leads to inadequate nutrition, anemia, and failure to thrive (Hodges & Hodges, 2000).

In addition to the standard preoperative history and examination, special attention must be provided in assessing associated anomalies such as: Pierre Robin Syndrome (with retrognathia, micrognathia, and lingual ptosis where recurrent hypoxemia and sleep apnea can lead to ventricular hypertrophy and Cor pulmonale), Treacher Collins Syndrome, Goldenhar Syndrome, congenital heart disease 5–10% and Down syndrome. Chronic rhinorhea, nasal regurgitation, and pulmonary aspiration might also be associated with cleft lip and palate (Nazer, 2005).

Clinical and anesthesia considerations

Our population included a total of 763 newborns, of which 439 had unilateral complete cleft lip, 324 had bilateral complete cleft lip, and 114 were secondary cases. Gender distribution was 39.6% female and 58.7% male. The mean age for lip and nose reconstruction was 4 months and the average weight was 6.3 kg. The palate repair was completed at a mean age of 10 months with an average weight of 9.1 kg. Regarding revisions, the age varied between 2 to 29 years, with a predominance of 71.7% being female patients.

Preoperative anesthesia assessment included: fasting for 6 hours for solids, 3 hours for breast milk, and 2 hours for clear fluids (water and apple or orange pulp-free juices). Routine presurgical lab tests included complete blood count, (hemoglobin of 9 g/dl in 2–5 months of patients due to transient physiological infant anemia), blood studies, and cardiac assessment.

Induction of anesthesia was safely performed by inhalation anesthesia with a gradually increasing dose of halothane or sevoflurane. Intravenous access was secured when an adequate depth of anesthesia was achieved and endotracheal intubation was performed under deep volatile anesthesia with a hydration protocol. The hydration protocol included 13 ml/kg/hour with 0.85% NaCl physiological solution. A neuromuscular blocking agent was used to relax muscles: atracurium besylate at doses between 0.–0.4 mg/kg, fentanyl citrate 1–3 ug/kg, or nalbuphine hydrochloride 30 ug/kg (Figure 7.1).

Regional anesthesia of both the face and palate were performed using superficial safe techniques by slowly infiltrating small volumes of local anesthetic with epinephrine to obtain a good and persistent neurosensory block.

Anatomical description

The arteries that supply the palate are branches of the sphenopalatine and the descending palatine vessels. The pterygoid plexus of veins and lymphatics drains into the internal jugular chain. Innervation is from the trigeminal or Vth cranial nerve and its upper maxillary branch.

Cleft Lip and Palate Management: A Comprehensive Atlas, First Edition. Edited by Ricardo D. Bennun, Julia F. Harfin, George K. B. Sándor, and David Genecov.
© 2016 John Wiley & Sons, Inc. Published 2016 by John Wiley & Sons, Inc.

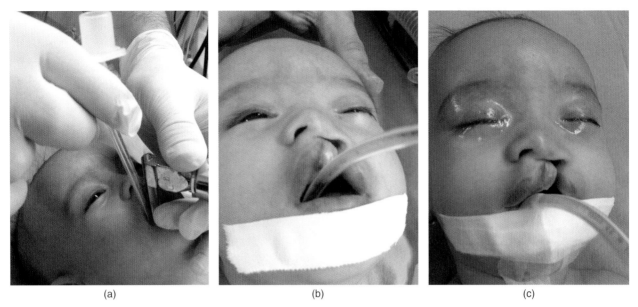

(a)   (b)   (c)

Figure 7.1 (a–c) The inferior lip can be fixed to avoid eversion and extubation during surgery.

The branches of the nasociliary nerve are: the infratroclear posterior ethmoidal nerve, and the ethmoidal nasal or former internal nasal nerve which, in turn, divide into two branches: internal and external. They innervate the skin of the nose below the bones and the nasal tip with the exception of the nostrils and wing areas, which are innervated by the descending infraorbital nerve.

For the blocking technique of the extraorbital nerve, there are two sites to make injections. The first is in the nasal root at the medial angle of the eye in the direction of the nasal base, and the second is on the nasal groove with a direction toward the cheek. The injection is performed with 2% lidocaine chlorhydrate with epinephrine 1:50.000 in a 1-cc syringe, at each anatomic location, slowly. Complications of the injections are perforation of a vein or artery, and injury by lifting of the periosteum (which results in a painful postsurgical recovery).

The infraorbital nerve appears as the main terminal branch of the maxillary nerve, emerging through the infraorbital foramen. The palpebral branches anastomose with the facial and the zygomaticofacial nerves. The nasal branches innervate the alae of the nose, nostrils, and the upper lip towards the cheek (Pulcini *et al.*, 2007) (Figure 7.2).

Both the infraorbital nerve and artery emerge some 4 to 7 mm from the edge of the orbit, through the infraorbital foramen. This superior alveolar branch is palpable and can be located by ultrasound techniques. This foramen is centered at the pupillary line, although the axis of the foramen is oriented toward the nasal wing; the infiltration must be directed toward the nasal root. The technique is easy, and arterial puncture is uncommon. Other ways to block the maxillary nerve also can be used (Pulcini *et al.*, 2007; Mesnil *et al.*, 2010).

Anesthetic and surgical results

Repair of cleft lip and palate involves sharing of the airway by the anesthesiologist and the surgeon. Therefore, adjustment of the endotracheal tube (ETT) is most relevant to the safety of the anesthetic. A tape should be placed over the lower lip and chin, without covering both corners of the mouth, in order to provide less mobility of tissue. Then, above this layer, another layer of tape is responsible for the fixation of the ETT. The procedure is performed using hypoallergenic paper tape, which is more resistant to wetting by either povidone-iodine and/or other secretions such as blood. In cleft lip surgery, we use ordinary uncuffed endotracheal tubes. If necessary, cuffed endotracheal tubes can also be used (should be 0.5 mm smaller in internal diameter), when using wet gauze with saline irrigating solution. Preformed guarded oral endotracheal tubes and reinforced ETT are used in cleft palate repair (Jaeger & Durbin, 1999).

Usually, there are no ventilation problems, but occasional problems may arise during direct laryngoscopy due to a lack of support of the straight blade of the laryngoscope. One useful maneuver is to fill the slot with gauze to serve as support for the laryngoscope blade. Intra-operative mechanical ventilation is controlled by pressure.

At the end of the surgical procedure, we cease administering anesthetics, and proceed with ventilatory recovery, administering antagonists (atropine-neostigmine in doses of 10 and 30 ug/kg respectively). Extubation is performed in forced inspiration and the patient is transferred to the Post Anesthesia Care Unit, where the baby recovers with its parents.

Surgical intervention time was between 49 ± 13 minutes for unilateral cleft lips and cleft palate repair, compared to 75 ± 28 minutes for bilateral cleft lip, and 68 ± 31 for revisions.

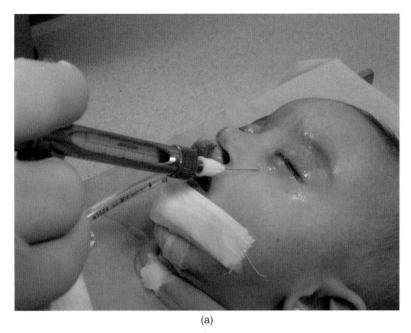
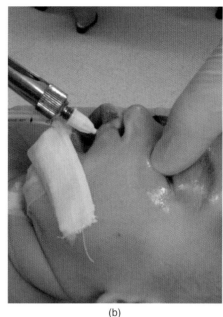

(a)   (b)

Figure 7.2 (a, b) Two different ways to perform regional anesthesia of the infraorbital nerve are shown.

Feeding starts approximately 30 minutes following the surgical procedure, beginning with the administration of breast milk or water to test gastric tolerance. If tolerated, then after 10 minutes we start with ice water or gelatin.

Discharge from the Post Anesthesia Care Unit is allowed after 120 minutes, with satisfactory gastric tolerance and recovery, requiring clear indications and fast communication contact with the surgical team.

Only two patients in this group of 739 patients required overnight hospitalization. The rest were discharged on the same day. The first overnight case was due to persistent vomiting, and the other because of social deficiencies.

Conclusions

Oral clefts represent the congenital malformations with the most stable frequencies over time. The most common post-operative complications are bleeding and airway obstruction (Chandy *et al.*, 2010).

Facial and palatal regional anesthesia is key in general anesthesia to allow the use of fewer central nervous system depressant drugs, allowing for a faster recovery and facilitating the possibility of moving these procedures to outpatient surgeries.

Ambulatory surgery is increasing worldwide, reducing hospital stays, lessening family separation, lowering costs in health insurance, and thus in the long run providing the desired results (Maestre, 2000).

Understanding the physiopathology of these malformations facilitates the reduction of risks in nutrition. These maneuvers

lead to the implementation of better policies in healthcare (Kundra *et al.*, 2009; Paine *et al.*, 2014).

References

Carreño, H., Paredes, M., and Tellez G. (2000) Estudio de asociación entre fisura labiopalatina no sindrómica y marcadores de microsatélite ubicados en 6p. *Rev Méd Chile* **127**:1189–1198.

Chandy, T. T., Pragasam, A. A., and Joselyn, A. S. (2010) Anestesia para Fisura Labial y Reparación del Paladar. *Entendiendo la anestesia pediátrica* **22**:209–215.

Hodges, S. C. and Hodges, A. M. (2000) A protocol for safe anesthesia for cleft lip and palate surgery in developing countries. *Anesthesia* **55**:436–441.

Jaeger, J. M. and Durbin Jr., C. G. (1999) Special purpose endotracheal tubes. *Respir Care* **44**:661–683.

Kundra, P., Supraja, N., Agrawal, K., and Ravishankar, M. (2009) Flexible laryngeal mask airway for cleft palate surgery in children: A randomized clinical trial on efficacy and safety. *Cleft Palate Craniofac J* **46**:368–373.

Maestre, J. M. (2000) Control de calidad en cirugía mayor ambulatoria. *Rev Esp Anestesiol Reanim* **47**:99–100.

Mesnil, M., Dadure, C., Captier, G., *et al.* (2010) A new approach for perioperative analgesia of cleft palate repair in infants: The bilateral suprazygomatic maxillary nerve block. *Ped Anesth* **20**:343–349.

Nazer, J. (2005) Fisuras orales. En Hübner Guzman ME, Ramírez Fernandez MC, Nazer Herrera J. *Malformaciones congénitas. Diagnóstico y manejo neonatal.* Ed. Universitaria. 91–5.

Paine, K. M., Tahiri, Y., Wes, A. *et al.* (2014) Patient risk factors for ambulatory cleft lip repair: An outcome and cost analysis. *Plast Reconstr Surg* **134**:275e–82e.

Pulcini, J.-P., Guerin, S., Sibon, *et al.* (2007) Bloqueos faciales. *EMC - Anestesia-Reanimación* 1–15 [Article 36–326–L–10].

CHAPTER 8

Developmental field reassignment cleft surgery: reassessment and refinements

Michael H. Carstens

Saint Louis University and Universidad Nacional Autónoma de Nicargua, Nicaragua

Introduction

All plastic surgeons involved in the care of cleft-affected children and adults experience first-hand both the rewards and the limitations of our craft. This work requires a certain mindset characterized by four qualities: an intense curiosity about cleft biology, a relentless pursuit of good technique, an unflinching assessment of results (both good and bad), and humility in the constant search for better ideas. Of all these characteristics, humility is perhaps the most important. It leads us to constantly search out and appreciate the work of other surgeons. Superior concepts or protocols should be embraced, not rejected.

In this chapter I shall discuss how my thinking about developmental field reassignment has morphed over the years. The focus will be restricted to problems related to lip clefts (complete or incomplete) combined with complete clefts of the alveolus and palate (the unstable dental arch). The principle sources for change stem from long-term observations of the outcomes of surgical interventions (my own and those of others) and intellectual contributions of colleagues that make so much biologic sense to me that they demand to be incorporated. The organization of this chapter is built around four sets of issues that I have found most perplexing. We shall consider each of these in turn.

Medial wall dissection: Certain aspects of the DFR design produced results that were not ideal or did not make sense. (i) In some cases I observed *flattening of the cupid's bow* at the intersection of the white-roll and the cleft-side philtral column. (ii) Since 2003 I have been advancing the cleft-side medial crus into the nasal tip using an *anterolateral columellar incision*. Although this design worked well (with excellent scars) I had the nagging suspicion that a simpler design would accomplish the same goals. (iii) I realized that the intranasal extension of the prolabial incision was an *embryologic challenge* because it would have to conform to the neurovascular field map of the medial nasal wall. What were the precise boundaries between skin of forebrain neural crest origin and skin originating from the hindbrain neural crest?

Lateral wall dissection: Nasal airway expansion, a top priority in DFR surgery, was difficult to maintain, despite the near-perfect fit of the non-philtral prolabium flap into the lateral wall releasing incision. Why should the cleft-side nasal airway arrive at its particular shape? What cause or causes could explain the functional limitations of breathing on the cleft side? There seemed to be a missing piece to the puzzle. What was it?

Dental arch management: Coming to clarity regarding the surgical-orthodontic sequence with respect to the alveolar arch was a very frustrating problem for me. The long-standing debate regarding presurgical orthopedics has been characterized by loudly stated opinions and a near-total lack of developmental biology. Understanding the cleft maxilla and its reconstruction requires the juxtaposition of new input from developmental field biology, with a surgical and orthodontic protocol in functional agreement with basic science. Above all, a biologic protocol should be backed up by long-term results.

Microform cleft: It has long been observed that a small number of patients have a nasal deformity characteristic of cleft lip but a minimal to absent affectation of the lip itself. The literature on this subject is limited but very consistent. All such patients have asymmetries of the nasal floor/alar base; some degree of septal deflection is always present. The microform cleft is truly the "*form fruste*" in the problem. It demonstrates most elegantly that the source of the pathology lies within the piriform fossa, not the lip. In addition, the microform cleft demonstrates how differences in the fluid mechanics of fetal ventilation cause deformation of the septum.

Cleft Lip and Palate Management: A Comprehensive Atlas, First Edition. Edited by Ricardo D. Bennun, Julia F. Harfin, George K. B. Sándor, and David Genecov.
© 2016 John Wiley & Sons, Inc. Published 2016 by John Wiley & Sons, Inc.

Of late, I have been able to find more satisfactory answers to these questions. And herein, at risk of being a bit informal, I'd like to include some personal details as to how these have emerged. No craniofacial surgeon works in a vacuum. The contributions of long-term work by David Matthews, Jean Claude Talmant, Jean-Pierre Lumineau, and Luis Monasterio are essential components in the evolution of the developmental field model. What is remarkable is that each of us, coming from different experiences, has arrived at a very similar set of priorities and techniques. My purpose here is to bring these perspectives together into a single unitary philosophy based on the developmental field model of cleft formation. As Victor Veau put it so well "the surgery of clefts is merely experimental embryology." This chapter intends to prove him right.

Embryology and neurovascular anatomy of the premaxilla and prolabium

Understanding the development of the premaxilla and prolabium is fundamental for cleft lip surgery. Paired premaxillae with four incisor teeth comprise the "keystone" of the dental arch. Each premaxilla is a relatively simple structure consisting of mucosa, membranous bone, and two incisors.

Prolabium refers to the non-mucosal soft tissue coverage of the premaxillae. Its anatomy is "more than meets the eye"

because the prolabium is a *composite of tissues* that originate from *different locations in the embryo*. Under normal conditions the original prolabium fuses with the lateral lip elements. Its lateral embryonic components become tucked inside the nose as the soft tissue coverage of the lateral incisor and the frontal process zones of the premaxilla. We tend to forget that they exist. Thus, the best way to study the embryology of the prolabium is in its "native" state: the complete bilateral cleft. We will then discuss how the prolabium in unilateral cleft patients contains extra tissues belonging to the first and second pharyngeal arches.

Where exactly do these tissues originate? Let us quickly review the salient facts. Recall that craniofacial mesenchyme (fascial, cartilage, bone, fat, dermis, submucosa, sclera, etc.) is derived from neural crest, not mesoderm. Only striated muscle and the chondral bones of the cranial base posterior to the pituitary (basisphenoid, basioccipital, and exoccipital) are mesodermal. Anterior to the four occipital somites that flank the hindbrain, paraxial mesoderm is segmentally organized into seven somitomeres (Sms). Extraocular muscles come from Sm1, Sm2, Sm3, and Sm5. The muscles of mastication arise from Sm4, facial muscles from Sm 5, Sm6, and the muscles of the third arch come from Sm7. All these muscles are innervated by cranial nerves; as these pass through the meninges they become ensheathed with neural crest cells.

Neural crest arises from the neural folds and begins to migrate into outlying embryonic tissues quite early, prior to neurulation.

The focus of this chapter is practical: to present technical in novations in cleft surgery based upon principles of developmental anatomy. The final configuration of a cleft is the result of tissue deficiency or fusion failure during in embryogenesis leading to displacement and distortion of otherwise normal adjacent structures. It has long been my conviction that understanding why and how this process occurs would provide the key to surgical strategy based on unraveling a mechanism rather than imposing a geometric design. DFR evolved as means to reassign developmental fields that had be come mismatched so that, with all fields restored into normal relationships, growth could proceed normally and relapse could be avoided.

My goal with these illustrations is to show exactly how to carry out DFR, including variations depending upon the philosophical goals of the surgical team. We will start with the original DFR design to point out what aspects proved to be of true functional value and what aspects could be either be discarded or used as an option. The sequence follows that of the surgery itself: medial dissection, lateral dissection, closure, and nasal splinting.

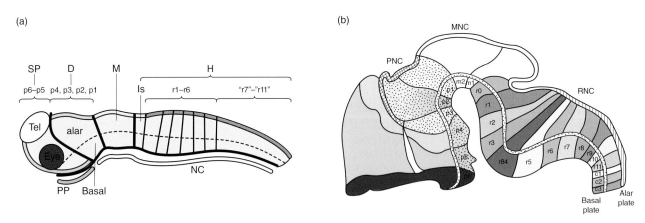

Figure 8.1 Review of neuromeric system and associated tissues. Colors represent source material of the skin and subcutaneous tissue. Red denotes vestibular mucosa epithelium derived from non-neural ectoderm (NNE) of prosomere p6. Blue denotes frontonasal epithelium from the non-neural ectoderm of prosomere p5. The submucosa and dermis of these zones respectively is likely derived from neural crest from prosomeres p4–p1 as it flows forward beneath the NNE. All structures derived from prosomeric (forebrain) neural crest or mesomeric (midbrain) neural crest are supplied by arteries of the stapedial system in association with sensory V1. All structures derived from anterior rhombomeric (hindbrain) neural crest, r0–r3, are supplied by arteries of the stapedial system in association with sensory nerves V2 and V3.

Neural crest cells carry with them an intrinsic segmentation system in genetic register with the developmental units of the underlying nervous system. The basis of CNS segmentation is a family of genes containing a 60-amino acid loop called a homeobox that unlocks DNA. A unique combination of Hox genes defines each developmental segment, or *neuromere*, along the anterior–posterior organization of the embryo. The original system of 38 homeobox genes has been conserved throughout evolution; we humans have an axis specification that is 75% concordant with *Drosophila* (Figure 8.1).

This original Hox system applies to the brain as far forward as the midbrain–hindbrain junction. More recent genetic analysis has demonstrated additional homeotic genes that define all sectors of the midbrain and hindbrain (Lumsden & Krumlauf, 1996; Rubenstein & Puelles, 1994; Flores-Sarnat *et al.*, 2007). The forebrain (prosencephalon) has 6 *prosomeres*, the mid-brain (mesencephalon) has 2 *mesomeres*, and the hindbrain (rhombencephalon) has 12 *rhombomeres*. Neural crest arising above any given neuromere will bear its genetic "tattoo." Thus, using a chick-quail chimera system, tissues derived from neural crest can be traced back to their neuromere of origin – conveniently that of the sensory innervation to that tissue (Le Douarin & Kalchiem, 1999). The neuroanatomic content of each neuromere (what nucleus or tracts are present) gives a very accurate idea of what tissue it will supply. This concept has been used to map out the developmental origins of craniofacial arterial systems (Etchevers *et al.*, 2002). Furthermore, we find pericytes within the basement membranes of blood vessels respond to VEGF produced by neural growth cones (Ribatti *et al.*, 2011). Thus we find that the mesenchyme producing structures supplied by the medial nasopalatine axis, that is vomer and premaxilla, are constructed from neural crest arising from the second rhomobomere. In sum, the neuromeric model of craniofacial development has many powerful applications for the understanding of craniofacial anomalies. For further information, the reader is referred to further work by this author (Carstens, 2002, 2008b, c) (Figure 8.2).

In anatomy, as in life, words can prove deceiving. Since these soft tissue fields of the "prolabium" are also paired in the midline, one should more properly use the term *prolabia*. To keep it simple, we will use the singular. But beware: *the idea of the prolabium as an isolated structure is a conceptual trap*, with consequences for the operating surgeon. This section is dedicated to helping us clear away misconceptions so that we can understand the embryology of the premaxilla and prolabium in simple terms of neurovascular anatomy.

The neuroembryologic model of cleft remains the same and has been well described (Carsten, 2008b). In broad brush-strokes, the spectrum of unilateral cleft lip alone or in combination with cleft palate results from defects along the axis of the *medial nasopalatine neuroangiosome*, the most medial of all the branches emanating from the sphenopalatine fossa. This neurovascular axis supplies two bone fields: the premaxilla and the vomer. Both bones are paired and for the

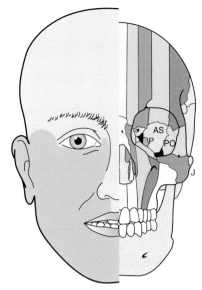

Figure 8.2 Tessier cleft zones. Skull bones on the left are color-coded for the origin of the neural crest mesenchyme: prosomeric (blue), mesomeric (white), rhombomeric (pink). On the right, individual cleft zones are depicted. The exact biologic relationship between orbital and maxillary cleft zones could be due to similarities in the homeotic code (or a different gene code) specifying their respective neurovascular axes. The following fields are all in register with rhombomere r2 and supplied by StV2 branches of the stapedial from the sphenopalatine fossa: *fluorescent* = medial nasopalatine axis, *tan/flesh* = lateral nasopalatine axis, *light green* = descending palatine axis (greater and lesser), *green* = medial infraorbital axis, *blue* = lateral infraorbital axis, *gold* = superior alveolar axis and *purple* = zygomatico-facial axis, and *pink* = zygomatico-temporal axis. Fields supplied by the non-stapedial external carotid system are colored *orange*. Fields supplied by StV1 branches are *light blue* for p5 and *red* for p6.

sake of simplicity, I am going to refer to them in the singular. The mesenchyme of the premaxilla and vomer is neural crest originating from the second rhombomere of the hindbrain.

Each premaxilla consists of three distinct zones (from oldest to newest): central incisor, lateral incisor, and a frontal process stretching upward from the lateral incisor all the way to the frontal bone. *When pathology strikes the premaxilla, the frontal process is the first to be affected* (causing the scooping out of the piriform rim). If the pathology is more extensive, the lateral incisor zone takes the hit. Very rarely, the entire field may be wiped out (Bartezko & Jacob, 2004).

Vomerine bones are triangular in shape. Because the vomer sits under the septum, its vertical height anteriorly is very small but, as one proceeds posteriorly, the height increases. Development of the vomer is: (i) anterior to posterior and (ii) dorsal to ventral. *When pathology strikes the vomer, the posterior height is affected first.* The deficient sector of vomer will fail to reach the plane of the palatal shelves.

Defects of the medial nasopalatine neurovascular axis can affect the premaxilla, the vomer, or both. As we shall see below, premaxillary deficiency always causes a contour deformity of the piriform fossa (the cleft lip nose). Depending upon its severity, isolated cleft lip or cleft lip plus alveolar defect can

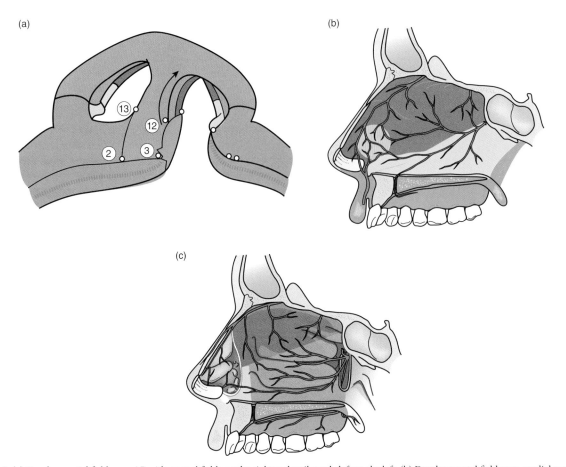

Figure 8.3 (a) Developmental field map, AP with normal fields on the right and unilateral cleft on the left. (b) Developmental field map, medial nasal cavity. (c) Developmental field map, lateral nasal cavity.

occur. Vomerine deficiency always affects the hard palate. When associated with premaxillary deficiency, the combination of cleft lip and cleft palate is observed.

The construction of the hard palate involves multiple neuroangiosomes. The *intranasal anterior ethmoid* and *posterior ethmoid* supply the perpendicular plate and septum. *The medial nasopalatine* supplies the vomer and premaxilla. The *greater palatine* supplies the oral surface of the secondary hard palate: the prepalatine bone and the palatine bone. The *lateral nasopalatine* supplies the nasal surface of the secondary hard palate and the inferior turbinate. Thus, the spectrum of cleft palate is more complex than that of cleft lip alone. Embryologic classification of cleft palate is a subject unto itself. In this chapter, we shall place our emphasis strictly upon the medial nasopalatine axis: the premaxilla and prolabium.

The connection between underlying bone field pathology and soft tissues is as follows. Whenever membranous bones are synthesized, BMP-4 is released. This protein diffuses upward through overlying soft tissues until it reaches the epithelium. There it encounters and inhibits a protein known as sonic hedgehog (SHH). The function of SHH is to stabilize epithelium. While it remains active, adjacent soft tissue processes

cannot fuse. BMP-4 is thus required for fusion of the lateral lip element to the prolabium. Premaxillary deficiency resulting in a reduction in [BMP-4] will reduce the inhibition of SHH and cause fusion failure. This mechanism is quantitative and directional. Defects in [BMP-4] affect the extent of downward diffusion. Thus, a minor reduction creates a cleft of the vermillion. The greater the reduction in [BMP-4], the higher the soft tissue cleft ascends (Zhang *et al.*, 2000, 2002; He *et al.*, 2014).

Neuroangiosomes are the functional basis of embryology and of facial clefts. Before we proceed onward with mapping out the prolabium and premaxilla let us get one concept straight. *Sensory nerves induce arteries.* As the face develops, various families of arteries arise, reorganize, and interact. How this takes place is a fascinating story beyond the scope of this chapter. However, the relationship between the intracranial and extracranial branches of the trigeminal nerve and stapedial arterial system is of such importance that we are going to take this on right now … and later on as well. Contrary to what is taught in Gray's Anatomy, both the ophthalmic artery and the external carotid artery are *composite systems!*

Nature never makes a structure without providing a blood supply to ensure its survival. Early in development, as soon as the optic apparatus emerges from the forebrain, the internal carotid provides blood supply to the globe. The terminal branches of the primitive ophthalmic system are the retinal artery, the long ciliary arteries, and the short ciliary arteries. At the same time, five (and only five) pharyngeal arches emerge, each one having an arterial axis known as an aortic arch artery. These arteries undergo rearrangements into what becomes the external carotid artery. The terminal branches of the external carotid are the superficial temporal and the external facial.

Later in development, just at the time of emergence of the cranial nerves, the *stapedial arterial system* appears. Its stem is the dorsal remnant of the defunct second aortic arch artery. It traverses the middle ear, where it divides, one part entering the skull and the other part exiting into the face. All branches of the stapedial system, both intracranial and extracranial, are programmed by sensory branches of cranial nerves (Diamond, 1991a, b; Georgiou & Cassell, 1992).

The intracranial stapedial produces the entire meningeal arterial system. A branch follows the greater petrosal nerve (a branch of cranial nerve VII) to the trigeminal ganglion. There it follows all the intracranial sensory divisions of the trigeminal system. Accordingly V1 takes it to the orbit via the superior orbital fissure. This branch of the intracranial stapedial system, the *supraorbital stapedial*, follows sensory branches of V1 to all extraocular structures. This makes sense. Structures surrounding the globe can be considered "new." Accordingly, they are supplied by the "new" arterial system. StV1 branches exit the orbit to supply frontonasal structures as well.

Shortly thereafter, the stapedial stem (now encased in the temporal bone) involutes. The only remnant is the carotico-tympanic artery. The intracranial stapedial arteries, like hungry fleas, eagerly pounce on neighboring arteries to make anastomoses. Thus, in the fetal (mature) state, the meningeal arteries are described as "originating" from branches of the external carotid system. In the orbit, the story is the same: supraorbital stapedial anastomoses with the ophthalmic. Evidence of this event is seen in a small "ring" of arteries around the optic nerve.

The extracranial stapedial is identical in its behavior. The artery follows chorda tympani (another branch of VII) until it arrives near the tip of V3 (lingual nerve). Here it "adds on" to the external carotid distal to external facial. (In another model, pharyngeal arch growth drags the stem of the stapedial forward until it reaches the extracranial root of V3 where it joins up with previous intracranial stapedial associated with the trigeminal ganglion.) The now-unified stapedial-ECA runs forward toward the sphenopalatine (pterygopalatine) fossa. This segment gives off four arterial branches prior to reaching the fossa. *Anterior tympanic* and *posterior tympanic* refer back to the middle ear. *Posterior meningeal* and *middle meningeal* communicate upward into the skull. Upon arrival in the sphenopalatine "switchyard," arterial branches follow all the sensory branches of V2 and V3 into the face. Involution of the stapedial stem leaves obliterates

the precursor state leaving us to conclude (falsely) that the external carotid artery is a single unitary structure.

The consequences of this neuroembryology were intuitively grasped by Paul Tessier when he developed his classification system of rare craniofacial clefts. *Orbital clefts* (zones 10–13) represent individual "knock-outs" of branches from the V1-induced supraorbital stapedial. *Maxillary clefts* (zones 1–8) represent individual "knock-outs" of branches from the V2 and V3-induced infraorbital stapedial. Zone 9 is the most rare because it receives blood supply from both systems. Zone 14 does not exist: it merely represents the failure of normal tissue involution (apopotosis) required to approximate the facial midline. Such patients have normal brains but large ethmoid complexes and widened interorbital dimensions (Tessier, 1976; Tessier *et al.*, 1977).

NB: For the curious, *there is no such thing as the sixth pharyngeal arch. There are five* (count them) pharyngeal arches. The sixth aortic arch artery is exclusively dedicated to the pulmonary circulation. The fifth aortic arch artery involutes, hence the fourth aortic arch artery takes over for both pharyngeal arches 4 and 5. Furthermore, pharyngeal arches 1–3 meld together. That is why, in the final configuration of the external carotid system: superior thyroid = arches 4–5; ascending pharyngeal = arch 3; and occipital, posterior auricular, lingual, superficial temporal, and external facial supply amalgamated structures of arches 1–2. The stapedial "add-on" to the ECA supplies the non-amalgamated structures of arch 1.

Having waded through the deep waters of vascular development, we are now in a position to "map out" craniofacial developmental fields using the tools of neuroembryology. Remember, arteries represent inductions from sensory nerves. Thus, *prolabium in the bilateral cleft can be "mapped" into four distinct embryonic zones.*

The **philtral prolabium**: In the center, paired *extranasal anterior ethmoid nerves and arteries* from the V1 stapedial system run down the columella about 4 mm apart. The anterior ethmoid fields make up the philtrum, that is, the Cupid's bow. The width of the philtrum = the width of the columella (as defined by the footplates of the inferior crura).

The **non-philtral prolabium**: Laterally, additional tissues flank the philtrum. These are supplied by the *medial nasopalatine neuroangiosomes*, from the V2 stapedial system (Ewings and Carstens, 2009; Moss *et al.*, 1981).

The skin and subcutaneous tissues of the philtral prolabium are unique: **ectoderm and mesoderm are not present**. Instead, all tissues arise from *p5 forebrain neural crest*. Recall that the forebrain is divided into six developmental zones called *prosomeres*. Neural crest arising from above each prosomere bears genetic markers associated with its zone of origin. Neural crest from p5 produces orbitofrontonasal skin. Neural crest from p6 produces the vestibular lining of the nose, from the septum to the roof and over to middle turbinate. Take a look inside your nose: the color difference between p6 and p5 is quite obvious.

The skin and subcutaneous tissues of the non-philtral prolabium are also nearly unique, but not quite. The epidermis *is* ectodermal but the dermis *is not* mesodermal (it comes from neural crest). Both are in register with the second rhombomere.

Let us repeat: prolabial skin, like all frontonasal skin supplied by V1 and the ophthalmic system, has a unique embryology. For this reason, it can manifest unique forms of *frontonasal dysplasia* not seen in the rest of the face. Facial skin supplied by V2 and V3 also differs from that of the rest of the body. Although its epidermis is ectodermal, its dermis comes from neural crest. One does not encounter true mesodermal dermis until dermatome level C2.

The deep layers of both the philtral prolabium and the non-philtral prolabium consist of mucosa and submucosa *associated with, but not in contact with, the premaxilla.* Mucosa arises from first arch ectoderm and submucosa is first arch neural crest. Again, both are in register with r2. The blood supply to these tissues is an extension from that of the premaxilla, that is, from the *medial nasopalatine axes.*

Septal circulation provides collateral blood supply to the isolated prolabium in complete bilateral clefts. Intranasal anterior ethmoid arteries course obliquely downward and forward, terminating in anastomoses with extranasal anterior ethmoid arteries in the membranous septum. For this reason, when aggressive bilateral dissection of the premaxilla takes place in the presence of pre-existing incisions in the membranous septum, necrosis of the premaxilla can occur.

Under normal conditions, unification between the premaxilla and the maxilla involves two sets of structures: the frontal process zone of the premaxilla fuses its maxillary counterpart. The lateral incisor zone of the premaxilla fuses with the canine zone of maxilla. This unites the medial nasopalatine neuroangiosome with the lateral nasopalatine neuroangiosome. In this way, the soft tissues covering the premaxilla become internalized within the floor of the nose.

Fusion of the lateral lip to the prolabium brings additional embryonic elements into the prolabium. Mucosal union is essential for this to happen. *Collateral blood supply* comes over from the medial infraorbital neuroangiosome (another branch of the StV2 system). *Myoblasts of both the deep and superficial orbicularis* arise from the sixth somitomere (as do all the muscles of facial expression). They are incorporated into the second pharyngeal arch and take up a position at the distal midline. Muscles destined for the upper lip lie in the distal zone of the second arch, just rostral to the midline. Their fascia likely arises from r4 neural crest. Muscles destined are similarly located, just caudal to the midline. Their fascia also arises from r5 neural crest. Amalgamation of arches 1 and 2 creates the lateral lip element.

Striated muscles are units of paraxial mesoderm that occupy spaces within a fascial envelope of neural crest from the same neuromeric level as that which gave rise to the myoblasts. *Fascia is primordial*: it recognizes binding sites that are "programs" that start within epithelium. These are shared with adjacent submucosa or dermis. Muscle-containing fascia forms an initial attachment to the first available proximal binding site(s) it encounters and thence, in an elegant game of "leapfrog," the fascia seeks out its secondary to the next available binding attachment site(s). These attachments are known as tendons.

When lip fusion occurs, the two layers of orbicularis oris do not "migrate," instead they passively accompany the epithelium with which they are associated. Deep orbicularis is associated with the r2 mucosa of the upper lateral lip element (medial infraorbital neuroangiosome). This mucosa fuses with the r2 mucosa of the prolabium (medial nasopalatine neuroangiosome). With muscle growth, DOO simply follows a new mucosal program. Under normal conditions DOO is continuous beneath the prolabium.

Superficial orbicularis follows different "rules." It develops in association with r2 skin of the upper lateral lip element (medial infraorbital neuroangiosome). This skin fuses with the p5 frontonasal skin of the philtrum (external anterior ethmoid neuroangiosome). These structures are biologically incompatible. SOO will not penetrate prosomeric mesenchyme. SOO-containing skin is inherently thicker than prolabial skin. The philtral column results from this discrepancy. A unilateral complete cleft philtrum demonstrates this nicely. Only one layer of muscle is encountered, the deep orbicularis oris.

In summation: the *non-philtral prolabium* (NP = non-philtrum) develops from hindbrain neural crest. It represents the distal extension of the medial sphenopalatine, originating as the terminal branch of the internal maxillary system in the sphenopalatine fossa. *Under normal conditions, NP represents the soft tissue coverage of the premaxilla within the nasal floor.* Tucked inside the nostril sill, it is difficult to appreciate. In cleft lip patients, NP is externalized and readily seen, being a lateral "add-on" to the true philtrum. Surgical separation of non-philtrum from the Cupid's bow makes use of this embryonic fusion plane. Reassignment of NP into the nasal floor and lateral nasal wall permits release and advancement of the lateral crus and expands the airway. Modifications of the DFR incisions based on the contributions of Matthew and Talmant make the surgical design embryologically accurate and (not surprisingly) give significant functional improvement.

Medial wall dissection: modifications

Ten years ago, I met David Matthews at the ASPS in Orland, Florida. Over the years we have developed a close professional cooperation. We found that, from a technical standpoint, our dissections were very similar. Several years ago Dr. Matthews began to incorporate the NPP flap into the nasal floor. However, when we compared long-term outcomes my cases demonstrated a flattening of the Cupid's bow at the junction of the white-roll and the cleft-side philtral column whereas my colleague's patients maintained eversion all along the Cupid's bow. Clearly, there was something amiss with the design of my straight-line incision as it approached the caudal margin of the Cupid's bow.

Matthews #1: The answer was the *preservation of the uppermost fibers of the deep orbicularis oris* by means of a small back-cut incision that drops the muscle into proper position with respect to that of the non-cleft side. Technical details of this modification will be described below.

Matthews #2: I also observed that the proximal limb of Matthews' NP incision could be nicely carried into the nasal floor just beneath the footplate. The trick was to incise *just the skin*, leaving the subcutaneous pedicle powered by intact MSP artery branches. The resulting NP flap rotates perfectly into the lateral nasal incision. Furthermore, the incision *permits access to the internal surface of the medial crus*. One simply inserts the curved scissors inward, locating the internal surface of the medial crus, and elevates. From the very moment I saw his approach it was obvious to me that *the misplaced medial crus could be corrected perfectly well without an external incision*. Simple is always better.

The embryologic implication of Matthews' incision is that the true width of the philtral prolabium was not (as I had previously thought) merely the width of the columella alone. Instead, *PP equals the distance between the alar footplates*. This adds 2–3 mm to the width of the Cupid's bow along the white-roll. As we shall see, the terminal point of Matthews' back-cut is aligned with the old definition for PP.

Medial wall dissection: embryologic lessons

A side benefit of Matthews' critique of the DFR incision design (not the concept) was that it forced me to rethink the embryologic boundaries between the columella, the nasal floor, and the lip. Landmarks were needed to define the junction between frontonasal skin (of forebrain origin) and facial skin (of hindbrain origin). To illustrate this point we have to discuss the embryologic origins of body skin, facial skin, and frontonasal skin. All three arise in a radically different manner. Here is a quick and dirty summary. Armed with this information, we can understand how the developmental fields of the lip and nose are laid out.

Body skin arises from two tissue sources. Epidermis comes from ectoderm whereas dermis is mesoderm. During gastrulation (the creation of a three-layer embryo) the mesoderm becomes segmented into somites. Each somite is supplied by a sensory nerve, the nucleus of which lies within the corresponding developmental unit of the CNS: the neuromere. These tissues are in genetic register with each other. T3-innervated dermis is genetically connected with the third thoracic neuromere. Each "swatch" of mesoderm is "assigned" to a zone of overlying ectoderm; together they share a common genetic definition. This skin unit is what textbooks refer to as a "dermatome" (sic).

Precisely where does body skin begin? The alert reader may ask, "Why is there no C1 dermatome?" All somites contain dermatomes, but those of the first four occipital somites and the first cervical somite are *unstable* and degenerate. Thus, the body skin

(dermatome-derived dermis) does not appear until the second cervical somite.

Facial skin arises from two different sources as well. The epidermis comes from ectoderm but the dermis arises from neural crest. Once again, neuroanatomy comes to our rescue. Facial skin is innervated by V2 and V3 whereas frontonasal skin is innervated by V1. Since the V2 nucleus resides within the second rhombomere it makes sense that the neural crest dermis of maxillary division skin arises from the neural fold just above r2. These tissues share a common genetic "signature." Mandibular dermis arises from the r3 neural crest.

Frontonasal skin is utterly different: it arises from a single source. Here, neural crest of the rostral prosencephalon (forebrain) gives rise to *both* epidermis and dermis. This part of the brain has six developmental units called prosomeres, p6–p1. Intranasal (vestibular) skin arises exclusively from neural crest of the sixth prosomere. Skin of the external nose, upper eyelid, and forehead arises from neural crest of the fifth prosomere.

For readers new to the subject of neuromeric mapping, the above description probably seem abstract. Let's convert this to anatomic terms understandable to all surgeons, that is, to *neuroangiosomes*. Vestibular skin (p6) and fronto-orbital-nasal skin (p5) are innervated by V1. Arterial supply to both these regions is from branches of the ophthalmic artery (internal carotid). Sixth prosomere "skin" consists of septal mucoperichondrium and lateral nasal wall mucoperiosteum. These tissues are supplied by the posterior ethmoid artery and by the anterior ethmoid artery, both of which send out nasal branches to their respective targets. Fifth prosomere skin is supplied by terminal branches of the anterior ethmoid. These exist from beneath the nasal bones and run downward to supply the distal (non-vestibular) internal nasal skin and the columella. The skin lying immediately beneath the alar footplates belongs to a separate developmental field, the r2 non-philtral prolabium.

Cartilages of the nose develop when neural crest mesenchyme comes in contact with, and is "instructed" by, an epithelial program. The size and shape of the upper lateral (triangular) cartilages are determined by p6 vestibular lining whereas the contours of the lower lateral (alar) cartilages are fixed by interaction with p5 skin. Thus the footplates of the medial crura are the landmark for where p5 skin ends *and where r2 upper lip skin begins*.

The whole idea of the DFR incision is field separation. By taking the prolabial separation incision up the side of the columella, I was combining two unrelated neuroangisomes. The flap was large: NPP skin (medial nasopalatine) in continuity with the entire ipsilateral columella (anterior ethmoid). It merited an equally awkward term: NPP-LCC (lateral columella chondrocutaneous) flap. This design did not achieve embryologic field separation but it seemed to work. I rationalized this compromise by convincing myself that the downward-displaced, cleft-side medial crus needed a surgical release in order to be repositioned correctly.

This concept proved to be unnecessary. Correct separation of p5 and r2 skin takes place just below the footplates. This permits elevation of the media crus *from below* just as effectively as the lateral columella incision with shorter time of closure.

Lateral wall dissection: modifications

In normal patients, the lateral nasal wall just in front of the inferior turbinate contains the soft tissues and bone of the premaxillary frontal process. In virtually all cleft patients this zone appears contracted. A prominent vertical fold or web is seen running downward from the distal margin of the lateral crus and terminating at the palatal shelf. Absence of the PMx subfield seemed to neatly explain the entrapment of the lateral crus. After working out the neurovascular anatomy of the prolabium in 2000, it seemed logical that this problem could be addressed by a mucosal releasing incision and addition of the NPP flap into the defect. As an adjunct, the nasal airway was supported by postoperative stenting for up to three months.

By 2010 I was convinced that this idea was insufficient. Although the initial release seemed to create a nearly perfect airway, in many patients the expansion was unstable. Airflow in these patients was reduced compared to the normal side. Furthermore, I noted a dynamic component to the cleft airway. Despite the addition of adequate soft tissues, forceful inspiration would be accompanied by an *inward contraction*. It was time to return to the drawing board: Gray's Anatomy and the work of Jean Claude Talmant. I was fortunate to meet Dr. Talmant in 2005 as invited faculty for the Indian Society for Cleft Lip, Palate and Craniofacial Anomalies in Guwahati, Assam. His emphasis on the nasal airway as a key to maxillary growth made biologic sense and his results were impressive. His concepts are well summarized in "Evolution of the functional repair concept for cleft lip and palate patients," published in *IJPS* 2006; 39(2):197–209. This article should be required reading for all cleft surgeons. This being said, I must confess that my initial review of Talmant's work was too superficial. I underestimated the physiologic significance of the nasalis muscle and I missed its embryologic relationship to the frontal process of the premaxilla (Talmant, 2006).

Four years later, Dr. Talmant's work came to my attention once again via David Matthews. After visiting Talmant in Nantes he brought back three key ideas: (i) reassignment of the nasalis muscle to its correct position; (ii) subperiosteal release and the internal nasal lining; and (iii) effective techniques to correctly reassign the nasal lining using packing and stenting. These three maneuvers made instant biologic sense. Cleft surgery without them is inconceivable.

Talmant #1: Like all muscles innervated by the facial nerve, the nasalis muscle originates from the paraxial mesoderm of somitomere 6. It flows forward within the substance of the SMAS along the trajectory of the buccal branch of VII. Upon reaching its destination it inserts at two distinct locations.

Under normal conditions, the muscle has two proximal sites of attachment, both of which are into the mucoperiosteum of the canine fossa. A lateral "head" lies over the root of the canine while the medial "head" is located above the lateral incisor. These proximal attachments require the correction position of the embryologic fields making up the piriform rim. First to develop is the frontal process of the maxilla, arising from just above the canine. Second to develop is the frontal process of the premaxilla arising from just above the lateral incisor. The proximal heads of nasalis form their insertions in the same sequence. The SMAS then migrates upward, tracking along the vestibular lining, carrying the remaining nasalis myoblasts upward into the nose. At the lateral crus, the cartilage-vestibular attachment forces the SMAS over the dorsal surface of the alar cartilage. Here it forms a distal insertion into the perichondrium of the lateral crus.

In cleft patients the frontal process of the premaxilla is missing. The proximal muscle mass is pathologically displaced into the piriform fossa. It is attached to the mucoperiosteum immediately in front of the inferior turbinate, *the exact location of the missing frontal process of the premaxilla*. Distal nasalis anatomy remains unaffected. At operation, the muscle is readily encountered, using the same type of releasing incision as for DFR. The proximal muscle mass is substantial, one simply has to look for it. It is detached from two points: (i) from the mucoperiosteal lining, using sharp dissection; and (ii) from the internal surface of the piriform margin using the subperiosteal plane. The distal muscle mass may be optionally released from the lateral crus using the subperichondrial plane. Reassignment of the displaced nasalis is accomplished by placing a mattress suture into the distal muscle mass and then suturing it to the alveolar mucoperiosteum just above the canine. This maneuver instantly corrects the pathologic vector of muscle contraction; it now acts functionally to *open the airway*, not to constrict it.

Talmant #2: Redistribution of the nasal lining is simple and elegant. It involves four maneuvers: (i) elevation of the septal mucoperichondrium all the way backward and upward to the nasal bone; (ii) subperiosteal dissection from the internal piriform margin all the way backward and upward to the nasal bone; (iii) subperiosteal dissection of the maxilla, external piriform margin and nasal bones; and (iv) optional subperichondrial dissection via a rim dissection. Note that (iii) and (iv) involve the sub-SMAS plane.

Nasalis detachment requires entry into the piriform fossa. Using a sweeping motion, the mucoperiosteal sleeve of the lateral nasal wall is elevated off the bone completely, all the way up to the nasal bone. Here, the lateral dissection becomes continuous with the medial dissection of the septal mucoperichondrium. The result of these maneuvers is the *complete liberation of the nasal lining*; the lateral wall rotates internally. Embryologic anchorage of the lateral crus to the underlying vestibular skin (its "program") ensures that it will be dragged into a correct position. At this juncture, the tip defining point is assessed. If additional medicalization is needed, the lateral crus can be freed up from its overlying nasalis attachment, using the *subperichondrial* plane. This requires a rim incision.

Talmant #3: Once separation of the nasal lining from the SMAS is achieved, how can one effectively reposition the lower lateral and upper lateral cartilages? A roll of thin silicone sheeting is placed into each nostril and secured with transfixion sutures. During this maneuver, the now mobilized lining can be physically manipulated and the position of the alar cartilage observed. The silicone stents are then packed with vaseline gauze. This expands the nasal cavity and effectively pushes the upper lateral cartilage into a new relationship with the nasal bone and with the septum.

Lateral wall dissection: embryologic implications

The shape of the piriform fossa dramatically affects the appearance of the nasal soft tissues. Recall that this structure is bilaminar. It is composed, externally, by the frontal process of the maxilla and, internally, by the frontal process of the premaxilla. The alar base is pinioned to the external rim. The vestibular lining contains the "program" of the lateral cartilages, determining their size, shape, and position. In cleft patients, deficiency or absence of the premaxillary frontal process causes the rim to be posteriorly recessed and inferiorly scooped out. The canine fossa is ablated. This causes pathologic displacement of the distal nasalis. A lateral vestibular "web" results. In the quantitative absence of PMxF soft tissue (r2 neural crest), p5 nasal skin and p6 vestibular lining are contracted into the defect. This flattens and displaces the lateral crus and with it the proximal nasalis.

Talmant's first contribution is the recognition of the physiologic role of the nasalis: to maintain a patent airway. By demonstrating over two decades the consistent displacement of the nasalis muscle inside the piriform fossa, his work explains observable anatomy long misunderstood, that is, the nasal "web." Moreover, it confirms the role of the frontal process in constructing the normal nasal vault.

Talmant's second contribution is supported by two important embryologic points. (i) Soft tissues produce membranous bone. Biosynthesis of the internal piriform fossa depends upon stem cells within an internal lining of adequate dimensions. When the lining is contracted (as in clefts), over time bone desposition and resorbtion of the piriform fossa cannot take place normally. *Freeing up the internal lining reassigns stem cells into a correct functional position*. Thus, growth over time creates a normal nasal cavity. The end result of Talmant's mucoperiosteal dissection is a *redistribution of the osteosynthetic envelope* into a developmentally correct position. (ii) The frontal process of the premaxilla is the missing Lego® piece of the piriform fossa. Its absence results from an absolute lack of premaxillary soft tissue immediately in front of the inferior turbinate. This deficit causes the "scooped

out" appearance of the piriform fossa in cleft patients. The soft tissues of the non-philtral prolabium (NPP) represent the "housing" of the missing lateral incisor and frontal process fields. The NPP flap (based on the medial nasopalatine artery) can be separated from the philtral prolabium and transferred into the floor of the nose and the lateral nasal wall. It fits into the releasing incision required for nasalis dissection. By replacing the missing frontal process field, NPP reassignment accomplishes two important goals: it potentiates Talmant's lining release; and it increases the surface area at the external valve.

Nasal breathing plays a vital role in shaping the nasal air passage. It determines, in no small measure, the physical dimensions of the nasopharynx and, by extension, of the maxilla itself. This is vital for speech because the functional position of the soft palate depends upon the bony platform to which it is attached.

Cleft patients have impaired nasal breathing for the following reasons. (i) Deficit of the soft tissues responsible for synthesis of the frontal process of premaxilla reduces the surface area of the vestibular lining, dragging the lateral crus downward. (ii) In the absence of the frontal process, the proximal attachments of nasalis are malpositioned. Muscle contraction restricts the airway rather than opening it. (iii) Contraction of the vestibular lining means that ongoing osteosynthesis of the piriform fossa cannot be normal. Its physical dimensions become abnormal. (iv) The lower and upper lateral crura provide support for the vestibular lining. In particular, correction of the upper lateral cartilage has been largely ignored in cleft surgery. The sum of these four factors is *increased turbulence at the external valve* and *reduced airflow*. Talmant's concepts provide an embryologically sound answer to these issues.

Microform cleft: premaxillary deficiency and Poiseiulle's law $\Delta P = 8uLQ/\pi r^4$

The underlying problem in the microform or "minimal" cleft is no different than in more explicit manifestations of cleft. The stigmata arise from a mesenchymal deficiency in the premaxilla. The frontal process zone deficit causes a warping of the piriform fossa. A deficit in the lateral incisor zone causes the nasal floor to be "scooped out." To the degree that the bone volume is reduced, the strength of the BMP-4 signal will also be diminished. Sonic Hedgehog, the protein within lip tissue that stabilizes the epithelium, will be less inhibited (Carstens, 2000b).

In sum, the spectrum of minimal clefting is absolutely quantitative, with the degree of soft tissue involvement proportional to the reduction in bone stock. Premaxillary deficits always affect the insertion of the nasalis muscle with consequent depression of the alar cartilage. Nasalis misinsertion, when significant, manifests itself as a "band" in the lateral nasal wall. That these factors should also cause a deviation of the anterior nasal septum is not intuitively obvious.

Talmant deserves credit for drawing our attention to the effect of hydraulic forces resulting from fetal ventilation of amniotic fluid upon the shape of the nasal fossae. As previously mentioned, sagittal real-time ultrasound studies demonstrate how the alar cartilages and septum respond to the influx and efflux of fluid through the nares. In the case of cleft lip associated with cleft palate, Talmant postulates a difference in pressure between the two sides, the non-cleft nostril having higher pressures than those within the labiomaxillary cleft. It is easy to conceive how the anterior septum could be warped.

The "fly in the ointment" of this argument is the minimal cleft. Here, the septal deformity is exactly the same yet the nasal floor remains intact. The answer, once again, lies in the reduction in bone volume within the frontal process and lateral incisor fields of the premaxilla. Poiseiulle's law predicts that minor increases in radius will significantly reduce the pressure drop (ΔP) in a linear tube of length L. Let us consider the nostrils as two tubes of equal length in parallel sharing a common wall (the septum). Fluid viscosity (u) and fluid flow velocity (Q) upon entry into the tubes stays constant. Although the piriform fossae are not circular, the premaxillary deficit increases the overall perimeter on the cleft side. This translates into a non-traditional "radius" that exceeds that of the non-cleft piriform fossa. Unequal pressures within the nostrils result, the difference being maximal at the level of the external nasal valve. Growth of the nasomaxillary complex and of the septum takes place in the fetal period. Unequal intranasal pressures during this time account for warping of the septum as seen in the microform cleft and in all other variants.

Finally, displacement of the lower and upper lateral cartilages in the microform cleft demonstrates the importance of epithelial-mesenchymal programming, a concept we have invoked previously. Nasalis in the microform is minimally displaced but the piriform fossa deformity remains. The finite deficiency of nasal skin from the defective premaxilla creates an insufficiency state within the lateral nasal wall. The vestibular lining, displaced downward, synthesizes a perfectly normal cartilage in the wrong place. A similar effect can be observed, on occasion, in microform clefts in which one notes an asymmetry of the nasal bones, with slight flattening on the side of the cleft. The effect can only be explained by an abnormally positioned epithelial program.

The surgical consequence of repairing the microform cleft using a Talmant intranasal subperiosteal dissection is that the biologically active vestibular "bone factory" will be repositioned into its normal state. As membranous bone synthesis continues over time one can expect progressive improvement in the shape and volume of the piriform fossa.

Dental arch management

The impact of cleft surgery on maxillary growth after surgery has been intensively studied. Blame in such cases is usually attributed to surgical intervention versus maxillary "hypoplasia." Nonetheless, multiple studies of *unoperated* CL(P) patients demonstrate two patterns of fundamental scientific importance. (i) The cleft-side maxilla has an *abnormal piriform fossa*; this can exert distal effects on the overall shape of the anterior maxillary wall. (ii) The cleft-side alveolar process has *normal growth potential*. We have already discussed the first phenomenon so we shall concentrate on the second. What is at the root of all this confusion?

Prior to the era of molecular embryology and stem cell biology, the mechanism of membranous bone growth was poorly appreciated. Textbooks would describe the maxilla as developing in membrane from a single ossification center. This model, based upon nineteenth-century descriptive embryology, is completely out of date.

We now know that osteoblasts arise from stem cells residing in the cambium layer of periosteum. The relationship between membranous bone and soft tissue is like butter and bread: the bread synthesizes the butter. More precisely, membranous bond develops when a unique population of neural crest cells organized as a *neuroangiosome* comes in contact with an epithelial surface (mucosa, skin, meninges) from which it receives a "program" determining the size and shape of the bone product.

Some membranous bones are *unilaminar*. The nasal bone is synthesized from forebrain neural crest (sixth prosomere). Its "program" is nasal mucoperiosteum supplied by the V1 anterior ethmoid neuroangiosome. Others membranous bones are *bilaminar*, with two sources of programming. Such bones are characterized by a *separation plane* occupied by *sinuses or bone marrow*. The prepalatine bone (sic. the horizontal plate of the maxilla) is synthesized from hindbrain neural crest (second rhombomere). It has two "programs." The upper (nasal) layer is the V2 lateral nasopalatine neuroangiosome. The lower (oral) layer is the V2 greater palatine neuroangiosome. Sinuses in the prepalatine bone are a well-described anatomic variant. Membranous bones of the calvarium, such as the parietal bone, arise from dual sources of mesenchyme (dermis and dura); these are programmed by skin and neuroepithelium. The interspace of the parietal bone contains marrow.

Let us now consider the membranous bones of the dental arch. The purpose of the alveolus is to house the dental apparatus. Two factors determine the size and shape of the arch: the *number of dental units present* and the *effective biosynthesis of its bony walls*. Both the upper and the lower dental arches are constructed in exactly the same way. They are "sandwiches." In the center is a dental field arising from neural crest cartilage. It has its own intrinsic neurovascular supply. The lingual wall is composed of three distinct bone fields: premaxilla, prepalatine, and palatine. The buccolingual wall is composed of an apparently single bone, the maxilla proper, divided into three developmental zones supplied by branches of the superior alveolar system. Stem cells of neural crest origin within these various neuroangiosomes lay down membranous bone on either side of the dental anlage, much like armor plating.

Table 8.1 lists the neurovascular territories of the three layers (see Table 8.1). Here are the main take-home points. (i) The

Table 8.1 Neurovascular territories

Premaxilla

Dental field (incisors and canines) = superior alveolar/dental br. + infraorbital
Lingual wall = medial nasopalatine
Buccolabial wall = superior alveolar/non-dental br. + infraorbital/medial br. + anterior ethmoid collaterals

Maxilla (palatoquadrate cartilage)

Dental field (premolars and molars) = superior alveolar/dental br. + infraorbital/lateral and medial
Lingual wall = greater palatine
Buccolabial wall = superior alveolar/non-dental br.

Mandible (Meckel's cartilage)

Dental field (all units) = inferior alveolar/dental br.
Lingual wall
Ramus (pterygoid) = 2nd part stapedial/pterygoid br.
Body, proximal (mylohyoid) = 1st part stapedial/inferior alveolar/mylohyoid
Body, mesial (anterior digastric) = ECA/facial/submental
Symphysis = ECA/lingual/sublingual
Buccolabial wall
Ramus
Body, distal (masseter) = 2nd part stapedial/masseteric br. + ECA/facial/masseteric br.
Body, mesial (platysma) = ECA/facial/submental br
Symphysis (mentalis) = ECA/facial/inferior labial br. + 1st part stapedial/inferior alveolar/dental/mental br.

Fates of mandibular bone fields

Dentary > alveolar housing of incisors + symphysis
Coronoids (2–3) > alveolar housing of canines, premolars, molars
Splenials (2) > mandibular body underlying the non-symphyseal dental arch
Pre-articular (lingual) > manubrium of malleus
Articular (lingual) > malleus
(buccal) > tympanic temporal bone

alveolar bones of both jaws are complex structures composed of multiple neuroangiosomes. (ii) Alveolar osteogenesis is utterly dependent upon the integrity of these fields. (iii) Malformations of the dental arch arise from abnormalities in the number or size of teeth, deficits in the alveolar housing, or both.

The nasomaxillary complex is a series of neural crest bones, each of which is innervated by a specific branch of V2. Using a VEGF mechanism each nerve induces an accompanying artery from the stapedial system (the internal maxillary). All these neuroangiosomes have a common point of origin: the pterygopalatine fossa. The maxilla *per se* has a partial role in the alveolus: it is responsible for the dental field and the external lamina. The prepalatine and palatine bones form the internal lamina. Although the premaxilla is an autonomous bone, under normal conditions, its external lamina receives mesenchyme of the maxilla.

The mandible is equally complex. In its primitive tetrapod form it consisted of multiple bones. The original dental lamina arose from Meckel's cartilage and consisted of a *dentary bone* plus two to three *coronoid bones*. The body of the mandible supporting the teeth had two splenial bones. The primitive ramus had four bones: pre-articular and articular were lingual. The fates of these bones are listed. The mammalian mandible bears muscle insertions corresponding to the genetic "idea" of these ancient bone fields.

Response of the dental arch in clefts to surgery

Clefts are experiments of nature. They present us with clues as to the mechanisms behind craniofacial embryology. Nowhere is this more apparent than in the completely divided palate. The cleft-side maxilla is dynamic; it responds to surgical intervention in two primary ways: *retroposition* (growth restriction) and *collapse* (cross-bite). We shall deal with these problems in sequence.

Retroposition

At birth, the cleft-side maxilla appears smaller and/or retropositioned when compared with its normal counterpart. This situation likely results from disruption of force vectors in utero. Forward, centric growth of the ethmoid, vomerine, and premaxillary fields is disconnected from the cleft-side maxilla (in bilateral clefts, from both maxillae). Nonetheless, multiple studies of *unoperated* CL(P) patients demonstrate two patterns of fundamental scientific importance. (i) The cleft-side maxilla has an *abnormal piriform fossa*; this can exert distal effects on the overall shape of the anterior maxillary wall. (ii) The cleft-side alveolar process has *normal growth potential*. We have already discussed the first phenomenon so we shall concentrate on the second. Why does the dental arch in cleft patients present as it does? Why does it self-correct over time (in the absence of surgery)? How does surgical intervention affect this process?

Recall that the *primary determinant of alveolar size is the number of teeth*. Assuming that the cleft-side alveolus has all six dental units, one can expect that it will eventually achieve normal proportions. Dental development involves the interaction between the epithelial program and the underlying mesenchyme. Although this process is delayed on the cleft-side, it eventually takes place. Assuming a normal mucoperiosteal envelope, the alveolar walls of the cleft maxilla will respond to accommodate the dentition. For this reason, patients with unoperated complete cleft palate can present with a dental arch of normal dimensions.

Restriction in maxillary growth after surgery has been intensively studied. Blame in such cases is usually attributed to surgical intervention versus hypoplasia intrinsic to the maxilla. Studies by Bardach (in the *supraperiosteal* plane) showed that increasing degrees of dissection were accompanied by increased growth reduction. At the same time, long-term work by Tessier and Delaire demonstrates that extensive *subperiosteal* dissection does not result in growth. What is at the root of all this confusion?

As previously discussed, biosynthesis of membranous bones is wholly dependent upon the vascular integrity of the neuroangiosomes from which they are constructed. These contain stem cells, located in the cambium layer of the periosteum. *Any surgical intervention that invades or falsely subdivides a neuroangiosome will potentially compromise the blood supply to the stem cell population* and negatively affect osteogenesis.

Traditional techniques of lip repair have mobilized the lateral lip element using the readily accessible *supraperiosteal plane.* As a consequence, cleft lip surgery disrupts blood supply to the stem cell rich cambium layer. Restriction in growth of the maxillary wall (Tessier zones 4, 5, and 6) can lead to malposition of the alveolus per se. Blood supply to the buccolabial mucoperiosteum can also be reduced. Bardach's findings in beagles, using the supraperiosteal plane, were originally interpreted as a caution against wide dissection (Bardach, *et al.*, 1993, 1994a, b). In point of fact, these papers demonstrate just the opposite: the use of the supraperiosteal plane violates the principles of embryology by devascularizing developmental fields. Because membranous bone is just a by-product of its soft tissue envelope, preservation of the resident stem cell population in the cambium layer of the periosteum requires the use of the subperiosteal plane. Applications of this concept to cleft surgery were described in detail with a detailed literature review by this author (Carstens, 1999a, c, 2000a).

In cleft palate repair, oral mucoperiosteal flaps are commonly elevated using an incision placed at the junction between the lingual alveolar wall and the horizontal palatal shelf. This maneuver disrupts blood vessels directly laterally from the greater palatine axis to the lingual mucoperiosteum of the alveolus. As a consequence, blood supply to the lingual mucoperiosteum becomes random, based upon collateral flow from the opposing buccolabial mucoperiosteum and upon the underlying alveolar bone.

Just as the whole is greater than the sum of its parts, the most negative effects on alveolar development are observed in patients having combined surgical interventions for cleft lip and cleft palate surgery. The resulting process, *sequential vascular isolation*, is the *primary cause of maxillary growth arrest after cleft surgery* (Carstens, 1999b).

Collapse: a reversible phenomenon

Unoperated patients with complete clefts of the lip and palate demonstrate a gap corresponding to the absence of the two premaxillary fields (lateral incisor and frontal process). In the growing child, lip repair re-establishes force vectors across the alveolar cleft that are unopposed by bone: collapse ensues. This situation is dynamic; it is easily reversed by orthodontic expansion. The Achilles' heel of this approach to cleft management is access to orthodontic care, a resource not readily available in many countries with a high volume cleft population.

In theory, primary alveolar stabilization would prevent collapse and reduce/simplify subsequent orthodontic management.

Inclusion of soft palate repair with the primary lip intervention ameliorates, but does not prevent, arch collapse. Long-term splinting and delayed repair of the hard palate lead to good size and position of the arch but poor speech. Over the years, various attempts have been made to address this problem using soft tissue procedures with or without some form of grafting. Early work suffered from soft tissue considerations stemming from use of the supraperiosteal plane. Observation of maxillary growth restriction led to a consensus that primary grafting should be abandoned in favor of secondary grafting at ages 6–9 (eruption of the canine).

This dogma was successfully challenged by Kernahan and Rosenstein at the University of Illinois (Rosenstein *et al.*, 2003; Rosenstein, 2003). Using extremely limited dissection and rib grafts, stabilization was achieved. Long-term growth studies (up to 30 years) in these patients demonstrated arch development without maxillary restriction. Of note, the grafts were placed as struts high up over the alveolar cleft, leaving the actual walls of the cleft site largely untouched. Rosenstein's final report is of great scientific importance for several reasons. First, it shows that primary arch stabilization is achievable. Second, and more importantly, the relationship between grafting and maxillary growth restriction reported in previous studies is an artifact of the surgical technique resulting from entry into the supraperiosteal plane.

More recently, gingivoperiosteoplasty (GPP) using local flaps at the alveolar cleft site has been reported with the hope that autologous bone would be generated at the cleft site (an idea dating back to Skoog (1967)). This approach is limited by the dimensions of the cleft site (wide clefts are not amenable). The dissection is technically demanding: flaps are taken directly over alveolar bone that is extremely delicate. The amount of bone generated by this technique has been disappointing. Elevation of the flaps may compromise the stem cell population within them. Furthermore, scar formation at the site may have consequences for dentition, such as tipping or rotation. Such problems are certainly amenable to orthodontic correction, but the limited benefits of GPP and its technical nuances do not recommend it.

Delaire's work demonstrates the surgical importance of the subperiosteal plane in cleft surgery (Precious & Delaire, 1992; Delaire *et al.*, 1993). Elevation and medicalization of such flaps from the face of the maxilla represents the transfer of bioactive stem cell-bearing mucoperiosteum into a correct midline position. This concept is of fundamental importance for DFR cleft repair because it corrects the displacement of soft tissues that is present on both sides of the cleft. Such displacement is asymmetrical in the unilateral cleft and symmetrical in the bilateral cleft.

As previously mentioned, an unintended side effect of the Delaire's dissection is that it draws the malpositioned nasalis into the midline along with the rest of the lateral lip musculature. This changes the function of the nasalis and constricts the airway. Talmant, having inherited many of Delaire's patients, recognized this problem and worked out how the nasalis could be repositioned to its natural attachment at the canine fossa. This simple dissection frees both heads of the muscle and passes them below the orbicularis complex. Technical details are provided in the addendum.

Using the Delaire dissection plus alveolar cleft closure as described by Demas and Sotereanos, in 1996 this author described use of an extended alveolar flap that can span a distance of two tooth units (Carstens, 1999c). This size of this flap permitted abundant tissue to be mobilized backwards from the alveolar margins for a secure soft tissue closure in larger clefts. The *sliding sulcus* technique was therefore more versatile than the GPP. It worked well for patients 2 years of age and up. In younger patients, the sliding sulcus had the same technical drawbacks of soft tissue manipulation at the alveolar cleft site. In 2004–06 the problem of inadequate stem cell response seen in the above techniques was addressed by placing rhBMP-2 in the alveolar cleft site. CT scans demonstrated bone formation that filled nearly the entire vertical dimensions of the cleft site. At the end of ten years of work and observation I came to the conclusion that *gaining alveolar cleft closure at the primary surgery was do-able but not worth the effort.* A simpler approach was required. As we shall see, my search for this better solution led eventually to the Talmant protocol.

The bottom line is this: *Only nature can make a dental arch … and only the orthodontist can set it right.* In the un-grafted complete cleft palate the dental arch is unstable; all forms of lip repair cause alveolar collapse. Fortunately, such perturbation is only temporary. Developmental field reassignment transfers stem cell populations into correct, centric positions such that they produce bone where desired. DFR is designed to assist the orthodontist in all other aspects of cleft palate development: airway, soft palate positioning, and achieving complete closure of the anterior hard palate.

Functional lip and palate repair: the five As

Let's put the dental arch into the overall scheme of the cleft problem. Patients with complete clefts of the lip and palate require a prioritized, functional approach characterized by the "five **A**s": **a**irway, **a**rticulation, **a**nterior fistula avoidance, **a**rch, and **a**esthetics. What is the rationale behind this order? There is no question that intelligible speech is the most important social benefit for these patients, so why prioritize the airway before articulation?

Airway
The anatomic and physiologic relationships between the hard and soft palate can be described by the *pinball machine* model. The soft palate is like the "*flipper*" in a pinball machine (a moveable lever that prevents the ball from escaping and keeps it in play). The hard palate is the *platform* to which the flipper is attached. The function of the soft palate flipper is to reach backward and upward to make contact with the pharynx; thereby

closing off the nasal airway during phonation. The ability of the soft palate to accomplish this goal depends on: (i) normal motor innervation from cranial nerves V3 and IX; (ii) normal muscle mesenchymal mass from somitomeres 4 (first arch) and 7 (third arch); and (iii) normal length of the bony platform to which the soft palate musculature is attached. In other words, one must be able to control the flipper. It must be of normal length and not be floppy. Above all, the flipper mechanism must be positioned on the platform in such as way that it closes off the escape of the ball.

The size and shape of the hard palate bones (prepalatine and palatine) determine the positioning of the soft palate. When these bones are deficient, soft palate musculature cannot make contact with the pharynx. In some patients, however, an apparently normal hard and soft palate complex is inadequate, causing velopharyngeal incompetence. What is the problem here? The secondary hard palate is not an isolated entity. It is part of a larger bone complex, the nasal chamber. The prepalatine and palatine bones are in anatomic contact with the frontal process of the maxilla, the inferior turbinate, the sphenoid. Thus, *the overall dimensions of the nasal airway determine the spatial relationship between the soft palate and the posterior pharynx* and consequently its function.

Surgical implications of the above are as follows. First, the vestibular lining of the cleft nose is malpositioned due to deficiency/absence of the premaxillary frontal process. If left in this state, the ongoing process of osteogenesis during the first years of life will produce a permanent deformity in the bony dimensions of nasal chamber. Although the primary determinants of soft palate position are the prepalatine and palatine bones, these in turn are affected by the spatial dimensions of the surrounding bones, that is, the nasal airway. Correction of the airway by reassignment of the internal lining field (and therefore the cartilages) and of the nasalis is required to achieve optimal hard palate dimensions.

When should nasal airway correction be undertaken? Talmant believes that if nasal breathing patterns are not established in the first six months of life, oral breathing patterns will develop. Mouth breathing has negative effects that are difficult to reverse. These include: head positioning, body posture, and maxillary shape. This logic is indisputable but it is unclear to me how rigid one should be on this issue. Children can present late, with wide clefts or with complications. The good news is that airway correction can be easily done secondarily, either concomitant with lip revision or as an isolated procedure. It seems thus reasonable to conclude that nasal breathing should be accomplished in all children by age 2.

A caveat to the reader here: technical details regarding intraoperative nasal packing and postoperative nasal stenting are of the utmost importance for airway correction. These accomplish the following: (i) a subtle, but very precise, control of alar cartilage position; (ii) upper lateral cartilage repositioning; and (iii) adequate diameter of the external nasal valve. These maneuvers will be described in the technical section that follows … stay tuned.

Articulation

Timing of palate closure is yet another area of cleft management that is rife with controversy. As we have previously seen, palate clefts can be classified by embryologic mechanism, depending on which components are affected. Cleft palate arises from faulty mesenchyme involving bones (neural crest from rhombomeres r1, r2, r3), muscles (paraxial mesoderm from somitomeres 4 and/or 7), or a combination of both. In the absence of such classification, studies relating surgical technique to speech are inherently unreliable; apples cannot be compared with oranges.

Nonetheless, some general concepts of cleft palate repair make sense. First, soft palate closure mechanically positions the tongue, helping to prevent the acquisition of motor patterns that are difficult to correct later. This can be done as early as 6 months, as in the Talmant protocol (see below). Soft palate repair establishes normal force vectors across the posterior midline. These balance against force vectors created by lip repair or lip adhesion. Any form of early lip closure exerts force vectors across the alveolar cleft leading to arch collapse and cross-bite. Thus, lip repair and soft palate repair are a rational combination at 6 months.

A quick review of the embryology of the soft palate musculature is required. Five sets of muscles are involved. First pharyngeal arch muscles arise from paraxial mesoderm of the fourth somitomere. The only Sm4 palatal muscle is tensor veli palatini. Third pharyngeal arch muscles arise from the seventh somitomere. These are: levator veli palatini, palatoglossus, palatepharyngeus, uvulus, and superior constrictor. These muscles can readily be tested using a Pena® muscle stimulator (Integra Life Sciences, Plainsboro, New Jersey). Normal function is graded as follows: normal = 2, hypotonic = 1, and no response = 0. Differences frequently exist between the left and right sides. Such information is valuable for classification of the palate cleft and for diagnosis of speech problems, if these should arise.

Soft palate muscles exist in two layers. *Nasal mucosa* provides the "program" for the tensor and levator. *Oral mucosa* is the "program" for the palatopharyngeus and palatoglossus. Uvulus is programmed by both mucosal surfaces. The *upper pharyngeal mucosa* contains the "program" for the superior constrictor.

Only the muscles of the nasal layer (tensor and levator) are responsible for palatal elevation/elongation. Only these muscles are directly attached to the palatine bone. These are the ones that need to be set back. The dissection plane between the nasal and oral layers is readily defined. *Extensive three-layer intervelar veloplasty is not embryologically rational and causes unnecessary scarring.* Soft palate repair is best viewed as a "first-pass" event. If the functional result is good, nothing more is required. If VPI is present, and the *elevation pattern is V-shaped*, secondary lengthening with a double-opposing z-plasty will readily resolve the issue.

Anterior fistula avoidance

The greater palatine neuroangiosome (GPA) supplies two bone fields: the horizontal shelf of the palatine bone and the oral lamina of the prepalatine bone. It runs all the way forward to the junction of the canine and lateral incisor. There it makes an anastomosis with the medial nasopalatine neuroangiosome (MNP). In traditional cleft palate surgery, hard palate incisions located at the junction of the palatal shelf and lingual alveolar wall constitute an *embryologically incorrect subdivision* of the greater palatine fields. Not only does this incision *interrupt blood supply* to the alveolar mucoperiosteum; it also creates *short flaps.* Troublesome anterior fistulae result from this design.

In the unoperated state, the length of the GPA field is designed to reach the premaxilla. Achieving a water-tight closure is simply a matter of using the entire neuroangiosome, using a pericoronal incision (or one just lingual to the teeth). The term *alveolar extension palatoplasty* (AEP) refers to the additional tissue gained by this flap. The anatomy and developmental biology of this procedure have been previously described. The AEP procedure is also useful in secondary cases. When enough time has elapsed after the primary palate repair, collateral flow is reestablished between the palatal shelf and alveolar mucoperiosteum. One can therefore use the AEP incision design to re-elevate the entire mucoperiosteum of the hard palate and lingual alveolus as a single flap. In unilateral clefts, the AEP flap from the non-cleft side always projects beyond the alveolar cleft, while that from the cleft side reaches the back-wall of the alveolar cleft. These flaps permit closure of anterior fistulae in virtually all situations.

Arch

Surgeons and orthodontists get along best when goals of each specialty are respected.

(i) Early lip closure (at 6 months) will cause the alveolar cleft to narrow down and may create a cross-bite of the primary dentition, but this is readily correctible. **Orthodontist to surgeon**: *Alveolar soft tissues over un-erupted teeth are delicate … **leave them alone**.*

(ii) Achieving a perfect closure of the entire nasal floor is a major goal of the primary surgical sequence. The most technically difficult site for this is the anterior floor, just over the alveolar cleft, exactly where the collapse has taken place. When nasal palatine mucoperiosteum is joined with that of the vomer, the *floor will always be short* in the anterior–posterior dimension. The NPP flap corrects this deficit: it is dissected out of the lip, transferred into the nasal floor, and sutured to the vomer-maxilla closure. **Surgeon to orthodontist**: *The anterior nasal floor is tight and tricky … can you **expand the alveolar cleft** prior to hard palate repair and then **keep it open** until I graft it?* What is required here is a means of palatal expansion that can be maintained over time. This also favors proper positioning of the lateral nasal wall. Such a *device cannot be fixed*; it must be capable of adapting to changes in the arch. As detailed below, the modified quad helix as designed by Lumineau fulfills these requirements and produces, often by age 4, a dental arch ready for bone grafting.

Developmental field reassignment: toward a rationale protocol

At the beginning of the chapter we set out to define a set of biologic goals for cleft repair. At this point, the protocol that comes closest to achieving them is that published by the Nantes group. Their results have been gained over 20 plus years. Credit should be given to Jean Delaire, from whose work Talmant's concepts have evolved. In any case, the outcomes of the airway and dental arch using this protocol not only are the best I have seen but have a sound basis in developmental biology.

Talmant–Lumineau protocol
Step 1. 6 months: soft palate repair plus full lip/nose repair. Wide bilateral subperiosteal dissection is carried out, both extrapiriform and intrapiriform. *In some countries, OR and anesthesia conditions may require that the soft palate repair be carried out separately.*

Step 2. As soon a primary dentition permits, a *modified quad-helix* is placed. The cleft site is expanded over a period of approximately one month and then maintained. Unlike traditional quad-helix designs, it is *not* fixed to the molars. Instead, it is secured with three wire ligatures. The expander has four "eyelets." These are 360 degree loops placed posteriorly at the level of the second molars (E) and anteriorly at the level of the canines. The expander is attached to each molar, with the "pull" of each wire loop placed in opposite directions. A third wire is passed through the posterior "eyelet" and over the second wire. The purpose of this wire is to prevent backward slippage of the expander. The third wire can be tightened to keep the device in place. In this way, the quad helix remains *in situ* but can be advanced forward to accommodate dental arch growth. Expansion is maintained until alveolar bone grafting is completed.

Step 3. 2 years: hard palate repair.

Step 4. 4 years: alveolar bone grafting. The timing for the procedure follows the extent of distraction: *the maxillary intercanine distance must exceed the mandibular intercanine distance by 6 mm.*

Step 5. 3–6 months later: remove quad-helix.

Comments
The Talmant lip repair accomplishes the following goals. (i) It establishes an adequate nasal airway in both the short and the long term. (ii) Subperiosteal elevation of the internal nasal lining elevates nasal cartilages into correct position, providing immediate support for the external nasal valve. (iii) Reassignment of nasalis into an anatomic insertion changes the force vectors of breathing, both immediately and in the long term. (iv) Lining release reassigns biosynthetic mucoperiosteum into a correct relationship with the developing bony cavity.

Talmant's lip/nose repair *does not touch the nasal mucosa of the hard palate*; furthermore, it *does not make use of a vomer flap*. The reader should be aware that some schools of thought (particularly in Europe) maintain that vomer flap closure to the nasal mucoperiosteum is to be avoided. Certainly, repair of the anterior nasal floor is not required to accomplish the four goals listed above. However, the decision to not unite the nasal floor completely, once and for all, may be technically disadvantageous.

Concomitant with the lip repair, soft palate repair helps with early tongue posturing, narrows the posterior palate cleft, and offsets the anterior forces created by the cleft lip repair. Talmant wants the hard palate cleft to narrow down in anticipation of palatoplasty at 2 years. He also knows that Lumineau's quad-helix will compensate for collapse.

Hard palate repair at 18 months has no particular drawbacks. As we shall see (below) the eruption of dentition and the quality of alveolar bone make *alveolar extension palatoplasty* flaps (when needed) simple to design and execute.

At age 4, the mucoperiosteum lining the (now fully expanded) cleft is easy to elevate. The alveolar bone is strong as well, protecting unerupted permanent dentition. Intervention at this age is rational because it does not pose a risk to the stem cell layer nor to the tooth buds.

DFR-modified Talmant–Lumineau protocol
Step 1. 6 months: DFR including complete nasal repair + soft palate

Step 1 option. Soft palate repair can be performed separately at 9–12 months.

Step 2. At eruption of dentition: Lumineau adjustable quad-helix.

Step 3. 18–24 months: hard palate repair. If lip adhesion or secondary case, DFR.

Step 4 and 5 as per Talmant–Lumineau.

Comments
Doing a full lip repair in isolation from the hard palate presents theoretical problems directly over the alveolar cleft site. (i) Prolabial tissue is brought into the nasal floor and remains isolated from hard palate mucoperiosteum. The NPP flap, to be most effective, brings with it periosteum from the lateral "shoulder" of the premaxilla. NPP is sutured under direct vision of the nasal palate closure, periosteum-to-periosteum. This type of continuity may be difficult to achieve at a second surgery. (ii) These authors do not subscribe to a "no touch" approach to the vomer. From a developmental standpoint, the nasal side of the floor of the nose is supplied by two neuroangiosomes: medial nasopalatine *from the vomer* and the lateral nasopalatine coming *from the lateral nasal wall below the inferior turbinate*. The oral side of the nasal floor is supplied by the greater palatine. Thus, in normal embryologic conditions, each vomer is united to the maxillary crest of the ipsilateral prepalatine shelf.

Achieving definitive nasal repair at 2 years versus 6 months represents an obvious trade-off. Do the requirements of cerebral "programming" demand nasal surgery at 6 months? Management of nasal stents is undoubtedly simpler in younger patients. Lip–nose surgery performed as a secondary procedure offers technical simplicity (the structures are larger and less delicate, have secure tissue planes, and a readily accessible continuity between the mucoperiosteum of the premaxilla, vomer, and septum). The length of the AEP (alveolar extension palato-plasty) flaps is such that the entire floor of the alveolar cleft will be covered. No oronasal fistula is produced. The technical design of doing a simultaneous lip and hard palate closure closes five of the six sides of the alveolar "box": roof, floor, sides, and back-wall. Thus, soft tissue closure of the alveolar cleft is possible at this stage. The relative merits of this are unknown.

Appendix 1: embryologic basis of occlusion and the lateral facial cleft

The maxilla and mandible develop within the confines of the first pharyngeal arch. In its initial state, PA1 hangs downward from the axis of the embryo like a saddle-bag. Pharyngeal arches are almost exclusively composed of neural crest. Running through the core of each arch is a mesodermal structure, known as an aortic arch. Let us explore how the first aortic arch develops.

Recall that the primitive embryonic vascular system consists of paired *dorsal aortae* running the entire length of the embryo. In the most anterior region of the stage 8 embryo (anterior to the brain) the dorsal aortae form a U-shaped loop. Here, the dorsal aortae take a different name, *primitive heart tubes*; these fuse to form the embryonic heart. The most distal (the most anterior) segment of the primitive heart is the atria, being connected to the vitelline veins. Stage 9 is characterized by three major events: embryonic folding, neural crest migration, and the appearance of the first pharyngeal arch. Brain growth is the driving force behind folding. The heart turns 180 degrees, brining it *ventral to the embryonic face*. The functional components of the heart also undergo a 180-degree reversal. As a result, the atria now are positioned posterior to the future ventricular outflow tract. The two vessels connecting the cardiac outflow tract with the dorsal aortae become surrounded by the neural crest mesenchyme migrating downward from rhombomeres 1–3 of the hindbrain. The connecting arteries acquire a new name: the first aortic arch arteries.

From an evolutionary and embryologic standpoint these bones are not single entities; maxillary bone fields arise from neural crest of the second rhombomere, whereas those of the mandible arise from neural crest of the third rhombomere. In its initial state, the first arch hangs down like a saddlebag. Its rostal half is all r2 while the caudal half is made from r3. Thus, maxillary and mandibular bone fields sit directly across from one another along the "neuromeric fault line." As we shall see, this situation explains their eventual occusal relationship.

Oral mucosa is an ectodermal tissue all the way back to the buccopharyngeal membrane (represented in the fetal state by Waldeyer's ring). Beyond that point, pharyngeal mucosa is endodermal in origin. Oral mucosa contains the "program" for each tooth. Neural crest mesenchyme simply responds, producing the appropriate dental units. For this reason, ectodermal dysplasias can result in malformed or absent teeth.

The premaxilla and the dentary bone (being formed from neural crest) merely "present" potential tooth germs to the epithelium.

In any case, all five pharyngeal arches are divided into quadrants by a set of *distal-less genes* (Dlx) genes: Dlx-1, Dlx-2, and so on. Recall that the first and second pharyngeal arches fuse together very early, probably by the time the third pharyngeal arch makes its appearance (Carnegie stage 11). It can be postulated that a nested set of genes related to, or controlled by, the Dlx system exists along the midline of each arch. This would ensure that a potential zone of apoptosis exists in the first arch running along the longitudinal midline from distal to proximal. Epithelium invading the apoptotic zone contains "mirror image" genes specifying opposing maxillary and mandibular dentition.

Under normal conditions, the apoptotic event is confined to the deep-lying bone fields of the first arch, not the skin. However, if the signals responsible for this division are also located in the second arch and/or in the overlying skin, a lateral facial cleft will be present. Such a cleft extends progressively proximal from the oral commissure to the external auditory canal, as successive Dlx fields are involved. Thus, the cleft described as number 7 has nothing whatsoever to do with Tessier cleft zone 7, that is, the jugal bone and overlying malar soft tissues.

Appendix 2 Technical details of developmental field reassignment cleft surgery

Children with CL(P) affecting the *primary hard palate* only (intact arch) are brought to the OR at 6 months of age for definitive repair (Carstens, 2008a).

When CL(P) affects both the *primary and secondary hard palate palate*, that is, when the cleft is complete (through the secondary palate) and narrow, DFR/Talmant lip–nose repair is done at 6 months.

In some cases cleft lip accompanied by a wide complete palate cleft may benefit from a passive splint or from a Dynacleft® device prior to surgery. Lip adhesion should not be considered a "failure." This procedure has a definite role; the resulting scar is not an issue because it will be relocated within the nose along with the non-philtral flap.

Embryologic definition of the philtral prolabium

As previously discussed, the lip incision in DFR cleft surgery divides the prolabium into two distinct embyologic components: a "true" *philtral prolabium* (PP) and a "false" *non-philtral prolabium* (NPP).

In normal patients, the central lip element (Cupid's bow) and the philtral prolabium are synonymous. The true philtral prolabium is the terminal extension of columella and nasofrontal skin, all of which (epidermis, dermis, and subdermal tissue) originate from p5 forebrain neural crest. The philtrum consists of two paired fields; both are supplied by a V1 sensory nerve and a terminal branch of the anterior ethmoid artery. The two AEA vessels run about 2–4 mm apart. The developmental field of the prolabium is therefore in continuity with the *entire columella, including the lateral walls* all the way to the pink p6 septal mucoperiosteum. Contained within the philtral–columellar fields are the medial crura and footplates of the lower lateral cartilages. In the Matthews model, the *philtral columns ascend from the white-roll to the footplates.* In this interaction, the width of the philtral prolabium is no longer considered just that of the columella; it is defined by the *transverse distance between the footplates.*

In cleft lip patients the prolabium contains additional tissue, the non-philtral prolabium (NP). This tissue is in continuity with the mucoperiosteum of the underlying premaxilla and vomer. The mesenchyme of the non-philtrum originates from r2 hindbrain neural crest. NP, premaxilla, and vomer share a common neurovascular axis: the medial sphenopalatine (nasopalatine) artery. Note that the mucoperiosteum of vomer and septum appears to be continuous, but these are actually embryologically separate fields. The soft tissue walls within which the septum is synthesized are derived from p6 forebrain neural crest. They are therefore innervated by branches of V1 and supplied by anterior and posterior nasal branches from the anterior ethmoid axis.

In normal patients, NP is never seen. It lies within the nasal floor as the skin cover for two premaxillary sub-fields: the lateral incisor field and the frontal process field. In the cleft situation, however, the neural crest bone elements of lateral alveolus and frontal process are gone. NPP becomes "shipwrecked," a lonely mass of mesenchyme is cast ashore alongside the pre-existing PP. In bilateral clefts the prolabium will therefore have four separate fields: two PP fields in the center and one NPP field on either side.

In sum, the normal prolabium consists of a tissue complex with four layers. The *skin* and the underlying *non muscle-bearing mesenchyme.* Both arise from forebrain neural crest (prosomere 5). These are supplied by the terminal branches of the anterior ethmoid artery. All remaining layers arise from the hindbrain. An *intervening layer of fat* conveys branches of the facial artery to the fascia and muscle of the *deep orbicularis oris.* The fascia is neural crest from rhombomere 5 while the muscle arises from somitomere 6. *The facial nerve* supplying the deep orbicularis has its nucleus in r5 as well. The *mucosa* is a neural crest structure arising from rhombomere 2. It is supplied by branches from the medial infraorbital artery.

Medial dissection: the non-philtrum flap, septum, the medial nasal fossa, and nasal tip

The DFR incision is designed to separate out tissues that are embryologically distinct. Recall that the purposes of the non-philtral flap are: (i) to add length to the nasal floor, that is replace the missing "housing" of the lateral incisor; (ii) to replace

tissue deficit resulting from release of the lateral nasal wall from the piriform fossa, that is, reconstruct the missing frontal process of the premaxilla; (iii) to release the alar footplate and permit advancement of the lower lateral cartilage into the nasal tip; and (iv) to create direct access to the septum from below.

In harvesting the NP flap, knowing the width of the philtral prolabium is critical. Previously, this author had described the transverse dimensions of the true philtrum as being equal to those of columella proper. Matthews' definition above is broader … and better. *The width of the true philtrum is equal to the transverse distance between the alar footplates.* This has two implications: (i) the resulting Cupid's bow is embryologically more accurate; and (ii) surgical dissection using these landmarks has technical advantages (Figures 8.4 and 8.5). Both these points will be discussed later.

The prolabial incision we are describing has implications for lip height and lip esthetics. Using the former (narrower) definition of philtral width (in which 2–3 equals columellar width) only lip height is almost uniformly equal. That is, the height of

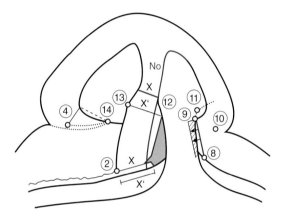

Figure 8.4 (a) Markings. This is based on the original numerical sequence popularized by Millard. The width of the "true" philtral prolabium (P) is the width of the columella at the level of the alar footplates at the tips of the medial crura). Let us call this distance x. Point 2 is the normal /non-cleft philtral column at the white-roll. The new philtral column on the cleft side, point 3, is 2-x. Point 1 in the Millard system, the visual "center" of the Cupid's bow, is therefore irrelevant. Points 4 and 10 are the centers of the alar bases on the non-cleft and cleft sides respectively, as defined by the light reflex. Point 5, the Millard back-cut, is irrelevant. Points 6 and 7 are the commissures. Point 8 is the tentative location of the cleft-side philtral column on the lateral lip element at the white-roll. This can be adjusted. Measuring distances 2–6 and 7–8 are rough guides to equality but not terribly useful. The height of the Cupid's bow is measured from the alar footplates, with point 13 on the non-cleft side and point 12 on the cleft side. Distance 13–2 is the true height of the lip and will equal 12–3 with the addition of the Matthew's triangle (discussed below). 13–2 will equal 8–9. Point 9 can be marked as the highest point on the skin margin of the lateral lip element. The alar base on the cleft-side is rotated inward and this translates the nostril sill internally. The nostril sill is a triangle defined on the non-cleft side by 4–14, with point 14 being the terminus of the sill. This is usually 3–4 mm. You can take the compass and measure across the sill from point 4 into the nose and find the other leg of the triangle. In similar fashion, the nostril sill on the cleft side can be marked out from point 10 based on the measurements on the normal side. The tip of nostril sill flap, point 11, is inserted at the base of point 12 to re-establish the normal width of the nostril floor.

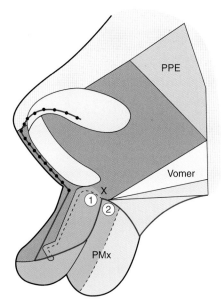

Red = anterior and posterior ethmoid axes (StV1)
Yellow = medial nasal palatine axis (StV2)
Orange = medial infraorbital axis (StV2)
Green = non-philtral prolabium skin and mucosa supplied from the most distal medial sphenopalatine axis

The subcutaneous pedicle is indicated by the number 1.

The anterior ethmoid supplies the distal 2/3 of the septum and the posterior ethmoid the proximal 1/3 of the septum and the perpendicular plate of the ethmoid. In the unilateral cleft the prefixal maintains this dual blood supply but in the bilateral cleft the premaxilla is completely isolated from the infraorbital; it depends strictly on the medial nasapalatine. The unilateral lip has infraorbital to the deep orbicularis and anterior ethmoid pink to the prolabium.

Figure 8.5 Markings of the older version of DFR. Here the incision separating the non-prolabium (NP) from the philtral prolabium (PP) sweeps upward along the lateral margin of the columella. A small counter-incision in the membranous septum helps lift up the medial crus like a boot strap. The lower paring incision of the NP flap is carried over the alveolus. If the alveolar cleft is complete, it can reach to the vomer to elevate an optional vomer flap and thus achieve closure of the nasal floor. A lateral nasal incision elevates tissues in front of the inferior turbinate. With the Talmant dissection of the nasalis complex, this lateral design is not useful. There may be situations in which the access gained by the lateral columellar incision justifies its use. The resulting scar behaves well and is inconspicuous. *Matthew's modification brings the incision underneath the alar footplate*. It can stop at point 1. Placing curved scissors through the incision beneath the footplate places the surgeon immediately beneath the medial crus. The dissection extends readily up to the tip, where it becomes superficial to the intermediate crus and to the lateral crus. Option 2 follows the alveolus backwards to the vomer permitting elevation of a vomer flap to close the floor of the nose. Complete closure of the nasal floor over an alveolar cleft is critical to avoid an iatrogenic fistula and for successful grafting at age 4. In the Talmant protocol, soft palate closure is achieved at the first surgery but nothing is done with the hard palate. Certain surgical situations, where recall is uncertain, may require closure on the nasal side because it will never be more readily accessible. The extension of the NPP flap incision can be readily carried backward on the vomer to accomplish this goal, leaving completion of the hard palate with mucoperiosteal flap mobilization to a later stage in the sequence. Note that the lateral columellar incision lifts up the entire medial crus and re-sets it into position *vis-a-vis* the normal side. This maneuver proved highly effective with exceedingly good scar but was superceded by Matthew's innovation.

the philtral column on the non-cleft side (13–2) equals the distance on the cleft side (12–3) equals the height of the lateral lip element (8–9). *The esthetic problem with this incision resides at the white-roll at the cleft-side philtral column.* The normal upper lip has natural pucker (a slight eversion) all along the white-roll. This esthetically important feature is caused by the presence of marginal fibers of the deep orbicularis oris (DOO). Recall that anatomic territory of DOO is biologically "programmed" oral mucosa. Thus, the distal margin of DOO follows the vermillion, curving upward in the form of a fishhook. It terminates at the mucosa–skin interface, that is, at the white-roll. In a non-cleft situation, these terminal fibers extend right across the philtral column. By lending bulk to the vermillion just below the while-roll, the terminal fibers are responsible for eversion.

Matthews has pointed out that that when a DFR incision is brought straight down based upon columellar width alone, *eversion at the white-roll is obliterated.* How can this be avoided and, at the same time, preserve lip height? Three simple steps will do the trick. (i) The definition of Cupid's bow width is expanded, marking it out using the transverse dimensions of the footplates and normal mucosal landmarks. (ii) The DOO fibers should be conserved all across the philtrum. (iii) A measured back-cut above the "ridge" of the DOO will preserve lip height. Over time this incision becomes a *straight line* and *conserves the esthetically important eversion* of the lip all the way across the repair.

In the Matthews modification of DFR, the philtral prolabium is mapped out as follows. Point 1 (the center of PP) is located *directly above the frenulum.* Point 2 is the non-cleft philtral column. Point 3 (the cleft-side philtral column) is marked out with distance 1–2 equal to 1–3. Remember that PP and columella share a common source of mesenchyme (forebrain neural crest) and a common neurovascular supply (V1 and the terminal branches of anterior ethmoid arteries). The width of these fields is the transverse distance between the footplates. In a unilateral cleft the non-cleft footplate is point 13 and the cleft-side footplate is point 12. Matthews' prolabial markings create a philtrum of the same width. Thus **2–3 = 13–12**. These medial markings will match those of the lateral lip element **8–9**.

The eversion (pucker) of the lip is marked all the way across the philtrum. Because the deep orbicularis follows the mucosa,

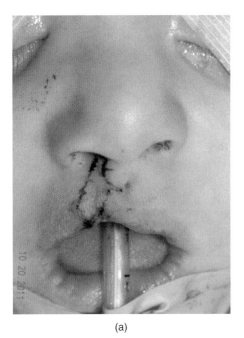
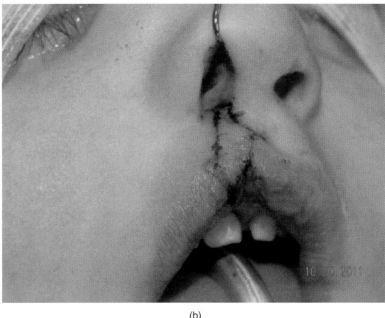

(a)   (b)

Figure 8.6 (a) Detail markings of DFR with Matthews' modification. The incision sweeps downward from the alar footplate and makes a 2 mm back-cut just above the white-roll. This provides for adjustment of what becomes essentially a straight line repair and allows for anchorage of a strong buried white-roll suture (5-0 PDS). (b) shows an additional back-cut to adjust height. It is located just beneath the footplate.

this will be observed to curve slightly upward. With our new definition, cleft-side lip height will fall short by 3–4 mm. One compensates for this by lengthening PP using a back-cut made *above the natural roll of the muscle along the margin of the Cupid's bow*. The back-cut will dart inward about 2 mm and then back outward by the same amount at a 45-degree angle, where it joints the original curve of the DFR incision. This gives two benefits: (i) parity of lip height; and (ii) a natural fullness of muscle at the base of the new philtral column (Figure 8.6).

The proximal component of the prolabium incision ascends toward the columella. It circles around the base of the columella, passing beneath the footplate of the medial crus. The incision terminates at the transition between the columellar skin and the septal mucosa. Initially, the depth of this incision is *skin only*.

The depth of the prolabial incision is important. Initially, it is entirely cutaneous. This permits elevation of the philtral skin from the underlying non muscle-bearing mesenchyme for about 5 mm. Once the initial incision and undermining are accomplished, the prolabial incision is deepened from the white-roll upward to the base of the columella (the underlying mucosa is spared). At the columellar base the incision remains cutaneous only. This is to preserve the underlying mesenchyme within which is contained the pedicle from the medial nasopalatine artery. This tissue is left intact. The cutaneous incision beneath the alar footplate permits entry into the columella with curved scissors. The tips of the scissors follow the medial aspect of the medial crus all the way into the nasal tip (Figure 8.7).

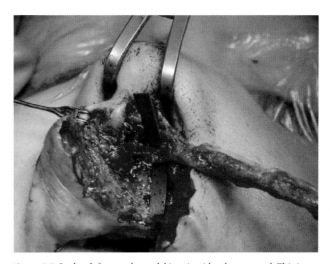

Figure 8.7 In the cleft state, the prolabium is wider than normal. This is because non-philtral tissue that should be assigned to the premaxilla becomes included. I have therefore considered the cleft "prolabium" to be a composite structure consisting of a "true" philtral component (supplied by the terminal branches of the StV1 anterior ethmoid axis) and a "false" non-philtral component (supplied by the StV2 medial nasopalatine axis). Thus, the incision that runs upward from point 3 separates the PP, philtral prolabium, from the NPP, non-philtral prolabium. Recall that the true position of the NPP is to provide soft tissue coverage over the lateral incisor, that is, the introitus of the nasal floor. The vessels supplying the NPP flap come from the vomer–premaxillary junction. These can be readily visualized, but blunt dissection in the subperiosteal plane is protective. Note here that the NPP flap has been dissected using a lateral columellar incision. The blue tape marks the pedicle. NPP flap is a skin flap. Note here the mucosal extension to the NPP flap.

A paring incision is now done from the white-roll up into the nose. Again, at the base of the columella, care is taken to make this incision cutaneous only. The non-philtrum flap is now elevated with a generous subcutaneous base. The flap is lifted off the premaxilla in the subperiosteal plane up to, but not beyond, the junction of the premaxilla with the vomer. This ensures mobility of the flap without compromise of the pedicle. In sum, the non-philtrum flap is a skin island supported by subcutaneous tissue supplied by the nasopalatine artery.

The disposition of the medial mucosa is at the discretion of the surgeon. The M flap can be dropped downward like a baby's diaper. It can be included with the non-philtrum flap for greater epithelial width. Finally, it can be inferiorly based and rotated. I prefer option 1 because it leaves option 3 open. The width of the non-philtrum flap is not strictly determined by the skin paddle. Subcutaneous tissue will readily epithelialize.

Septal mobilization is carried out next. This can be done by extending the incision like a hockey stick upward at the anterior septal border. A dental amalgam packer is very useful because its curved tip is flat and cross-hatched. It can rasp through the mucoperichondrium to the correct plane with great delicacy. The septum is completely dislocated.

Herein we encounter part 1 of Talmant's nasal fossa reconstruction: the dissection is extended upward to the nasal bone and the vestibular lining is freed in the subperiosteal plane from beneath the nasal bone. This frees up the upper lateral cartilage from beneath the nasal bone. Recall that the abnormal anatomy of the nasalis predisposes to a flattening of the nasal bone and entrapment of the upper lateral cartilage. This maneuver also lengthens the dimensions of the nasal fossa.

We have now completed the medial dissection. It is now time to ensure that the goals of our nasal dissection are accomplished. The nasalis complex needs to be freed in the subperiosteal plane from the underlying upper and lower lateral cartilages. A small infracartilagenous incision provides access to the nasal dorsum. It is a good idea to visualize the alara cartilage (once again, the amalgam packer proves helpful). A McComb dissection is carried out. One should drop downward to encounter the bone along the piriform fossa. Spatial limitations of the nasal incision limit what one can accomplish. We must await the lateral dissection to ensure that our subperiosteal nasal dissection is complete.

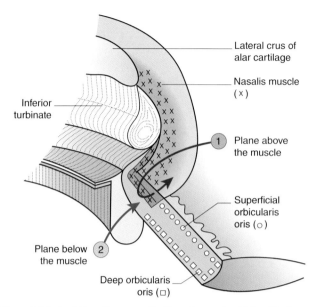

Figure 8.8 Lateral dissection opens the lip and separates: (i) the skin from the superficial orbiculars – about 5 mm; (ii) the superficial orbicularis (SOO) from the deep orbicularis (DOO); and (iii) the nasalis from both SOO and DOO. NB: actual separation of the nasalis is most easily accomplished after the muscle has been completely dissected out because it can be tensed away from the lateral lip element. Recall that the nasalis has two heads, both of which become displaced in the cleft condition. The superficial head should insert over the lateral incisor but instead becomes stranded beneath the nostril sill. The deep head should insert over the canine but instead it falls inside the piriform rim and attaches low on the wall. Dissection of the nasalis proceeds in two planes. First, the skin of the nostril sill is elevated off the muscle. Dissection is then extended up into the nose undermining the vestibular mucosa off the muscle, proceeding in front of the inferior turbinate, and extending all the way up to the edge of the lateral crus. Next, while grasping the muscle, one proceeds deep to it, separating it from the orbicularis and going directly to the rim of the piriform fossa. One then proceeds inward and, hugging the inner wall of the piriform rim, one elevates the deep head off the floor of the piriform. A McKenty or a Molt #9 elevator can prove useful as one "fishes out" the muscle from the piriform fish tank. Note here that the superficial plane of the nasalis (pink arrow) is dissected by proceeding just beneath the skin of the nostril sill and thence upward beneath the vestibular lining until one achieves the edge of the lateral crus. The deep plane of the nasalis (blue arrow) is achieved by following the mucosa down to the piriform fossa where one proceeds in the subperiosteal plane along both its internal aspect and upward to the nasal bones.

Lateral dissection: muscle separation, nasalis transposition, and the lateral nasal fossa

Paring incision proceeds from point 8 all the way into the nasal cavity. Recall that distances 8–9 = 13–2 = 12–3. Also recall that the width of the keratinized mucosa at point 8 should equal that at point 3. With the lateral lip element stretched, one immediately undermines the skin from the superficial orbicularis oris for a distance of about half a fingertip. This separation is continued upward to the nasal skin, involving both the lower

alar base and the nostril sill. The superficial and deep orbicularis muscles are separated by a fat pad analogous to that found in the prolabium. SOO and DOO are separated proximally all the way to the termination of the deep layer (Figures 8.8–8.13).

Nasalis and SOO are still confluent. Our next task is to separate them and gain control of the nasalis. This is most easily done using the concept of two planes: subcutaneous and subperiosteal. Recall that the medial head of the nasalis is inserted into the vestibular lining while the lateral head of nasalis resides in the piriform fossa, extending halfway up its

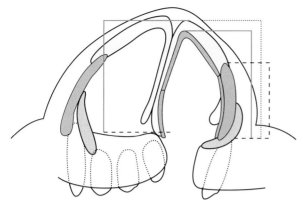

Figure 8.9 I could never get the lateral nasal wall right until I became aware of Talmant's findings. Formerly, I had tried lateral crus elevation using a V-Y incision, broad superiosteal freeing, and so on, all to no avail. Nasalis dissection is key but another maneuver worked out by Talmant is very helpful. Using a long curved elevator, one proceeds inside the piriform rim and frees it all the way to the nasal bones. Then you sweep downward – always in the subperiosteal plane – until you reach the nasal mucosa underlying the alar cartilage. Now, you do exactly the same maneuver outside the piriform fossa – again in the superiosteal plane – until you reach the nasal bones and then proceed downward bluntly separating the SMAS muscle layer from the underlying upper lateral (triangular) cartilage and thence to the lower lateral (alar) cartilage. The alar cartilage will be nicely mobilized. You will also fall into the dissection plane you previously created by the medial dissection with scissors up the columella. Recall Tessier's concept of blunt tissue dissection following embryonic planes. These maneuvers are simple and quick but a nicely sharpened elevator is a must.

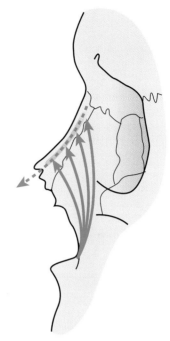

Figure 8.10 This brings me to a final detail regarding the lateral wall that is important if one wants to achieve a hermetic closure of the nasal mucoperiosteum. As we all know, elevating the lining away from the nasal/dorsal aspect of the palatal shelf can be challenging. Two maneuvers make this easier and safer. First, after making the incision along the edge of the palatal shelf, a small dental amalgam packer can be used to elevate off all fibers of periosteum. The head of this instrument is angulated and delicate. It can nicely lift up the edge without tearing it. Second, the incision to elevate the triangual nostril sill flap places one directly in front of the inferior turbinate – in the subperiosteal plane. Using a periosteal elevator or the amalgam packer, one proceeds straight backward beneath the turbinate, elevating the mucoperiosteum away from the vertical wall of bone. Then, at the horizontal palatal shelf, one simply proceeds in the same plane, elevating lateral to medial until one gains the cut edge of the palatal shelf.

vertical extent. We shall start with the medial head. Extension of the skin undermining into the nasal cavity now continues in a plane superficial to the medial head of the nasalis. The dissection should extend in front of the inferior turbinate and all the way up to the lower lateral cartilage. One now proceeds in the subperiosteal plane beginning at the entrance into the piriform fossa, that is, in the triangular zone corresponding to the nostril sill. One is now beneath the medial head of nasalis. The muscle is grasped and sectioned away from the bone. With the lateral lip once again on tension, the superficial orbicularis is divided away from medial nasalis at the level of the alar base. Tension placed on the nasalis at this point will transmit to the lateral nasal wall but will not be free (Figures 8.14 and 8.15).

The lateral rim of the piriform fossa is swept clean upward to the halfway point. One has now gained access to the lateral margin of the fossa. An elevator is passed upward along the lateral wall of the nose until it achieves the nasal dorsum. At this point one should switch to an elevator that is sharp and strong, with a broad and curved tip, such as a McKenty. A customized Molt elevator works well. The elevator is swept downward underneath the SMAS (including the nasalis) all the way to the nasal tip. The result of this *McComb* dissection should be a complete liberation of the dorsal nasal skin and SMAS from the underlying upper and lower lateral cartilages.

Recall that all unilateral cleft noses have an overall deviation of the soft tissue envelope on the non-cleft side away from the midline. This is an opportune moment to correct this problem and to centralize the entire midface envelope. Wide subperiosteal dissection is carried out over the face of the maxilla on both sides. *Care should be taken to free up the non-cleft alar base as well.* Because the mucoperiosteal envelope contains the stem cells required for future membranous bone synthesis, one has now "centralized the biosynthetic envelope" such that the external dimensions of piriform fossa (and the maxillae in general) will continue to auto-correct over time.

We now turn our attention to inside the piriform fossa to complete the dissection of the lateral head of nasalis. Using a curved elevator the nasalis muscle fibers lying within piriform are literally "scooped out" of the fossa. At this point the two heads are evaluated. They may appear distinct or as a single mass. The functionality of the muscle dissection is now tested. Traction is placed on the nasalis; motion along the lower lateral cartilages will be seen. The range is between 5–10 mm. If

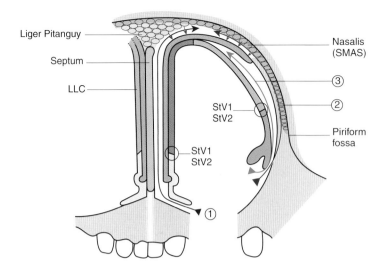

Liger Pitanguy

Septum

LLC

StV1
StV2

StV1
StV2

①

Nasalis
(SMAS)

③

②

Piriform
fossa

Turqoise = septum
Blue   = lower lateral cartilage
Red   = anterior ethmoid/medial nasal (StV1)
Pink   = anterior ethmoid/lateral nasal (StV1)
Yellow   = medial nasopalatine (StV2)
Brown   = lateral nasopalatine (StV2)
Green   = nasalis/SMAS
Dissection plane 1 (purple arrow) is subperichondrial; in the nasal tip it becomes sub-SMAS.
Dissection plane 2 (red arrow) is superiosteal outside the piriform fossa and over the nasal bones. As plane 2 descends beyond the nasal bones into the nasal dorsum and tip it becomes sub-SMAS and is therefore continuous with plane 1.
Dissection plane 3 is subvestibular. It begins high in the nasal vault beneath the nasal bone. As it descends beyond the nasal bone it lengthens the vestibular lining and fortress frees the lateral nasal cartilages.

Figure 8.11 Extent of the DFR/Talmant dissection planes. Columellar dissection just internal to the medial crus (blue) achieves the sub-SMAS plane – superficial to the nasal cartilages. Subperiosteal dissection internal to the piriform fossa goes below the nasalis and extends upward to nthe asal bones (green) and achieves the plane between the cartilages above and the vestibular lining below. The subperiosteal plane external to the piriform fossa is carried up to the nasal bones and then downward, once again in the sub-SMAS plane.

(a)

(b)

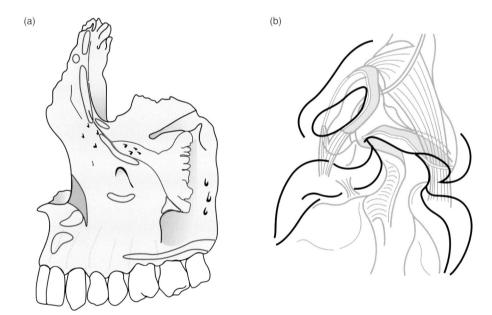

Figure 8.12 (a) Nasalis: Adapted from: Standring S. (ed.) *Gray's Anatomy* 40th edn. Elsevier, 2008, fig 32.3 also using Lews W. H. (ed.) *Gray's Anatomy of the Human Body*, 20th American edn, 1918, fig 157. Reproduced with permission of Elsevier. Note the older editions show the transverse head attaching just lateral to the piriform fossa. Here, the attachments are shown in blue. Nasalis has two components, both of which act immediately prior to inspiration. (1) Transverse nasalis or *compressor nasalis*, has its primary attachment along the lateral aspect of the piriform rim; and secondarily sweeps upward over the nasal dorsum to join its counterpart. The function of transversus is to tense the nasal vestibular soft against the piriform rim. (2) Alar nasalis or *dilator nasalis posterior*, has its primary attachment over the lateral incisor and canine – medial to transversus. Its secondary attachments are to the skin above the lateral crus and the membranous septum. Its functions are to tense the alar cartilage laterally and pull down on the membranous septum, thus making the nose longer. A third muscle, apicis nasi or *dilator naris anterior*, spans between the caudal margin of lateral crus and the upper lateral cartilage; its fibers are connected upwards with *dilator naris posterior*. These two muscles prevent collapse of the internal nasal valve during inspiration. (b) Illustration from Talmant's paper in IJPS, 2006 shows the nasalis mal-inserted into the nostril sill but does not depict the internalized position of the posterior (transverse) head within the piriform fossa itself.

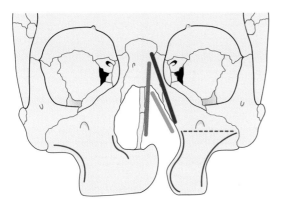

Figure 8.13 DFR achieves wide superiosteal undermining on the cleft-side without a buccal sulcus incision. A releasing incision up the buttress is connected with a medial incision along the alveolus. The non-cleft side is also released in the subperiosteal plane along the alar margin with the dissection extending into the piriform fossa. The three planes involving the nasal airway are shown. The medial columellar dissection plane (blue) connects with the external piriform fossa (pink) in the sub-SMAS plane. The internal piriform fossa subperiosteal plane (green) separates the vestibular lining from the nasal bones and from the cartilages. Note: the nasalis is repositioned using a mattress suture through the periosteum and the buccal sulcus over the canine fossa.

restriction is encountered, one can release the muscle further by first re-entering the piriform fossa to take down any residual attachments. One can then proceed along the external aspect of the muscle about halfway up, spreading it away from the overlying skin. Excessive external dissection will encounter blood supply to the muscle from the facial arcade.

Repositioning of the nasalis is done by anchoring the muscle to the mucoperiosteum of the canine fossa and the sulcus using a mattress suture of 4-0 vicryl. The suture is passed from the buccal sulcus upward behind the orbicularis. It loops through the muscle and is returned to the mouth where the suture is placed on a clamp. It will be approximated as the final maneuver of the surgery.

Having cleaned out the piriform fossa we are now in position to complete part 2 of Talmant's nasal fossa reconstruction. A curved elevator is passed anterior to the inferior turbinate and is then directed backward and upward until the nasal bone is reached. Using this combination of subperichondrial and subperiosteal dissection, a complete freeing of the mucoperiosteal lining of the nasal fossa is achieved. Once again, the biologic advantage of this maneuver is to reposition the stem cell envelope correctly such that osteosynthesis within the piriform fossa proceeds in a normal manner from 6 months onwards. The goal is normalization of the internal dimensions of the piriform fossa over the course of time (Figures 8.16 and 8.17).

Closure and nasal splinting

At this juncture, the dissection is complete. All cleft surgeons have their preferred sequence of steps to achieve closure. I will simply make note of a few maneuvers that I have found helpful over time. The closure sequence begins inside the nose. Access incisions to the septum and the nasal tip are addressed first. The non-philtrum flap is sutured to the release incision in the lateral

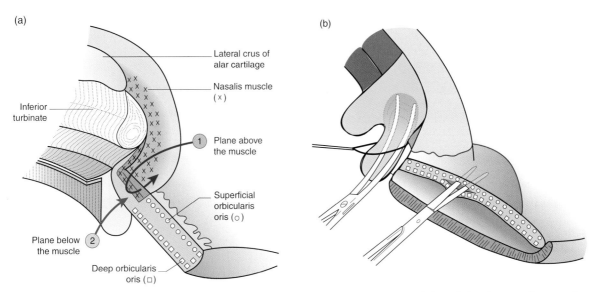

Figure 8.14 (a) Nasalis is dissected free from orbicularis oris complex. Mattress suture is placed, but not tied, through the sulcus over the canine fossa. Premature fixation may alter the geometry of the nasal floor. When lip closure is complete, then (and only then) is the nasalis anchored. (b) Elevation of the nasalis: (i) dis-insert pars alaris from the skin of the nostril sill and the vestibular lining; (ii) dis-insert pars dorsalis from the internal surface of the piriform fossa. (c) Left UCL incisions show the tip of the nostril sill flap internally rotated in the nasal cavity. When the nostril sill skin flap is elevated it will rotate externally to form the introitus of the nostril just external to the first valve. (d) The nasalis flap is substantial. Here it is being attached to its original insertion site. (e) Note the separation (of the nasalis) from the orbicularis complex of the lateral lip element.

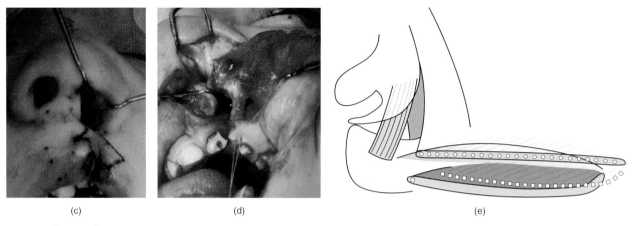

(c)   (d)   (e)

Figure 8.14 (*Continued*)

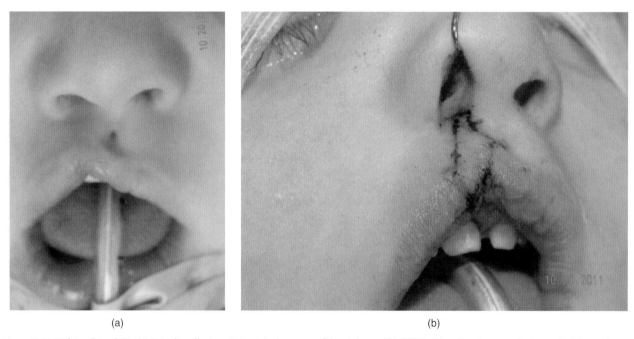

(a)   (b)

Figure 8.15 Right unilateral CL. (a) Prior lip adhesion. Note pit in the center of the philtrum. (b) DFR incision showing two adjustment incisions: (i) immediately above the white-roll; and (ii) just beneath the footplate. The incision extends below the footplate. At this point the scissors can separate the medial crura allowing advancement on the cleft-side. If an alveolar cleft and/or a cleft of the secondary palate is present, the incision can be extended inward and beneath the vomer to enlarge the NPP flap and elevate a vomer flap, if indicated. (c) NPP flap dissected away. Note the lengthening achieved with the white-roll back-cut. (d) NPP pulled forward. The nasalis complex is separated from the lateral lip element but is still in continuity with the skin of the nostril sill. (e) Here the pedicle to the NPP flap is demonstrated. (f) NPP flap inset in front of the nasal floor and into the space created by the releasing incision for the nostril sill flap. (g and h) Nostril tubes of thin silicon stent the nasal cavity. Through-and-through sutures compress the intranasal silicon sheet with that draped over the nasal dorsum.

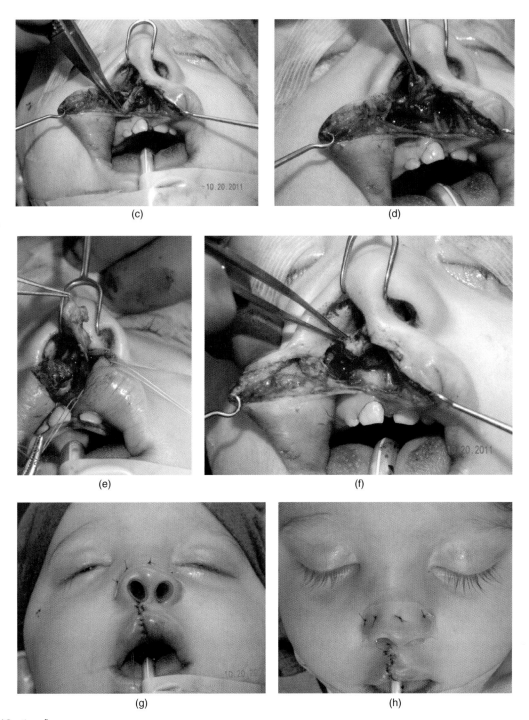

Figure 8.15 (*Continued*)

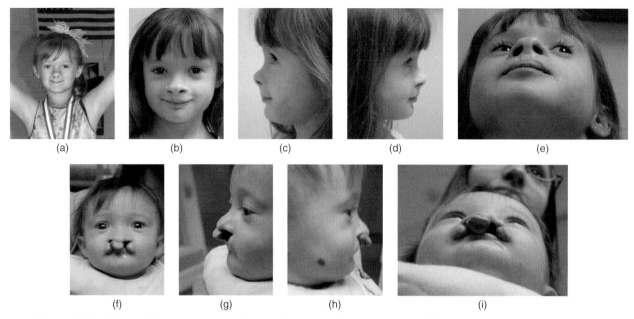

(a)   (b)   (c)   (d)   (e)

(f)   (g)   (h)   (i)

Figure 8.16 (a–i) BCL with 5-year follow-up and 8-year follow-up. Subperiosteal dissection preserves midface growth.

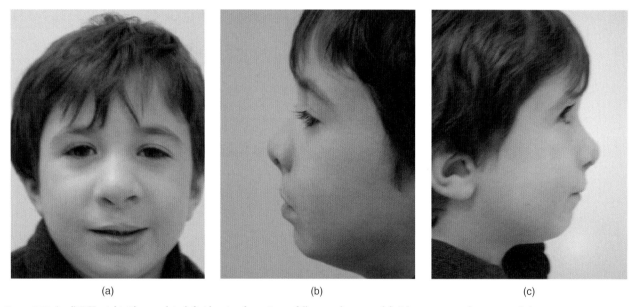

(a)   (b)   (c)

Figure 8.17 (a–d) BCL, right side complete, left side microform: 5-year follow-up shows good facial symmetry and patent nasal airways.

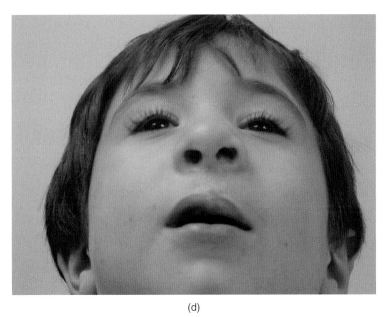

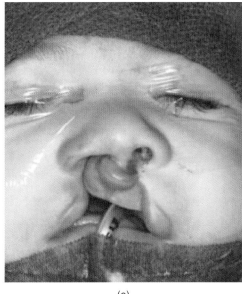

(d)   (e)

Figure 8.17 (*Continued*)

nasal wall. If a vomer flap has been raised, the NP flap is sutured on its back side to the vomer flap. Otherwise, the nostril sill flap created by the releasing incision previously described is brought along the front side of the NP flap and sutured with 5-0 vicryl sutures taking care to maximize the "fit" between the two flaps. A double hook is then placed in the nose and gently lifted. The posterior margin of the NP flap is sutured to the footplate of the alar cartilage. In this way one strives to re-establish the elusive "shoulder" of the columella (Figure 8.18).

Lateral lip height is first established by suturing the extreme tip of the deep orbicularis to its counterpart at the anterior nasal spine. Alignment of the white-roll is carried out using 4-0 or 5-0 vicryl in the DOO where it curls upward toward the white-roll. A confirmatory suture of 5-0 monocryl is placed at the dermal–epidermal junction of the white-roll. An additional vicryl suture is placed at the wet–dry mucosal junction. With the lip on traction, the remainder of the mucosa and deep orbicularis is closed as a single layer. Final decisions regarding the M and L flaps are taken at this time. The use of the L flap as a "diaper" to cover the raw area of the medial lip vermillion often makes sense.

The extreme tip of superficial orbicularis (sometimes referred to as the oblique head of the SOO) is attached by a mattress suture through the columella just below the footplate of the lateral crus on the non-cleft side. The suture is tightened to check the position but not tied. The superficial orbicularis is then sutured to the non muscle-bearing mesenchyme of the prolabium with three to four vicryl sutures. This helps to achieve some bulkiness beneath the new philtral column. Several sutures of 6-0 monocryl (or nylon, if nothing else is available) carefully placed at the dermal–epidermal junction seal up the skin. A running 6-0 vicryl suture completes the closure.

Ophthalmic 6-0 is particularly good because of its dissolution characteristics.

Suspension of the nasal cartilages is not a part of the Talmant technique. Nonetheless, I think that tip projection is improved by suturing the medial crura together in their new position with two sutures of 5-0 vicryl/monocryl. The unified crura can then be elevated and sutured to the septum with 4-0 vicryl/monocryl. Luis Monasterio has a very ingenious tip graft which is shaped like the number 1 with the upper limb pointing backwards. The *number 1 graft* is placed through a lateral columellar incision exactly the way I used to do if for the non-philtrum flap. The incision falls just anterior to the medial crus. The graft is harvested from the septum. Closure of the incision with 6-0 chromic is virtually unnoticeable. For simplicity and versatility, the number 1 graft is my first choice for secondary rhinoplasty or in adult cleft cases. The graft is fixed in place using the same suture sequence: medial crural unification followed by fixation to the septum.

Silicon stents cut from 0.5 mm sheeting are then placed (Figure 8.18). The initial two stents are only temporary. They are curled up like snails inside each nasal cavity. An additional sheet of silicon is placed over the dorsum and the tubes are secured with two sutures of 4-0 prolene, beginning with the non-cleft side. When one places these sutures on the cleft side, a very important phenomenon takes place. On the second pass from the nasal cavity back to the dorsum, the tip of the needle is engaged with the silicon sheeting. Moving the sheeting further repositions the alar cartilage. The needle is then thrust upward through the sheeting, fixing the cartilage in its final position.

Vaseline gauze or Xerofrom® gauze is then used to pack the nose. This further expands the nasal airway. During the packing phase, antibiotics are given. At one week, both the packing and

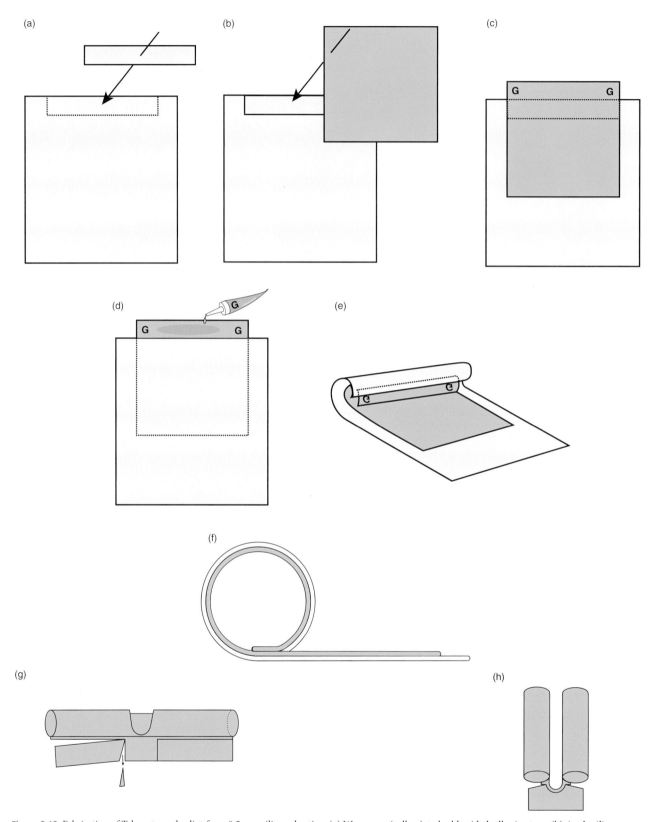

Figure 8.18 Fabrication of Talmant nasal splint from 0.5 mm silicon sheeting. (a) Wax paper (yellow) + double-sided adhesive tape. (b) Apply silicon sheeting (fluorescent yellow/orange) to the adhesive tape –1 cm excess. (c) Topology: wax paper down on the table; silicon sheeting faces you. (d) Flip over (silicon sheeting is on the table) and apply the glue. (e) Flip over once more (the wax paper is now on the table) and roll up. (f) Glued sector = orange to orange. (g) Trim the excess, avoid the glued sector inside. (h) Tube inserted. The "diaper" can be placed over the nasal dorsum or the nasal tip.

the temporary silicone stents are removed. Nasal stenting is then continued for four months using the design as illustrated. Once again 0.5 mm silicon sheeting is used. In countries where this is not available, intravenous solution bags can be cut up instead.

Acknowledgments

The author wishes to credit the following individuals for their intellectual and technical contributions to developmental field reassignment cleft surgery: Paul Tessier, M.D. (deceased) – for his pioneering work in facial cleft classification; Jean Delaire, M.D., D.M.D. – for his demonstration of wide subperiosteal dissection in cleft surgery; David Matthews, M.D. – for his refinements in the design of the non-philtral prolabial flap; Jean Claude Talmant, M.D – for his discovery of the nasalis muscle and the importance of correct nasal airway restoration; Jean-Pierre Lumineau, M.D., D.M.D. – for his unique technical advances in the management of the alveolar cleft; and Luis Monasterio, M.D. – for demonstrating the importance of the developmental field approach to cleft palate repair using the alveolar extension palatoplasty to treat or prevent fistulae and maintain dental development.

References

Bardach, J., Kelly, K. M., and Salyer, K. E. (1994a) Effects of lip repair with and without soft tissue undermining and delayed palate repair on maxillary growth: An experimental study in beagles. *Plast Reconstr Surg* **94**(2):343–351.

Bardach, J., Kelly, K. M., and Salyer, K. E. (1994b) Relationship between sequence of lip and palate repair and maxillary growth: An experimental study in beagles. *Plast Reconstr Surg* **93**(2):269–278.

Bardach, J., Kelly, K. M., and Salyer, K. E. (1993) Comparative study of facial growth following lip and palate repair performed in sequence and simultaneously. *Plast Reconstr Surg* **91**(6):1008–1016.

Bartezko, K and Jacob, M. (2004) A re-evaluation of the premaxillary bone in humans. *Anat Embryol* **207**:417–437.

Carstens, M. H. (2008a) Developmental field reassignment in unilateral cleft lip: Reconstruction of the premaxilla. In: Losee, J. E. and Kirschner, R. E. (Eds) *Comprehensive Cleft Care*. Lippincott, chapter 15. Note: the description given in this paper departs from the Losee chapter but it contains valuable material and references.

Carstens, M. H. (2008b) Neural tube programming and the pathogenesis of craniofacial clefts, part I: the neuromeric organization of the head and neck. *Handb Clin Neurol* **87**:247–276.

Carstens, M. H. (2008c) Neural tube programming and the pathogenesis of craniofacial clefts, part 2: Mesenchyme, pharyngeal arches, developmental fields, and the assembly of the human face. *Handb Clin Neurol* **87**:277–339.

Carstens, M. H. (2002) Development of the facial midline. *J Craniofac Surg* **13**(1):129–187.

Carstens, M. H. (2000a) Correction of the bilateral cleft using the sliding sulcus technique. *J Craniofac Surg* **11**:137–167.

Carstens, M. H. (2000b) The spectrum of minimal clefting: Process-oriented cleft management in the presence of an intact alveolus. *J Craniofac Surg* **11**:270–294.

Carstens, M. H. (1999a) Correction of the unilateral cleft lip nasal deformity using the sliding sulcus procedure. *J Craniofac Surg* **10**:346–364.

Carstens, M. H. (1999b) Sequential cleft management with the sliding sulcus technique and alveolar extension palatoplasty. *J Craniofac Surg* **10**:503–518.

Carstens, M. H. (1999c) The sliding sulcus procedure: Simultaneous repair of unilateral clefts of the lip and primary palate – a new technique. *J Craniofac Surg* **10**:415–434.

Delaire, J., Precious, S., and Gordeef, A. (1993) The advantage of wide superiosteal exposure in primary surgical correction of labial maxillary clefts. *Scand J Plast Reconstr Surg* **22**:710.

Diamond, M. K. (1991a) Homologies of the meningeal artery of humans, a reappraisal. *J Anat* **178**:223–241.

Diamond, M. K. (1991b) Homologies of the stapedial artery in humans, with a reconstruction of the primitive stapedial artery configuration in euprimates. *Am J Phys Anthro* **84**:433–462.

Etchevers, H. C., Couly, G., and Le Douarin, N. M. (2002) Morphogenesis of the branchial vascular sector. *Trends Cardiovasc Med* **12**(7):299–306.

Ewings, E. L. and Carstens, M. H. (2009) Neuroembryology and functional anatomy of craniofacial clefts. *Indian J Plast Surg* October Suppl. S19–S34.

Flores-Sarnat, L., Sarnat, H. B., Hahn, J. S., *et al.* (2007) Axes and gradients of the neural tube form a genetic classification of nervous system malformations. *Handb Clin Neurol* **83**:3–11.

Georgiou, C. and Cassell, M. D. (1992) The foramen meningo-orbitale and its relationship to the development of the ophthalmic artery. *J Anat* **180**:119–125.

He, F., Hu, X., Xiong, W., *et al.* (2014) Directed BMP4 expression in neural crest cells generates a genetic model for the rare human bony syngnathia birth defect. *Dev Biol* **39**(2):170–181.

Le Douarin N. M. and Kalchiem, C. (1999) *The Neural Crest*, 2nd edn. Cambridge: Cambridge University Press.

Lumsden, A. and Krumlauf, R. (1996) Patterning the vertebrate neuraxis. *Science* **274**:1109–1115.

Moss, M. L., Vilman, H., Das Gupta, G. and Sklak, R. (1981) Craniofacial growth in space-time. In: Carlson, D. S. (ed.) *Craniofacial Biology*. Ann Arbor, MI: University of Michigan Center for Human Growth and Development.

Precious, D. and Delaire, J. (1992) Surgical considerations in patients with cleft deformities. In: Bell W. H. (ed.) *Modern Practice in Orthognathic and Reconstructive Surgery*. Philadelphia, PA: Saunders, pp. 390–425.

Ribatti, D., Nico, B., and Crivellato, E. (2011) The role of pericytes in angiogenesis. *Int J Dev Biol* **55**:261–268.

Rosenstein, S. W. (2003) Early bone grafting of alveolar cleft deformities. *J Oral Maxillofac Surg* **61**(9):1078–1081.

Rosenstein, S. W., Grassechi, M., and Dado, D. V. (2003) A long-term retrospective outcome assessment of facial growth, secondary surgical need, and maxillary lateral incisor status in a surgical-orthodontic protocol for complete clefts. *Plast Reconstr Surg* **111**(1):1–13, discussion 14–16.

Rubenstein, J. L. R. and Puelles, L. (1994) Homeobox gene expression during development of the vertebrate brain. *Curr Top Dev Biol* **29**:1–64.

Skoog, T. (1967) The use of periosteum and Surgicel® for bone resotration in congenital clefts of the maxilla. *Scand J Plast Reconstr Surg* **1**(2):113–130.

Talmant, J.-C. (2006) Evolution of the functional repair concept for cleft lip and palate patients. *Indian J Plast Surg* **39**(**2**):197–209.

Tessier, P. (1976) Anatomical classification of facial, craniofacial, and latero-facial clefts. *J Maxillofac Surg* **4**:70–92.

Tessier, P., Hervouet, F., Lekieffre, M. *et al.* (1977) *Plastic Surgery of the Orbit and Eyelids.* Translated by S. Anthony Wolfe. Paris: Masson (distributed by Year Book Medical Publishers).

Zhang, Y., Zhang, Z., Zhao, X., *et al.* (2000) A new function of BMP4: Dual role for BMP4 in regulation of *Sonic Hedgehog* expression in the mouse tooth germ. *Development* **127**:1431–1443.

Zhang, Z., Song, Y., Zhao, X., *et al.* (2002) Rescue of cleft palate in Msx-1 deficient mice by transgenci Bmp-4 reveals a network of BMP and SHH signaling in the regulation of mammalian palatogenesis. *Development* **129**:4135–4146.

CHAPTER 9

Unilateral cleft lip and nose repair

Ricardo D. Bennun[1] and David Genecov[2]
[1] Asociacion PIEL, Maimonides University and National University of Buenos Aires, Argentina
[2] International Craniofacial Institute, USA

Introduction

Surgical treatment of cleft lip and palate has been documented since 317 AD, when Chinese General Wei Yang Chi had his cleft lip corrected by cutting and stitching the edges together. Since then, various authors have described the different surgical techniques for correction of cleft lip (Franco, 1556; Pare, 1575; Tennison, 1952; Millard, 1960).

Unilateral cleft lip and palate is much more than an alteration of the lip and palate; it is a defect of the middle one-third of the face. In treating this deformity, it is essential to address the different elements of the problem: the bony defect of the maxilla, the nasal deformity, and the dynamic force of the lip – the muscle – which is responsible for much of the distortion of the nose and maxilla.

We also have to keep in mind that the orbicularis muscle has a very significant effect on the growth of the maxilla. Muscular reconstruction is key to balancing the forces acting on the maxilla, the nasal tip, and the lip. The lip has to be symmetrical not only at rest, but also on animation, and it has to grow symmetrically. Usually when reference is made to the orbicularis oris muscle of the upper lip only the horizontal bands of muscle are mentioned. This muscle also comprises oblique fibers (orbicularis externus) that are of very great importance in lip movements. The balance of the lip derives from the activity of the two types of muscle fiber (Huffman, 1949).

The lip can thus perform, at the same time, a movement of compression of the underlying structures and projection movements whereby these structures are freed. These different modes of action are well demonstrated by selective electromyography. There is also, in the middle of the upper lip, a medial cellulo-fibrous septum forming a prolongation of the septum and penetrating into the median inter-incisive suture and ending at the frenulum of the upper lip. This medial septum seems to play a very important physiological role in the growth of the premaxilla.

"Do not touch the nose in primary repair of the unilateral cleft lip and palate!" In the past, this dogmatic attitude caused functional and esthetic (psychological) problems for the child until secondary corrections during adolescence were performed (Millard, 1990; Jackson & Fasching, 1990). In the 1950s, surgeons started to correct at least a few features of the nasal deformity and to develop radically corrective measures (Salyer et al., 2009; Vyas & Warren, 2014).

The addition of rhinoplasty to primary cheiloplasty for cleft lip improves not only the postoperative state but also, by re-establishing the equilibrium of all the cartilaginous and musculoperiosteal structures, benefits maxillary growth.

Placing the affected alar cartilage symmetrical to the normal side can be done before lip closure – before the columella and nostril base are brought together – because they are interdependent structures.

Finally, during the muscular reconstruction, the lateral orbicularis attached to the caudal portion of the septum is beneficial to equalize the force of traction and gradually centralize the columella preventing septal deviation. The correct muscular placement is also helpful in rebuilding the nasal floor and preventing oronasal communication.

Cleft lip and palate remains the most common congenital facial anomaly and requires the coordinated care of many specialists from birth to adulthood in order to achieve proper function and esthetic outcomes. Since the late fourth century, surgeons around the world have worked diligently to identify the best procedure. Since Millard (1958) introduced his rotation advancement technique, stability and predictability have been much easier to achieve.

To provide consistent results that not only repair the congenital defects, but also achieve symmetry and esthetic balance,

Cleft Lip and Palate Management: A Comprehensive Atlas, First Edition. Edited by Ricardo D. Bennun, Julia F. Harfin, George K. B. Sándor, and David Genecov.
© 2016 John Wiley & Sons, Inc. Published 2016 by John Wiley & Sons, Inc.

proper education, training, and a constant flow of patients is necessary (Gillies & Millard, 1957).

The techniques outlined in this atlas are the result of almost 30 years of education, practice, and experience as cleft surgeons. We are indebted to the work of numerous surgeons, and the technique described below brings together knowledge gathered over many years, emphasizing a one-unit concept.

The approach to the lip and nasal repair provides the flexibility and improvisation that is often needed with the diversity and complexity of cases presented (Da Silva Freitas *et al.*, 2012).

In patients where the modality of presurgical orthodontics has not been used, an extensive mobilization of the lateral lip and nose elements will be necessary.

Goals of primary cleft lip and nasal reconstruction

(1) Close the lip defect and create a competent lip closure.
(2) Regain muscle continuity.
(3) Reposition the displaced nasal elements and closure of the floor of the nose.
(4) Restoration of the lip and facial balance with recreation of the Cupid's bow and philtral columns.
(5) Elongation of the cleft-side columella and establishment of nasal tip projection.
(6) Stability of correction limiting future interventions.
   See Figures 9.1 to 9.14.

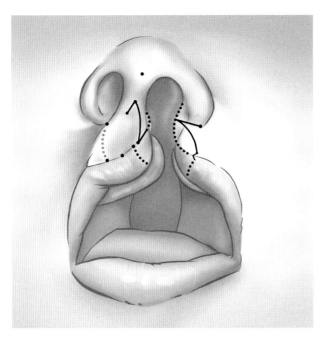

Figure 9.1 The first step with any lip repair is to identify the normal features of the lip. The anatomic points are designated using standard anthropometric marks and a modified rotation advancement flap is drawn.

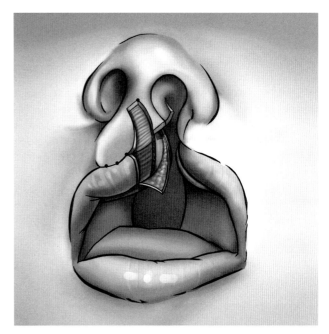

Figure 9.2 On the medial segment, the incision of the rotation flap is kept straighter and longer than originally described by Millard. Lengthening of this incision also opens the possibility of inserting a back-cut, up in the columella. The incision of the mucosa and periosteum is carried posteriorly along the edge of the cleft at the junction of the oral and nasal mucosa. This allows elevation of a medial flap, based superiorly. This flap is advanced laterally to provide a two-layer closure of the floor of the nose.

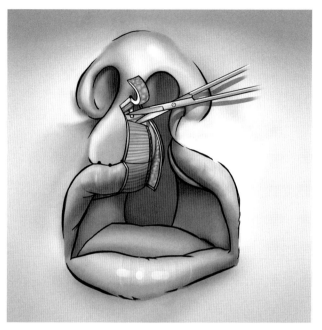

Figure 9.3 Subcutaneous dissection of the medial lip element is kept to a minimum so that the normal midline dimple is not disrupted. However, the medial muscular attachment to the columella is completely released to level the Cupid's bow. The relaxing incision, when needed, can be done after the muscle and mucosa have been completely released.

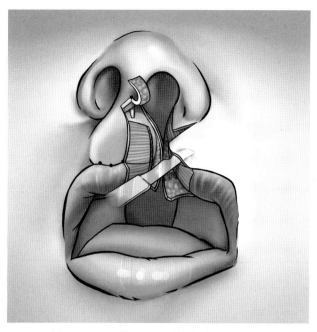

Figure 9.4 Subcutaneous and submucosal blade dissection of the lateral lip is performed conserving the vermillion portion attached.

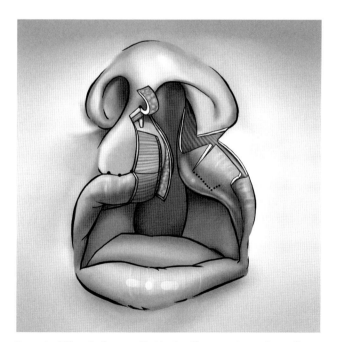

Figure 9.5 When the intranasal bridge is still present, it must be totally released, to allow an open dissection and liberation of all the elements causing the nasal distortion. An inferior pedicle mucosal flap is left to be posteriorly transposed to the raw intranasal area to prevent stenosis.

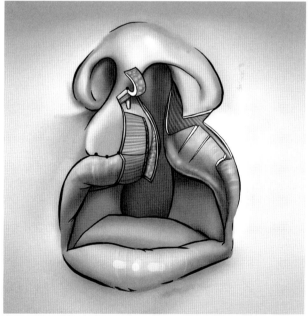

Figure 9.6 A second inferior pedicle mucosal flap, similar to the C mucosal flap described by Noordhoff, is planned to close the floor of the nose in very wide cleft cases.

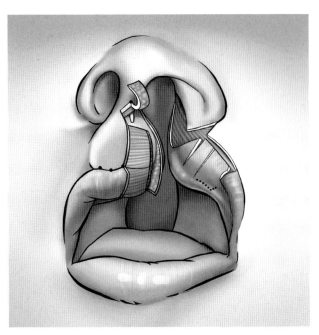

Figure 9.7 A supraperiosteal cheek detachment and liberation of muscular insertions around the pyriform aperture is achieved.

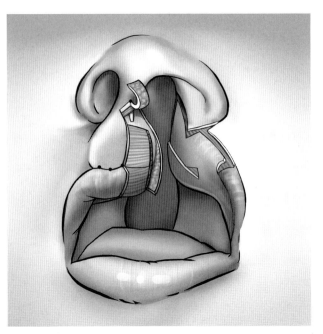

Figure 9.8 The mucosal incision on the underside of the lateral element is extended distally, on the anterior side of the gingivolabial sulcus. A back-cut of the mucosa is done to allow better advancement.

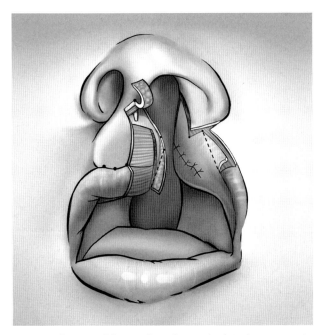

Figure 9.9 The mucosal flap must be undermined only in the upper portion of the lip, never on the free edge, to avoid thickening of the lower lip border.

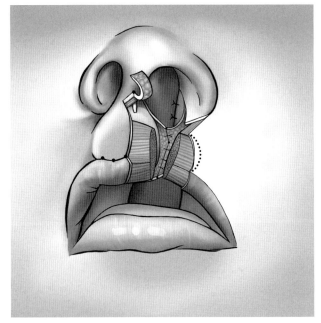

Figure 9.10 Closure of vestibular sulcus, nasal floor, and posterior wall of the lip, is completed by suturing both sides of the mucosal flaps. The last millimeters of the alveolar gap are not touched. Lateral skin resection reproduces the normal philtrum pillar.

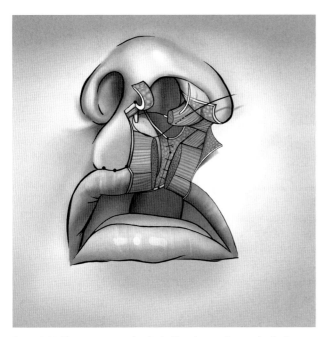

Figure 9.11 The common tendon including the nasalis muscle, the levator labii superioris alaeque nasi and the zigomaticus head is fixed to the caudal portion of the septum. Repositioning of these muscles prevents oronasal fistulas and helps gradual septal correction.

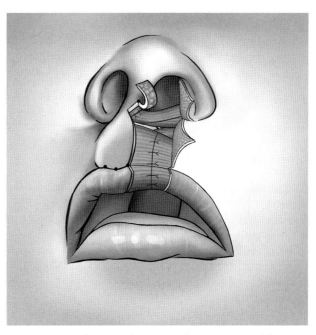

Figure 9.12 Normal anatomical situation and reconstruction of the orbicularis oris and the zygomaticus minor leads not only to better appearance and good mobility of the lip, but also to an enhanced growth of the underlying bony structures.

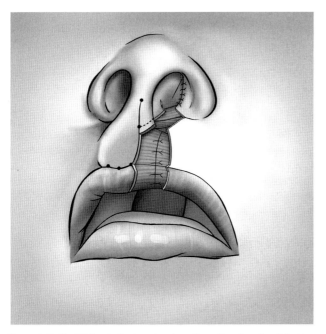

Figure 9.13 The 'C' flap is shortened and positioned to allow the cleft side of the collumella to be elongated, placing the scar in a non-visible area.

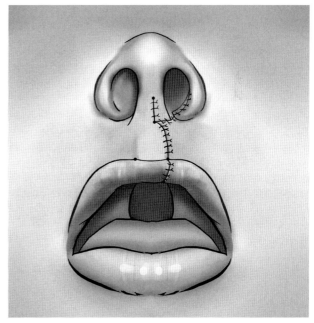

Figure 9.14 Millard's original technique has also been modified to reduce the length of the incision around the base of the nostril. The scar has reduced dimensions and is correctly emplaced from an esthetic point of view.

Surgical technique

The first step with any lip repair is to identify the normal features of the lip: the midline and Cupid's bow at the cutaneous vermilion junction (white-skin roll), and the vermilion–mucosa junction (red line) (Fisher, 2005).

On the medial segment, the incision of the rotation flap is kept straighter and longer than originally described by Millard to avoid an excess of tissue in the middle of the lip and a tight closure at the level of the white-skin roll. Straightening of this incision also keeps more tissue on the 'C' flap that can be used at the base of the nose, elongating the columella and keeping the lip down. Superiorly, the rotation flap does not cross the midline to avoid lengthening the normal side.

Lengthening of this incision also gives the possibility of inserting a back-cut, up in the columella, having the scar placed in a less visible place (Mulliken & Martínez-Pérez, 1999). This relaxing incision, when needed, can be done after the muscle and mucosa have been completely released. Subcutaneous dissection of the medial lip element is kept to a minimum so that the normal midline dimple is not disrupted. However, the medial muscular attachment to the columella is completely released to level the Cupid's bow. (See Figure 9.15.)

Simultaneous release of the mucosa and frenulum is completed. This allows, if the surgeon selects to do it, easy access to the base of the columella and pyriform aperture for simultaneous closure of the primary palate and nasal tip correction.

Scissors are introduced bluntly between the two medial crura of the alar cartilages and both sides of the nasal tip are undermined subcutaneously. Then, the pyriform aperture and the floor of the nose are closed to provide a stable base for the lip repair and to avoid an oronasal fistula.

A cut of the nasal mucosa, over the intranasal bridge, is performed to facilitate an open and better muscular dissection and liberation of all the shortened elements that produce alar nose distortion and retention. Similar to Noordhoff and Chen's (2006) strategies, a triangular inferiorly based flap of oral mucosa is designed, to be transposed into the nose to prevent nostril stenosis or functional alteration.

The lateral lip mucosa is incised over the sulcus to create a mucosal flap that is brought medially. The lateral mucosa is undermined only in the upper portion of the lip, never on the free edge, to avoid thickening of the lower lip border.

The incision of the mucosa and periosteum is carried posteriorly along the edge of the cleft at the junction of the oral and nasal mucosa. This allows elevation of a medial mucoperiosteal flap, based superiorly. This flap is advanced laterally to narrow the pyriform aperture to a normal size and to provide a two-layer closure of the floor of the nose.

In cases in which the maxilla and the base of the ala on the cleft-side are retrusive in comparison with the premaxilla and normal alar base, we can use a second inferior pedicled mucosal flap to allow the base of the nostril that is anchored to the lateral flap to advance anteriorly at the same level as the contralateral alar base; avoiding in this way extended external mucosal incisions.

Once the skin incision has been made, the muscle is undermined laterally more extensively than on the medial side. The muscle is completely freed from the alar base and the periosteum along the pyriform aperture. The deforming force of the orbicularis oris on the nasal tip (lateral and superior pull on ala) is therefore released and nasal tip correction is easier. This allows for a substantial amount of muscle fiber to be brought medially to be reattached at the base of the septum, centralizing the columella, lengthening the lip, giving support to the alar base, and preventing oronasal fistulas.

Once the muscle is released from the ala nasi, it gives easy access to undermine the nasal tip subcutaneously over the alar cartilage. Blunt scissors are used to reach the nasal tip already dissected through the medial lip incision.

The total reconstruction of the orbicularis oris muscle is complete.

Millard's original technique has also been modified to reduce the length of the incision around the base of the nostril. A scar in this area is often more noticeable, and the muscular dissection and repositioning of the alar base can effectively be done subcutaneously.

The 'C' flap is shortened and positioned to allow the cleft-side of the collumella to be elongated, placing the scar in a non-visible area.

The incision along the cleft can also be rounded to gain some extra length in wide clefts with short vertical height, and to provide a wider tip to the flap to insert above the medial lip flap.

The nasal floor is completely closed using U stitches.

The vermilion and mucosa along the cleft are retained based on the inferior border of the lip until the final mucosal adjustment at the end of the lip closure.

As described by Mulliken *et al.* (2003), the nasal procedure can be carried out using a little incision in the nostril rim, dissecting superiorly over the alar and upper lateral cartilages on the cleft-side, and extending over to the normal side in the tip area only. No dissection is performed over the nasal bones and the cartilage is left attached to the mucosa. To properly realign all the structures, the first step should be to obtain symmetry of the nasal domes. A little portion of skin can be resected if necessary. Transfixed stitches are used to fix the alar cartilage and nasal mucosa in the right position. (See Figure 9.16.)

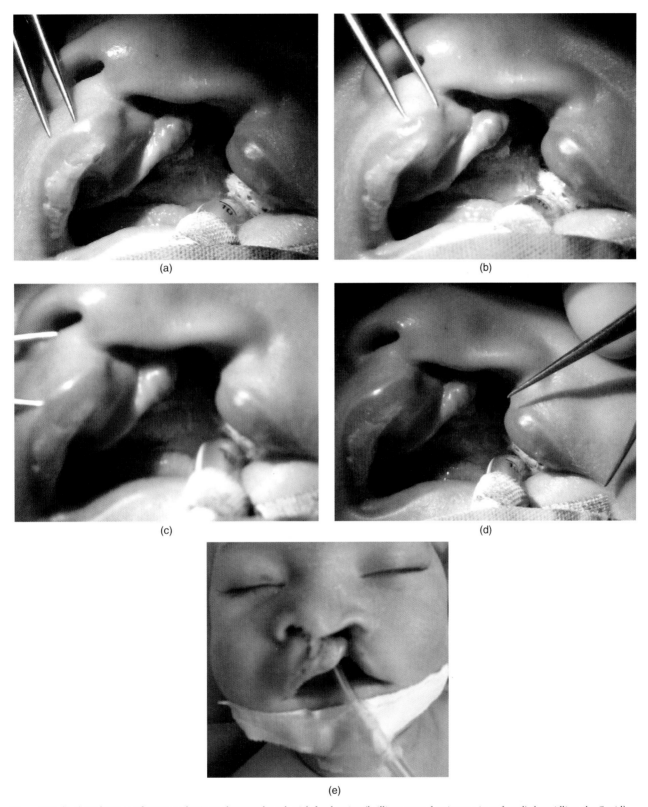

(a)

(b)

(c)

(d)

(e)

Figure 9.15 (a–e) Under magnification and using a sharpened tooth-pick for drawing (brilliant green dye tincture is preferred) the midline, the Cupid's bow, the philtrum, the cutaneous vermilion junction (white skin roll), and the vermilion–mucosa junction (red line) must be identified.

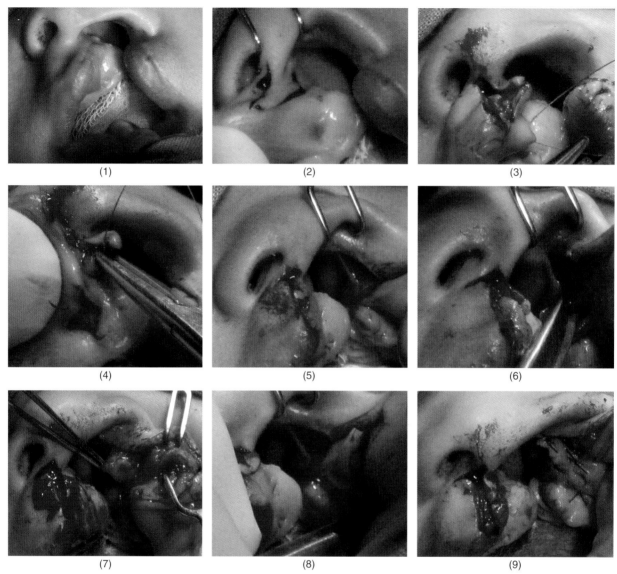

Figure 9.16 (1) An intraoral sponge is placed to fix the tube and prevent blood passage to the air way. (2) Straightening of the medial incision also keeps more tissue on the 'C' flap that can be used at the base of the nose, elongating the columella and keeping the lip down. (3) Superiorly, the rotation flap does not cross the midline to avoid lengthening the normal side. (4) Simultaneous release of the mucosa and frenulum is completed. This allows the surgeon easy access to the base of columella. (5) An incision at the nasal mucosa, over the intranasal bridge, is performed. (6) Open dissection facilitates the liberation of all the shortened elements producing alar distortion (nasalis, levator labii superioris alaeque nasi and zygomaticus head common tendon). (7) A substantial amount of muscle fiber can be obtained, in the lip and nose, to be brought medially. (8) A triangular inferiorly based flap of oral mucosa is left, to be transposed into the nose to prevent nostril stenosis or functional alterations. (9) The triangular flap is sutured to the nasal mucosa. (10) The mucosal incision on the underside of the lateral element is extended distally, on the anterior side of the gingivo labial sulcus, creating a mucosal flap to be brought medially. (11) The lateral mucosal flap is avanced to find the inferiorly based medial mucoperiostal flap. Total vestivular sulcus and floor of the nose closure is achieved. (12) Total posterior mucosal wall of the lip is completed. (13) Muscular nasal bundles are identified. (14) A 'U' stitch fixation to the caudal septal portion is done. (15) Orbicularis oris repair is initiated. (16) Labial muscular reconstruction is finalized. (17) Subcutaneous dissection of the medial lip element is kept to a minimum so that the normal midline dimple is not disrupted. (18) The 'C' flap is shortened and positioned to allow the cleft-side of the collumella to be elongated. (19) The scar is placed in a non-visible area. Lateral skin flap resection to reproduce the philtrum pillar. (20) A mattress stitch suture of the nasal floor is achieved. (21) White line continuity is supervised. (22) The skin closure is finished and the vermilion borders are appositioned using matress stitches. (23) A minimal rim incision allows a semi-open exposure of the lower lateral cartilage. Careful scissor separation in the upper vestibule helps display the splayed and dislocated cartilages. (24) Minimal resection of redundant skin is performed. (25) The aim is to reproduce the normal collumelar side and to obtain more tip protection over the cleft side. (26) Occulted stitches are utilized to fix the alar cartilage in a new position. (27) Inferior view of the finalized procedure. (28, 29) Preop and postop frontal views. (30, 31) Preop and postop inferior views.

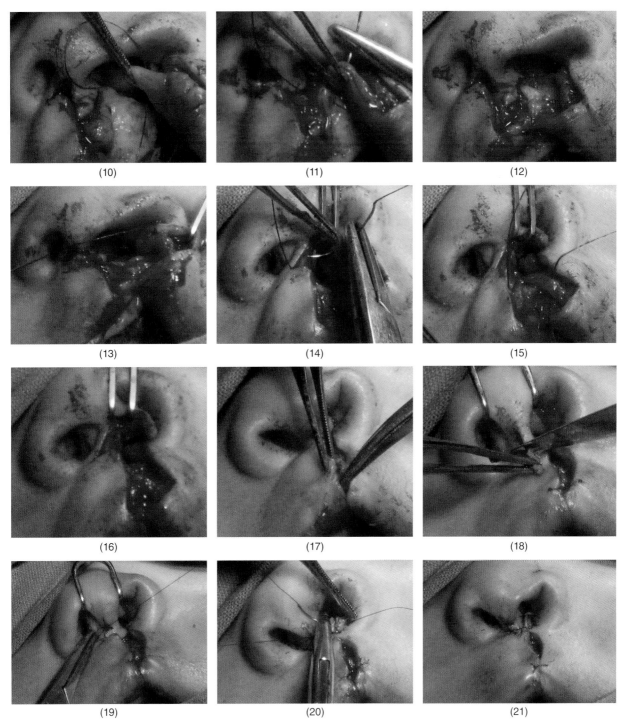

(10)   (11)   (12)

(13)   (14)   (15)

(16)   (17)   (18)

(19)   (20)   (21)

Figure 9.16 (*Continued*)

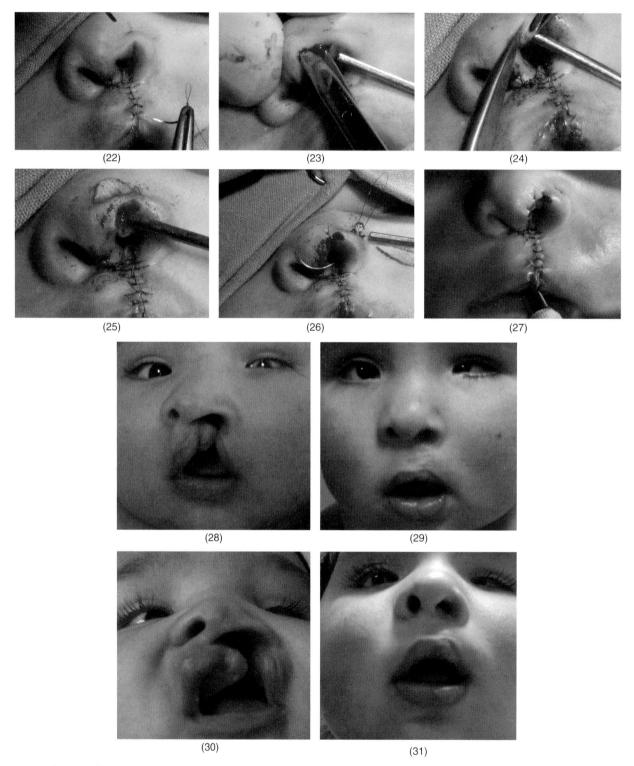

(22)

(23)

(24)

(25)

(26)

(27)

(28)

(29)

(30)

(31)

Figure 9.16 (*Continued*)

Discussion

These combined procedures are generally performed at 3 months of age (Laberge, 2007). The size of the airway is drastically changed after lip closure and nostril reshaping, and there is more resistance to breathing. In these young babies, airway monitoring and specialized nurses are essential in the immediate postop. Fortunately, if the baby is awake and without pain the adapting process is very short and the patient can initiate breast or bottle feeding after 30 minutes.

Symmetry of the nasal tip can be obtained with the subcutaneous dissection of the nasal domes or with nasal incisions depending on the severity of distortion, but is not perfect in all cases. Results are certainly acceptable so as to avoid secondary corrections before growth completion. The nasal tip subcutaneous undermining (Anderl et al., 2008) is less extensive than the original technique proposed by McComb, in which the undermining was carried over the nasal bones. The use of shorter traction (Salyer et al., 2005) is different from other authors' proposals; the alar cartilages are dissected free from the skin and the mucosa. Long-term results with primary nasal tip corrections have been published (McComb & Coghlan, 1996; Mulliken & LaBrie, 2012).

Since many approaches to the closure of the cleft lip have not satisfied the hopes placed on them, the author has gone back to the principles stated by Veau (1935). Careful dissection of all muscles involved, anatomical repositioning of all structures of the lip and the nasal entrance (Delaire, 1978; Talmant & Talmant, 2014) does not seem to have a risk of affecting innervation and blood supply.

The muscular insertions on the lateral nostril, pyriform aperture, and the columella must certainly be free and cautious reconstruction of a normal anatomical situation leads not only to better appearance and good mobility of the area concerned, but also to an enhanced growth of the underlying bony structures. Correction of septal cartilage deviation must be gradually obtained by means of correct function and reposition of muscles in the nasal floor.

Presurgical orthopedics is now widely used to reduce not only the width of the cleft before surgery but also for better nose conformation at the time of reconstruction. Our program has used the nasoalveolar remodeling technique for 15 years (Bennun et al., 1999) and then we changed to the DPNR technique over the last 10 years (Bennun & Figueroa, 2006). It is interesting to note that the surgical correction is easier in the presence of a narrow cleft, and the surgical results, after the introduction of presurgical orthodontics, have improved. In fact, in some children, flare of the nostril has been easier to correct in case of secondary procedure necessity.

Concept of gingivoperioplasty

Vomer mucoperichondral flaps to close the primary palate have been used for many decades. An extensive study on maxillary growth following unilateral cleft lip and palate repair, showed that alveolus repair using soft tissue without the addition of a bone graft did not influence the anterior–posterior growth of the maxilla but may have had some minor effect on the vertical height (Ross, 1987).

The main difference in the Campbell (1926) technique, as opposed to the Veau technique (1935), is that the vomer flap, based inferiorly, provides a two-layer closure adaptable to wide clefts without any tension because the flaps can slide on each other, leaving more or less raw area laterally or medially.

The surgical bridging of the cleft alveolar process with periosteal flap was initially described as a means of stabilizing the separated segments of the maxilla. It has been suggested that repair of the cleft lip is incomplete without the simultaneous reconstruction of bone defects of the maxilla by gingivoperioplasty, as there will be the risk of collapse of the lateral segments of the maxilla due to the pressure exerted by the repaired lip (Skoog, 1965). Furthermore, it is advocated that it coordinates the growth at the growth centers as the maxillary discontinuity is restored (Liao et al., 2014). However, controversies exist regarding the conduct of gingivoperioplasty in cleft patients because of its potential to impair maxillary growth. It is important to recognize that state of art gingivoperioplasty has changed since the time of its introduction (Skoog, 1967).

Skoog's technique necessitated wide mucoperiosteal dissection to mobilize the flaps enough to allow for approximation of the cleft alveolus, as he did not perform presurgical nasoalveolar molding. The current technique of gingivoperioplasty introduced by Millard and Latham (1990) is performed after the patients undergo presurgical orthopedic closure of the cleft alveolar gap. Strict association of presurgical nasoalveolar molding and alveolar gap closure allows conservative gingivoperioplasty to be performed.

Studies have indicated that there is no need for an alveolar bone graft if gingivoperioplasty is performed during infancy. Also it has been indicated that there are greater cost savings in patients undergoing nasoalveolar molding combined with gingivoperioplasty as there is no need for further bone and nasal revision surgeries (Pfeifer et al., 2002). Several studies have shown the high osteogenic potential of periosteum depositing bone without subsequent resorption in patients undergoing gingivoperioplasty procedures (Smith et al., 1995). However, some other studies have quoted a higher frequency of anterior cross-bite in patients treated with gingivoperioplasty (Berkowitz et al., 2004; Hsieh et al., 2010; Phillips et al., 2012).

To avoid bad effects, the surgeon/orthodontist should take into consideration the extent of palatal osteogenic deficiency and the presence or absence of teeth. At present if any doubt exists, a wide mucoperiosteal dissection will certainly produce growth alterations. In this way, a conservative high gingivoperioplasty (vestibular sulcus closure), with muscular nasal floor reconstruction, to prevent oronasal fistula is recommended. But the alveolar gap closure, in the area of dental germens, is not necessary.

Results

See Figures 9.17 to 9.23.

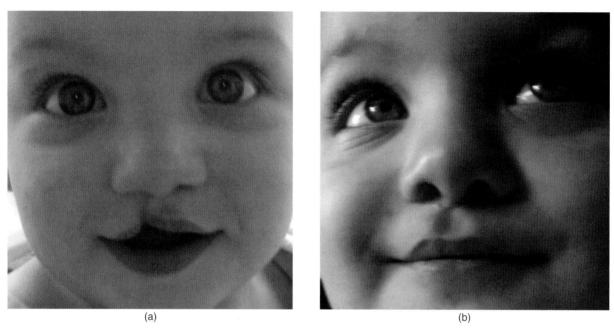

(a)   (b)

Figure 9.17 (a, b) Minimal forms force the surgeon to obtain superior results. In cases without alar cartilage distortion the nose must not be touched.

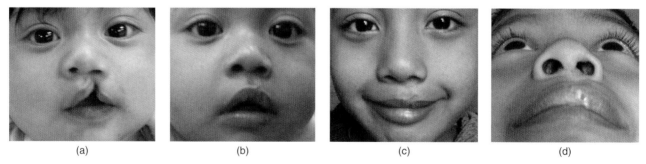

(a)   (b)   (c)   (d)

Figure 9.18 (a–d) Incomplete case preop views, one year, and three year follow-up. Small initial mistakes such as white-line discontinuity become more noticeable as the patient becomes older.

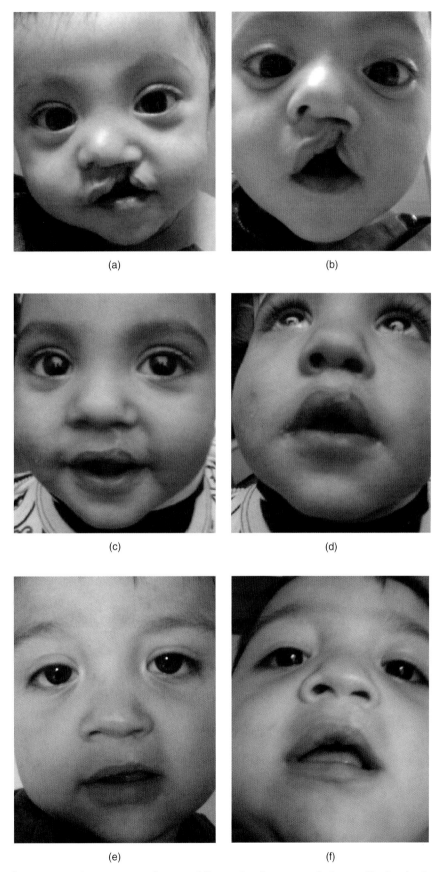

Figure 9.19 (a–f) Incomplete case preop views, one year, and two year follow-up. Local massage to obtain wound healing decoloration and scar compresion in the case of hypertrofic scars are a routine indication.

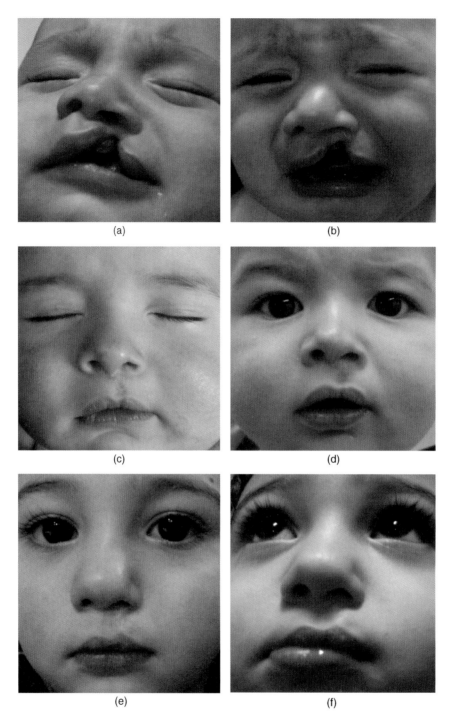

Figure 9.20 (a–f) Incomplete case preop views, one month, one year, and three year follow-up.

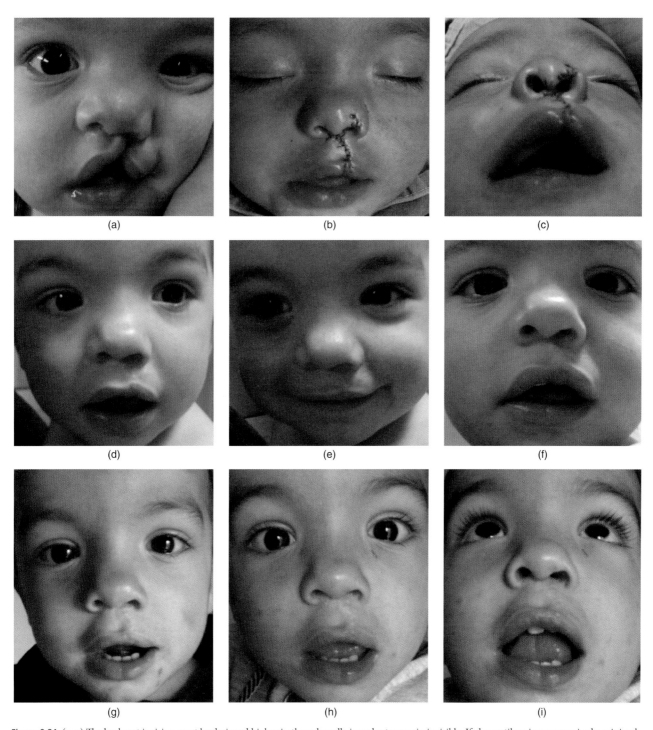

Figure 9.21 (a–c) The back-cut incision must be designed higher in the columella in order to remain invisible. If alar cartilage is compromised a minimal alar rim incision may be necessary. (d–i) Same patient one year and two year follow-up.

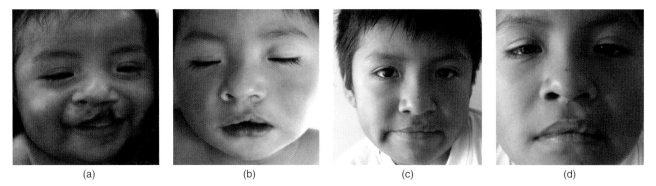

Figure 9.22 (a–d) Front preop view, one year, and five year follow-up. Short vertical lips result in a great challenge for expert surgeons.

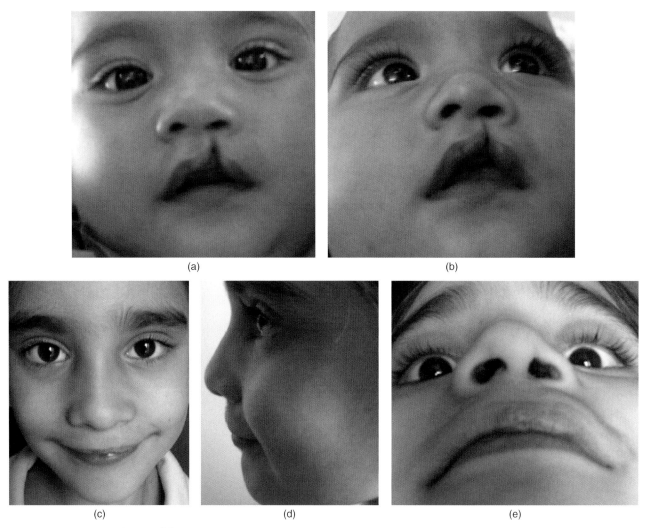

Figure 9.23 (a–e) Preop and six year follow-up views.

Presurgical treated series

See Figures 9.24 to 9.36.

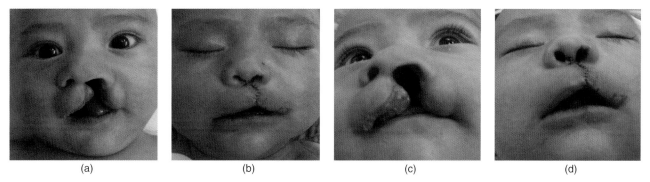

| (a) | (b) | (c) | (d) |

Figure 9.24 (a–d) Frontal and inferior preop and postop of a presurgically treated patient. Millard's original technique has been modified to reduce the length of the incision around the base of the nostril. Minimal labial incision and no nose repair needed. Excellent nose symmetry can be observed.

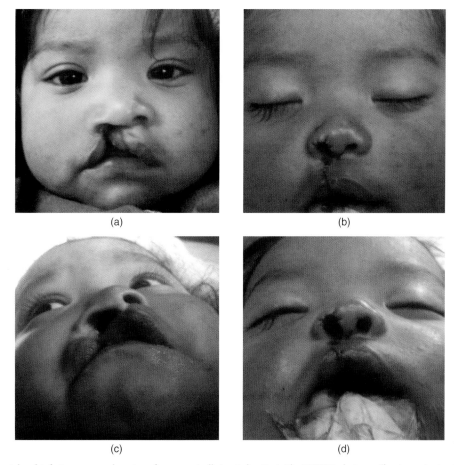

| (a) | (b) |
| (c) | (d) |

Figure 9.25 (a–d) Frontal and inferior preop and postop of a presurgically treated patient. The DPNR technique offers important and permanent advantages in surgical reconstruction of these patients. Maxillary, nostril, and alar base distortions have been solved with a correct muscle reconstruction and alar rim incision.

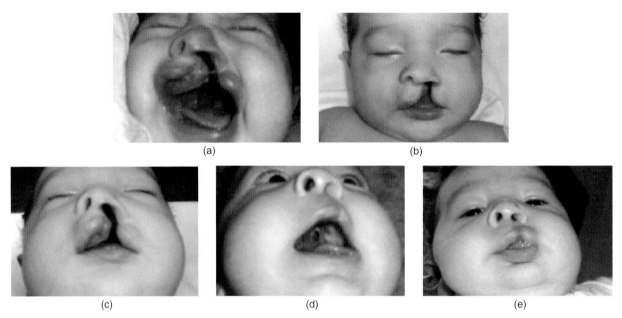

Figure 9.26 (a–e) Unilateral complete cleft lip and palate case previously treated by DPNR technique. Arch and nose distortion and vertical labial height have been improved. Six month postop shows nasal and labial symmetry without touching the nose.

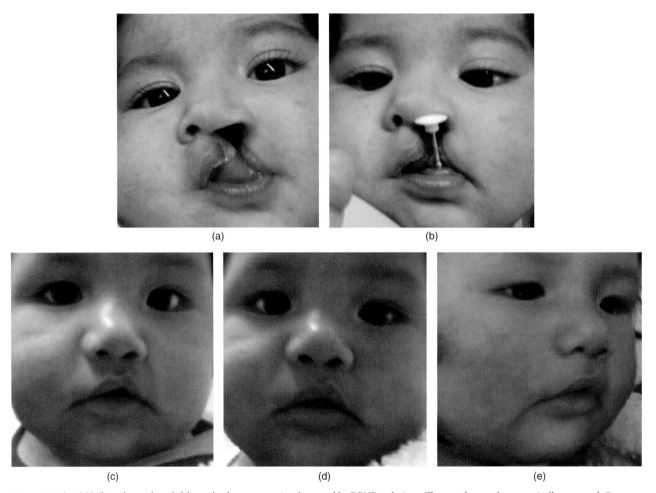

Figure 9.27 (a–e) Unilateral complete cleft lip and palate case previously treated by DPNR technique. The nose has not been surgically corrected. One year postop different views.

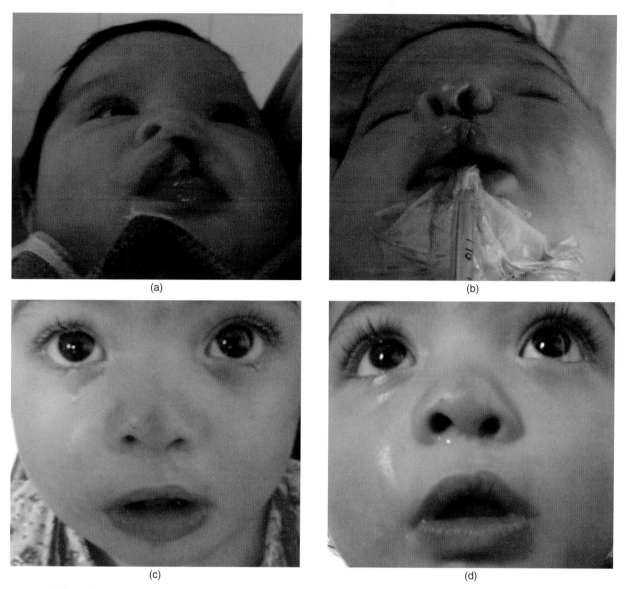

(a)

(b)

(c)

(d)

Figure 9.28 (a–d) Unilateral complete cleft lip and palate case previously treated by DPNR technique. The nose has not been surgicaly corrected. Two year postop frontal and inferior views.

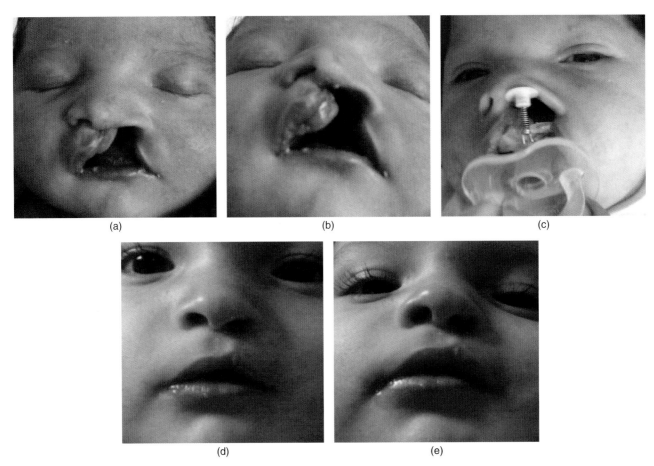

(a)   (b)   (c)

(d)   (e)

Figure 9.29 (a–e) Unilateral complete cleft lip and palate case previously treated by DPNR technique. The nose has been treated using a rim incision. Six month postop frontal and inferior views.

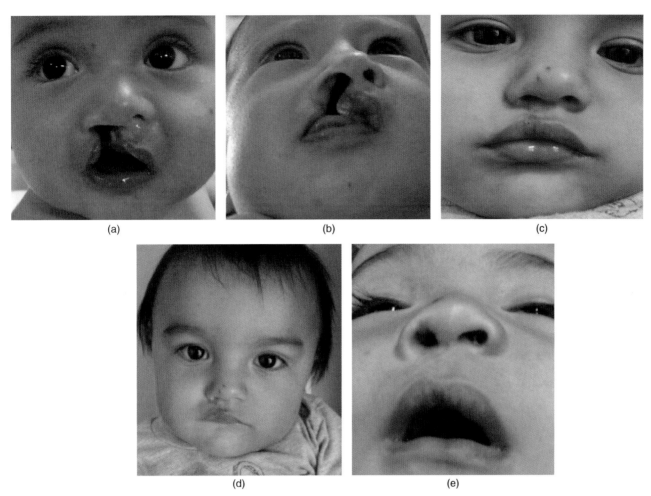

(a)   (b)   (c)

(d)   (e)

Figure 9.30 (a–e) Unilateral complete cleft lip and palate case previously treated by DPNR technique. The nose has been treated using a rim incision. One year postop frontal and inferior views.

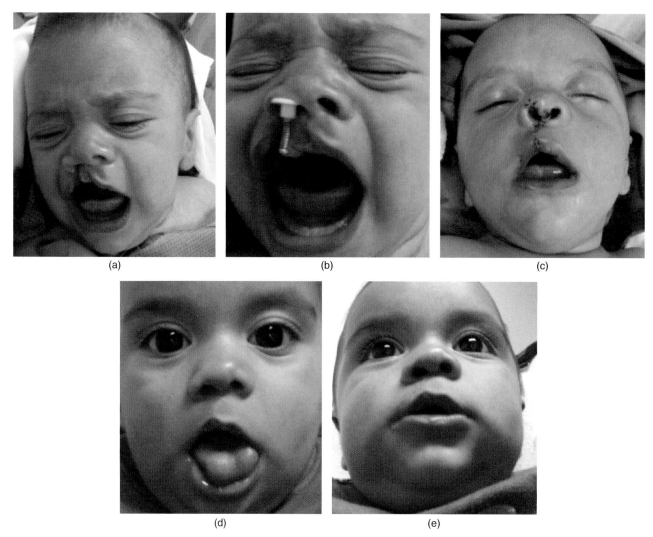

(a) (b) (c)

(d) (e)

Figure 9.31 (a–e) Unilateral complete cleft lip and palate case previously treated by DPNR technique. The nose has been treated using a rim incision. Two year postop frontal and inferior views.

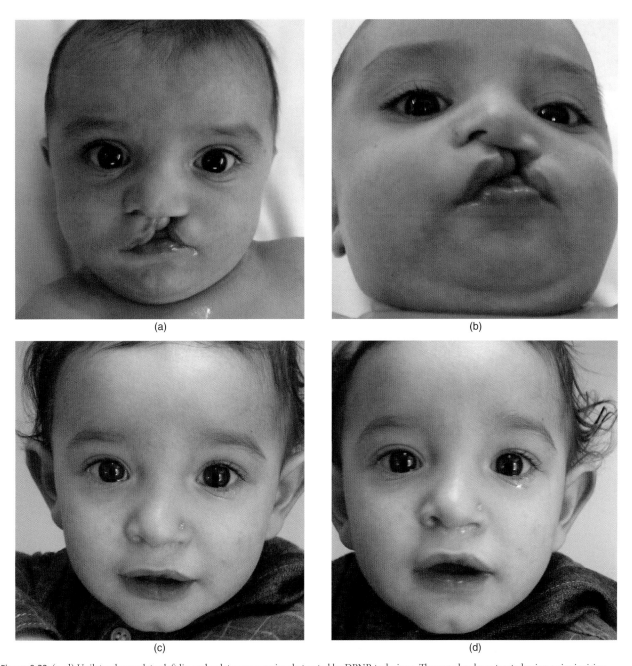

Figure 9.32 (a–d) Unilateral complete cleft lip and palate case previously treated by DPNR technique. The nose has been treated using a rim incision. Two year postop different views. If the scar is correctly placed and closure results without tension, a high percentage of patients have excellent esthetic results.

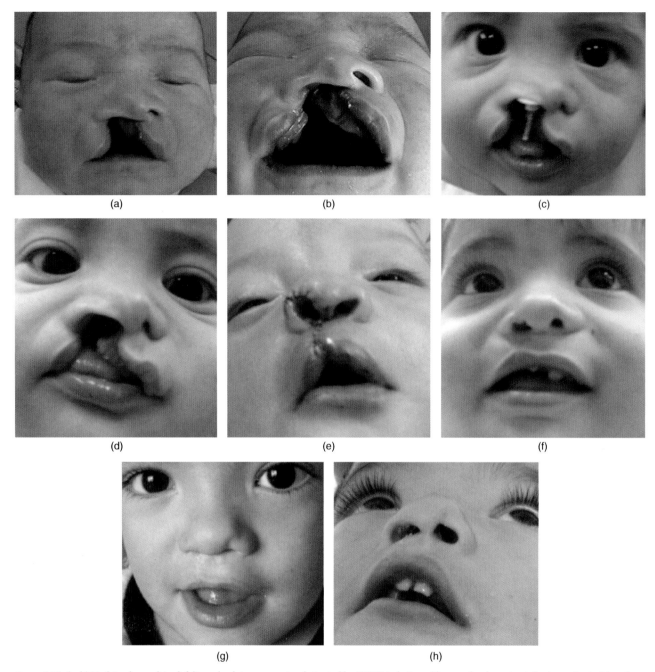

(a)   (b)   (c)

(d)   (e)   (f)

(g)   (h)

Figure 9.33 (a–h) Unilateral complete cleft lip and palate case previously treated by DPNR technique. The nose has been treated using a rim incision. In some cases we decide to make an overcorrection. One and three year postop frontal and inferior views.

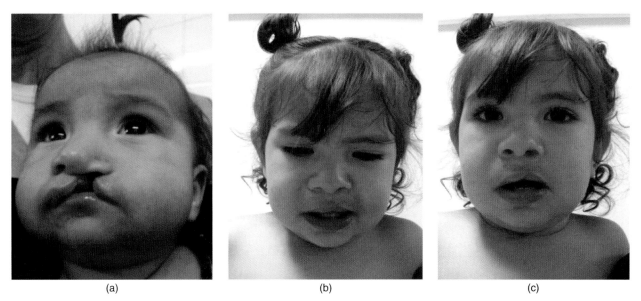

Figure 9.34 (a–c) Unilateral complete cleft lip and palate case previously treated by DPNR technique. The nose has been treated using a rim incision. Three year postop frontal and inferior views.

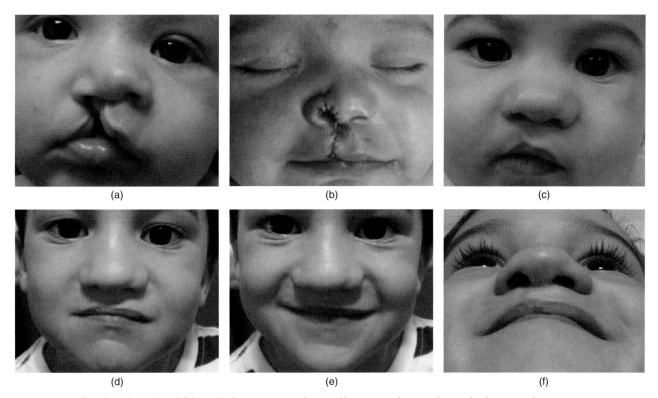

Figure 9.35 (a–f) Unilateral complete cleft lip and palate case previously treated by DPNR technique. The nose has been treated using a rim incision. Five year postop frontal, showing proper function and inferior views. Nose primary correction continuous and symmetrical with facial growth and development.

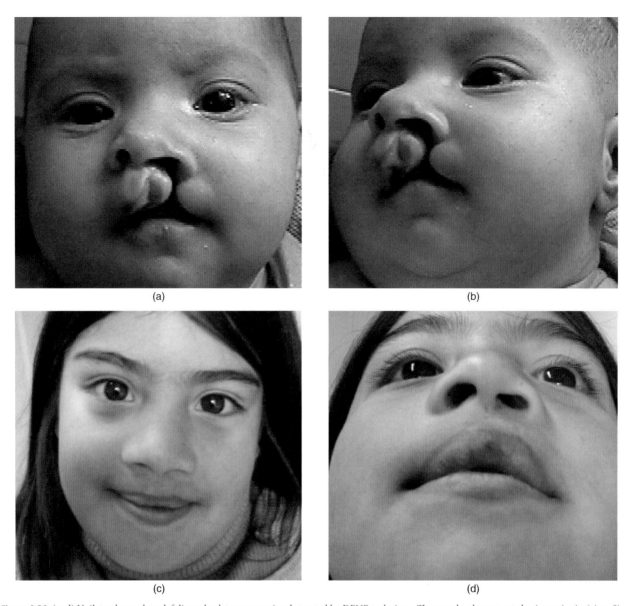

(a)

(b)

(c)

(d)

Figure 9.36 (a–d) Unilateral complete cleft lip and palate case previously treated by DPNR technique. The nose has been treated using a rim incision. Six year postop showing proper function and an inferior view presenting an alar relapse that can be treated with a minimal surgical revision.

Without presurgical treatment series

See Figures 9.37 to 9.39.

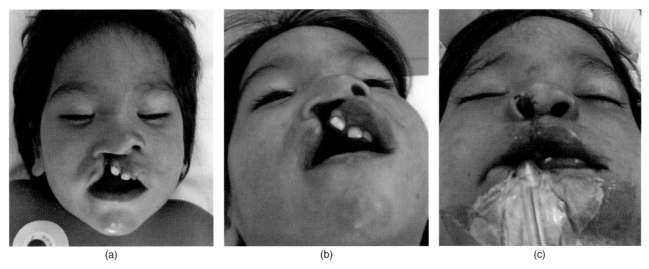

Figure 9.37 (a–c) Older patient simultaneous lip and nose reconstruction with good results is also possible. The correct muscular reconstruction will complete the correct maxillary segment traction and alineation. Although growing patients can modify the initial result, a primary reconstruction correctly executed will need few revisions of minor magnitude.

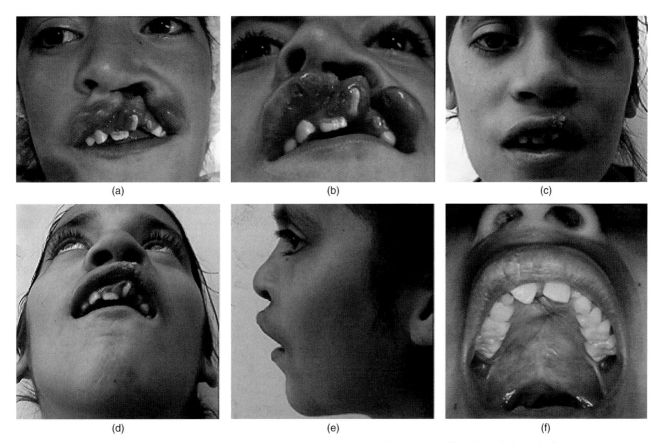

Figure 9.38 (a–f) Adult patients also present an opportunity. Using more aggressive procedures it is possible to finish the lip and palate reconstruction with only two surgeries. But you must know that this is the exception and not the rule, as its chances are incredible small.

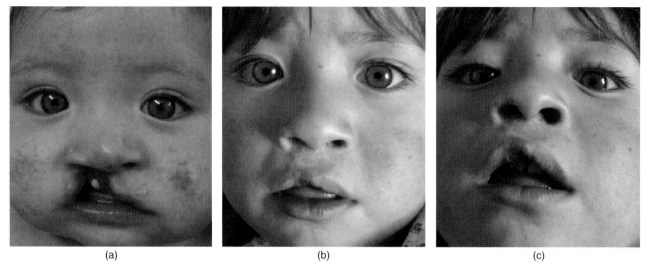

(a)   (b)   (c)

Figure 9.39 (a–c) Unilateral complete cleft lip and palate case without previous presurgical treatment. Three year postop frontal and inferior view.

Immediate complications

Dehiscence is not very common in unilateral cleft lip repair. The main reason is either tension in the repair or improper suturing of the orbicularis muscles. Trauma or infection also may be possible causes.

UNI scarring depends on three factors:

- Intrinsic strain, which depends on the tightness of the suturing.
- Extrinsic strain, which is the tension with which the tissues are brought together.
- The inherent reaction of the individual to surgical trauma.

The surgeon has control over the first two factors, but not over the third.

Deficiency in the height of the lateral vermillion on the cleft-side

It is probable that by bringing the medial and lateral bony shelves in alignment, the discrepancy in lateral vermillion height is overcome. Teams utilizing presurgical orthodontics like nasoalveolar remodeling do not seem to encounter such a problem.

Orovestibular fistulas

These happen because of a breakdown of the nasal floor repair at the vestibular sulcus, or because the nasal floor has not been repaired.

Final recommendations

Here follows some suggestions that the authors feel could be useful for new surgeons.

- Remember that the best surgeons will be those who can obtain superlative results with the minimum of aggression.
- Preserving blood supply, innervation, and growth centers is a moral obligation to protect newborn patients.
- Prepare your case in the best way you can to make your labor easier.

- Surgery must be performed ideally between 2 and 4 months.
- Entering the operating room should switch your mind to 3D mode.
- Regional and local anesthesia helps avoid bleeding and posterior pain.
- Employ the technique you are most comfortable with.
- Avoid using wide incisions and dissection.
- The first step, if you have not used presurgical orthopedic, will be nose relaxation by liberating the abnormal muscular insertions.
- To prevent stenosis, do not leave drawn areas in the interior of the nose.
- Carefully close the oral mucosa to avoid oronasal fistula and touching the alveolu.
- Muscular reconstruction comprises two steps: the floor of the nose and the lip.
- Attaching the muscle to the septum is a good option to prevent caudal septum deviation.
- If distorted, the nose must be treated during the primary reconstructive procedure.
- Not considering the mechanisms implicated in the deformity process is a cause of recidivated cases.
- Use magnification and select the best atraumatic suture you have available.
- When finishing the surgery you must be happy with the end result obtained, and remember that nothing will improve your outcome.

Conclusions

We believe that presurgical nasoalveolar remodeling with a complete reconstruction of the lip and nose, in one setting, is a better option for children presenting with a unilateral cleft lip and palate. The majority of children will require only this early surgery at 3 months of age, one for complete palate closure before 1 year of age, and eventually one at the end of growth for septal and nose asymmetry correction when needed. Primary bone graft and alveolar gap closure, in the area of dental germens, do not seem to be necessary. A conservative high gingivoperioplasty, with muscular nasal floor reconstruction, to prevent oronasal fistula is recommended. Fewer revisions mean less scarring and more predictable results. The first team definitely has the best chance of a good result.

References

Anderl, H., Hussl, H., and Ninkovic, M. (2008) Primary simultaneous lip and nose repair in the unilateral cleft lip and palate. *Plast Reconstr Surg* **121**:959–970.

Bennun, R. D., Perandones, C., Sepliarsky, V. *et al.* (1999) Non surgical correction of nasal deformity in unilateral complete cleft lip: A six years follow up. *Plast Reconstr Surg* **104**(3):616–630.

Bennun, R. D. and Figueroa, A. A. (2006) Dynamic presurgical nasal remodeling in patients with unilateral and bilateral cleft lip and palate: modification to the original technique. *Cleft Palate Craniofac J* **43**(6):639–648.

Berkowitz, S., Mejia, M., and Bystrik, A. (2004) A comparison of the effects of the Latham-Millard procedure with those of a conservative treatment approach for dental occlusion and facial aesthetics in unilateral and bilateral complete cleft lip and palate: Part I. Dental occlusion. *Plast Reconstr Surg* **113**(1):1–18.

Campbell, A. (1926) The closure of congenital clefts of the hard palate. *Br J Surg* **13**:715–719.

Da Silva Freitas, R., Bertoco Alves, P., Shimizu, G. K. *et al.* (2012) Beyond fifty years of Millard's rotation-advancement technique in cleft lip closure: Are there many "Millards"? *Plast Surg Int* **2012**:731029. doi: 10.1155/2012/731029. Epub 2012 Dec 6.

Delaire, J. (1978) Theoretical principles and technique of functional closure of the lip and nasal aperture. *J Maxillofac Surg* **6**(2):109–116.

Fisher, D. M. (2005) Unilateral cleft lip repair: An anatomical subunit approximation technique. *Plast Reconstr Surg* **116**:61–71.

Franco, P. (1556) *Petit traite contenentune des parties principals de chirurgie*. Lyon: Antoine Vincent.

Gillies, H. and Millard, D. R., Jr. (1957) *The Principles and Art of Plastic Surgery, Vol. 1*. Boston: Little Brown, p. 49.

Hsieh, C. H., Ko, E. W., Chen, P. K., and Huang, C. S. (2010) The effect of gingivoperiosteoplasty on facial growth in patients with complete unilateral cleft lip and palate. *Cleft Palate Craniofac J* **47**(5):439–446.

Huffman, W. C. and Lierle, D. M. (1949) Studies on the pathologic anatomy of the unilateral harelip nose. *Plast Reconstr Surg* **4**(3):225–234.

Jackson, I. T. and Fasching, M. C. (1990) Secondary deformities of the cleft lip, nose and palate. In: McCarthy, J. G. (ed.) *Plastic Surgery*, Philadelphia, PA: Saunders, pp. 2803–2814.

Laberge, L. C. (2007) Unilateral cleft lip and palate: Simultaneous early repair of the nose, anterior palate and lip. *Can J Plast Surg* **15**(1):13–18

Liao, Y. F., Lee, Y. H., Wang, R., *et al.* (2014) Vomer flap for hard palate repair is related to favorable maxillary growth in unilateral cleft lip and palate. *Clin Oral Investig* **18**(4):1269–1276

McComb, H. K. and Coghlan, B. A. (1996) Primary repair of the unilateral cleft lip nose: completion of a longitudinal study. *Cleft Palate Craniofac J* **33**(1):23–30; discussion 30–1.

Millard, D. R., Jr. (1958) A radical rotation in single harelip. *Am J Surg* **95**:318–322.

Millard, D. R., Jr. (1960) Complete unilateral clefts of the lip. *Plast Reconstr Surg* **25**:595–605.

Millard, D. R., Jr. (1990) Unilateral cleft lip deformity. In: McCarthy, J., (ed.) *Plastic Surgery*, Vol. **4**. Philadelphia, PA: WB Saunders Company, pp. 2639.

Millard, D. R., Jr. and Latham, R. A. (1990) Improved primary surgical and dental treatment of clefts. *Plast Reconstr Surg* **86**(5):856–871.

Mulliken, J. B. and Martínez-Pérez, D. (1999) The principle of rotation advancement for repair of unilateral complete cleft lip and nasal deformity: technical variations and analysis of results. *Plast Reconstr Surg* **104**(5):1247–1260.

Mulliken, J. B., Wu, J. K., and Padwa, B. L. (2003) Repair of bilateral cleft lip: Review, revisions, and reflections. *J Craniofac Surg* **14**(5):609–620.

Mulliken, J. B. and LaBrie, R. A. (2012) Fourth-dimensional changes in nasolabial dimensions following rotation-advancement repair of unilateral cleft lip. *Plast Reconstr Surg* **129**:491–498.

Noordhoff, M. S. and Chen, K. T. (2006) Unilateral cheiloplasty. In: Mathes, S. J. (ed.) *Plastic Surgery* 2nd edn., Vol. **4**. Philadelphia: Saunders, pp. 165–216.

Pare, A. (1575) *Les oeuvres de M. Ambroise Pare*. Paris: Chez Gabriel Buon.

Pfeifer, T. M., Grayson, B. H., and Cutting, C. B. (2002) Nasoalveolar molding and gingivoperiosteoplasty versus alveolar bone graft: an outcome analysis of costs in the treatment of unilateral cleft alveolus. *Cleft Palate Craniofac J* **39**(1):26–29.

Phillips, J. H., Nish, I., and Daskalogiannakis, J. (2012) Orthognathic surgery in cleft patients. *Plast Reconstr Surg* **129**(3):535e–548e.

Ross, R. B. (1987) Treatment variables affecting facial growth in complete unilateral cleft lip and palate. Part 3: Alveolus repair and bone grafting. *Cleft Palate J* **24**:33–44.

Salyer, K. E. (1990) Unilateral cleft lip and cleft lip nasal reconstruction. In: Bardach, J. and Morris, H. L. (eds) *Multidisciplinary Management of Cleft Lip and Palate*, Philadelphia, PA: Saunders, pp. 179–180.

Salyer, K. E., Rozen, S. M., Genecov, E. R., *et al.* (2005) unilateral cleft lip: Approach and technique. *Semin Plast Surg* **19**(4):313–328.

Salyer, K. E., Xu, H., Genecov, E. R. (2009) Unilateral cleft lip and nose repair; closed approach Dallas protocol completed patients. *J Craniofac Surg* **20** Suppl **2**:1939–1955.

Skoog, T. (1965) The use of periosteal flaps in the repair of clefts of the primary palate. *Cleft Palate J* **2**:332–339.

Skoog, T. (1967) The use of periosteum and Surgicel for bone restoration in congenital clefts of the maxilla. A clinical report and experimental investigation. *Scand J Plast Reconstr Surg* **1**(2):113–130.

Smith, W. P., Markus, A. F. and Delaire, J. (1995) Primary closure of the cleft alveolus: A functional approach. *Br J Oral Maxillofac Surg* **33**(3):156–165.

Talmant J. C. and Talmant J. C. (2014) Cleft rhinoplasty, from primary to secondary surgery. *Ann Chir Plast Esthet* **59**(6):555–584.

Tennison, C. W. (1952) The repair of the unilateral cleft lip by the stencil method. *Plast Reconstr Surg* **9**:115–20.

Veau, V. (1935) Bec-de-lievre. Hypotheses sur la malformation initiale. *Ann Anat Pathol* **12**:389.

Vyas, R. M. and Warren, S. M. (2014) Unilateral cleft lip repair. *Clin Plast Surg* **41**(2):165–177.

CHAPTER 10

Bilateral cleft lip and nose repair

Ricardo D. Bennun[1] and George K. B. Sándor[2]

[1] Asociacion PIEL, Maimonides University and National University of Buenos Aires, Argentina

[2] Tissue Engineering, University of Oulu, and Institute of Biosciences and Medical Technology, University of Tampere, Finland

Introduction

The bilateral cleft lip and nasal deformity presents a complex and often frustrating challenge for surgical repair. It has a wide degree of variability with regard to the severity of the cleft (incomplete vs. complete) (Mulliken & Kim, 2013). There is also the complex three-dimensional dynamics and position of the prolabium and lateral maxillary segments that challenge the surgeon. The deformity is characterized by a protruding maxilla, prolabium lacking muscle fibers with a blunted white-roll, vertically long lateral lip elements widely spaced due to discontinuity of the orbicularis oris, short columella, flattened nose, and abnormally positioned alar cartilages.

Multiple secondary deformities may arise leading to poor results. Cleft surgeons may opt to deal with the secondary deformities in planned revisions. However, multiple revisions will result in increased scarring and contracture. Therefore, a single-stage bilateral cleft lip and nose repair to correct the deformity and allow for proper growth is believed to be better for future appearance and function.

This chapter is based on two major advances in the surgical management of bilateral cleft lip over the past quarter century. First is the understanding of the need for preoperative remodeling of the cleft maxillary segments and nasal/labial tissues. Second is the recognition of the principles of bilateral labial repair, especially the significance of simultaneous correction of the nasal deformity.

Principles

Surgical principles, once established, usually persist; whereas surgical techniques continue to progress. From the literature and analyses of residual deformities, the authors are agreed upon the following principles to repair a bilateral complete cleft lip (Mulliken, 2004).

- Maintain nasolabial symmetry because even the smallest differences become magnified with growth.
- Secure orbicularis oris continuity to construct the muscular ring and minimize philtral distortion.
- Design proper philtral size/shape because it rapidly elongates and widens.
- Construct the median tubercle using the lateral labial elements because retained prolabial vermilion lacks white-roll and normal coloration and fails to grow to ample height.
- Position and secure the displaced lower lateral cartilages (this point can also be partially or totally achieved using the presurgical orthopaedics protocol) to establish normal nasal projection and columellar length.

It is unnecessary to drag up labial tissue to elongate the columella. "The columella is in the nose"– can be exposed by anatomic positioning, apposition, and fixation of the lower lateral cartilages, and sculpting the excess (expanded) skin in the nasal tip.

Third and fourth dimensions

"During repair of the bilateral cleft lip and nasal deformity, like the sculptor working in marble, the surgeon must conceptualize the three-dimensional features. But different to the sculpture, the repaired lip and nose in a newborn change with time. For that reason, the surgeon must also understand the normal nasolabial variations as well as the particular facial distortions that occur with growth and development, in a child with a repaired bilateral cleft lip" (Mulliken, 2009). Normal nasolabial growth patterns in Caucasians aged 1–18 years have been documented using anthropometry (Farkas & Lindsay, 1971).

Cleft Lip and Palate Management: A Comprehensive Atlas, First Edition. Edited by Ricardo D. Bennun, Julia F. Harfin, George K. B. Sándor, and David Genecov.
© 2016 John Wiley & Sons, Inc. Published 2016 by John Wiley & Sons, Inc.

Preoperative dentofacial orthopaedics

Alignment of the maxillary segments and improvement of nasolabial distortions sets the stage for synchronous, bilateral, nasolabial repair (Mulliken, 1995). Symmetric and malleable tissues with normal placement of the premaxilla as well as the lateral maxillary segments allow better reconstruction and repositioning of muscles, design of the philtral flap in proper sizes, facilitates nasal repair, and allows soft tissue closure of the alveolar clefts, which stabilizes the maxillary arch and prevents oronasal fistulas. Furthermore, controlled postop premaxillary retropositioning prevents descent and minimizes the nasolabial distortion that occurs during the rapid growth of early childhood.

Surgical procedure

Bilateral cleft lip presents in four major anatomic variants: bilateral incomplete (25%), asymmetrical bilateral (complete/incomplete) (25%), bilateral symmetrical complete (40%), and bilateral asymmetrical complete (10%); the technical steps are described from the easier to the most complicated case (Figure 10.1).

A one-stage procedure to reconstruct complete and incomplete unilateral/bilateral cleft lip and nose deformities is presented. Emphasis was made on closure of the lip muscles, correction of the nostril floor, correction of the alveolar cleft as well as reconstruction of the nose through an intranasal approach (Figure 10.2).

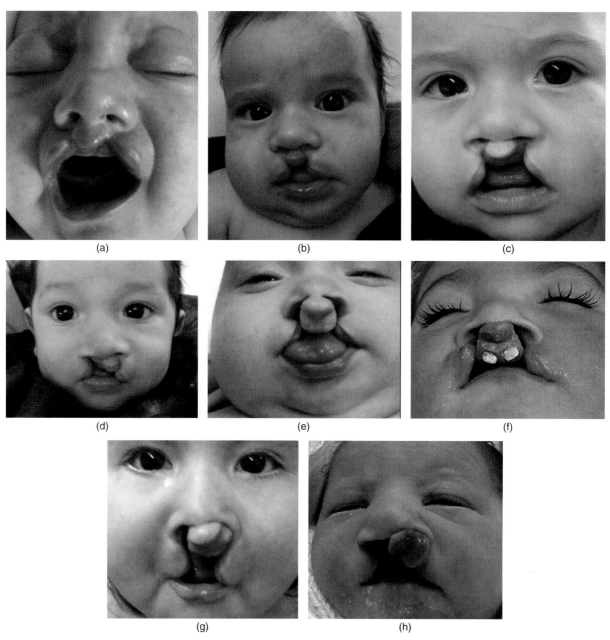

Figure 10.1 (a–h) Eight different variants of bilateral cleft lip.

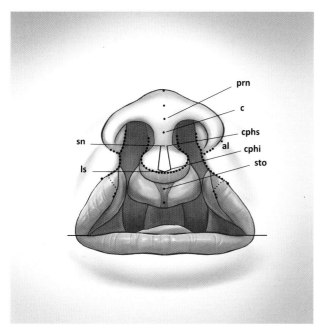

Figure 10.2a Anthropometrics points for sequential repair of bilateral complete cleft lip and nasal deformity: prn = pronasale; al = alare; c = columella; sn = subnasale; cphs = crista philtri superior; cphi = crista philtri inferior; ls = labiale superius; sto = stomion.

The anatomic points are designated using standard anthropometric marks (Farkas *et al.*, 1992). The philtral flap is drawn first while the nostrils are held upward with a double-ball retractor. Under magnification and using a sharpened tooth-pick for drawing; brilliant green dye (tincture) is preferred. The

dimensions are determined by the age of the child and ethnicity. The average age at primary repair is 4 months. Philtral flap width is set at 3 mm at the columellar–labial junction (cphs–cphs) and 4–5 mm between the proposed Cupid's bow peaks (cphi–cphi). The sides of the philtral flap should be drawn slightly concave because the scars tend to bow. The dart-like tip of the philtral flap should not be overemphasized. A thin rectangular flap is drawn on each side of the philtral flap. These side flaps will be de-epithelialized and will come to lie beneath the lateral labial flaps in an effort to simulate the elevation of philtral columns (Mulliken *et al.*, 2001).

First, all labial incisions are lightly scored. The flaps flanking the philtral flap are carefully de-epithelialized conserving venous return. Vertical incisions are made on each side of the premaxilla.

At the nasolabial angle and preserving prolabial blood supply, a tunnel is built. Prolabial flap elevation is not recommended (Cutting, 2006).

The white-roll–vermilion–mucosal flaps are incised (just short of the tattooed lateral Cupid's bow point) and the lateral labial elements are disjoined from the alar bases.

An incision on the intranasal bridge is performed to allow an open dissection and liberation of the muscles producing nasal distortion. The basilar flaps are freed from the pyriform attachments. An inferior pedicle triangular flap is planned to be transposed intranasally, as a Z-plasty to the intranasal raw area. The mucosal incisions on the underside of the lateral elements are extended distally, on the anterior side of the gingivolabial sulcus. With a double-hook on the muscle layer, the lateral labial elements are dissected off the maxilla in the supraperiosteal

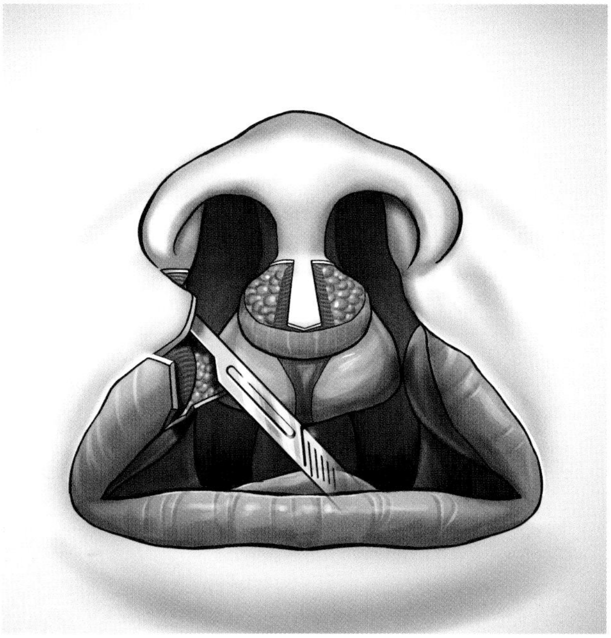

Figure 10.2b The skin is dissected from the orbicularis oris muscle. Two lateral white-roll–vermilion–mucosal flaps are created. Vertical incisions are made on each side of the premaxilla and the flaps flanking the philtrum are carefully de-epithelialized conserving venous return.

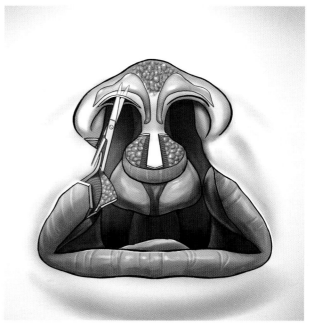

Figure 10.2c Semi-open exposure of the alar cartilages through rim incisions and displaying of the splayed and dislocated cartilages.

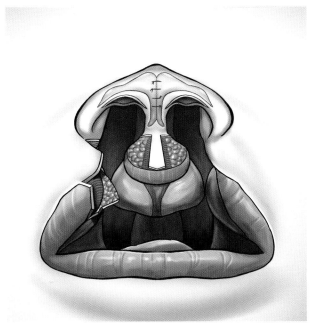

Figure 10.2d Placement of an interdomal mattress suture, previous subtraction of the interdomal fat.

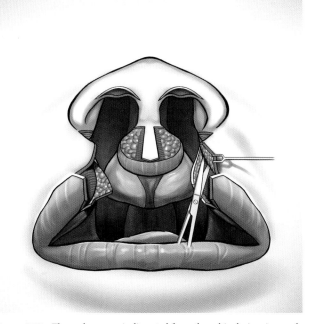

Figure 10.2e The oral mucosa is dissected from the orbicularis oris muscle. The muscle is completely freed from both the alar base and the periosteum along the pyriform aperture. This allows for a substantial amount of muscle fiber to be brought medially to be reattached with the muscle of the opposite side.

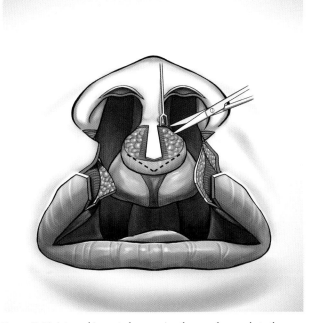

Figure 10.2f A tunnel is created preserving the vascular supply to the prolabium. Prolabial flap elevation is not recommended. Redundant premaxillary vermilion mucosa is trimmed.

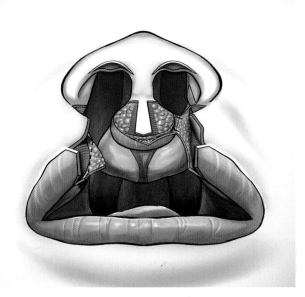

Figure 10.2g Bilateral gingival sulcus and nasal floor closure are accomplished. Alveolar closure is not recommended.

plane. This permits greater advancement of the cheek than is possible using subperiosteal dissection. Releasing the lip from the maxilla is a critical maneuver; this is required to minimize tension on the muscular closure and permit tension-free cutaneous closure. The orbicularis oris bundles are dissected in both the subdermal and submucosal planes.

Using a semi-open approach, to dissect under vision – through bilateral rim incisions – the anterior surface of the slumped and splayed lower lateral cartilages is exposed by scissor detachment. This dissection continues superiorly over the upper lateral cartilages and across the dorsal septal junction. Interdomal fatty tissue is elevated and partially excised to visualize the medial

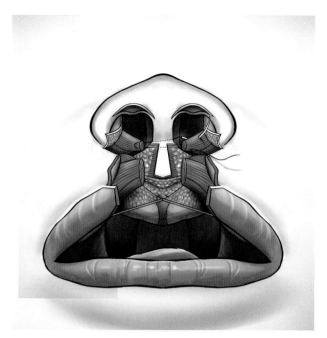

Figure 10.2h 'U' stitch tacking the nasal muscle bundles from both sides and going through the tunnel.

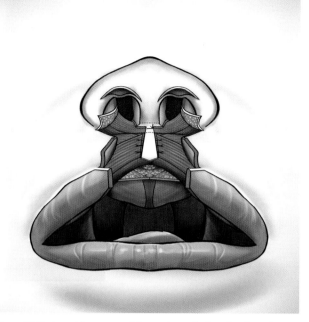

Figure 10.2i Apposition suture of the nasal muscles bundles, from the sides, going through the tunnel. Narrowing of the interalar width observed through the skin is a way to check the correct reposition of the nasal muscles. Bilateral fixation of the orbicular muscle bundles to the periostium on both sides of the prolabium.

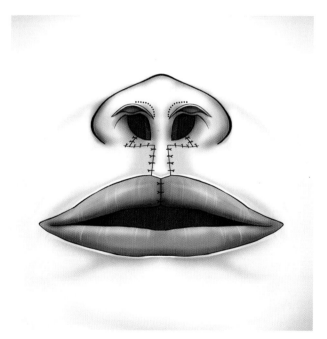

Figure 10.2j Redundant upper columella skin trimmed before the alar rim is closed. Alar base flaps sutured side-to-end to columellar 'C' flaps and trimmed after the sill is closed. Lateral white-roll–vermilion–mucosal flaps used to construct Cupid's bow and full median tubercle. Redundant vermilion-mucosa trimmed to form median raphe.

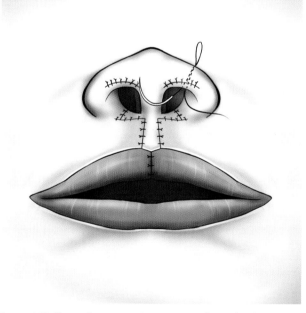

Figure 10.2k Two or three suspension sutures are always placed to join cartilage to the skin in the new position.

crura; perichondrium-to-perichondrium heals more securely without intervening soft tissue. An interdomal suture, to project and narrow the nasal tip, is performed. Two or three suspension sutures are always placed to join cartilages to the skin in the new position.

Alveolar gingiva and nasal floors are closed using a lateral mucosal flap and a medial flap from the premaxilla. The vermilion component of the premaxillary mucosa is trimmed and the remaining mucosal flange is secured above the premaxillary periosteum to construct the posterior side of the central gingivolabial sulcus.

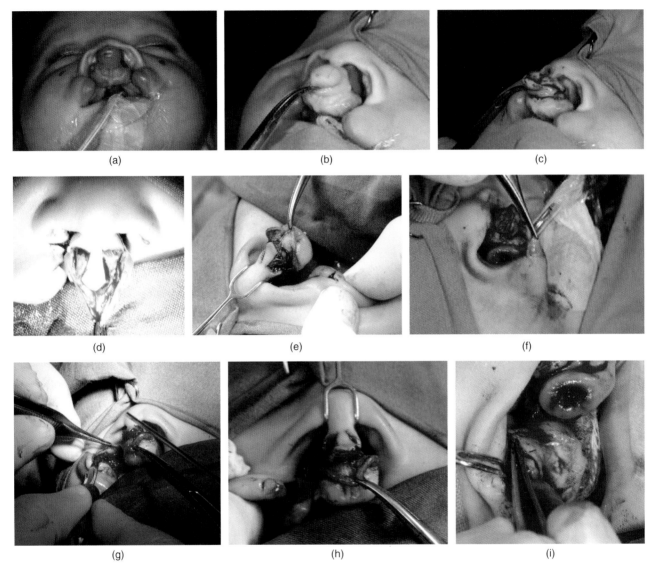

(a) (b) (c)

(d) (e) (f)

(g) (h) (i)

Figure 10.3 (a–c) Local and regional anesthesia is injected 10 minutes before surgery. The philtral flap is drawn first while the nostrils are held upward with a double-ball retractor. First, all labial incisions are lightly scored. The flaps flanking the philtral flap are carefully de-epithelialized conserving venous return. Vertical incisions are made on each side of the septum. (d–f) The white-roll–vermilion–mucosal flaps are incised (just short of the tattooed lateral Cupid's bow point). (g–i) The lateral labial elements are disjoined from the alar bases. An incision on the intranasal bridge is performed to allow an open dissection and liberation of the muscles producing nasal distortion. The basilar flaps are freed from the pyriform attachments. An inferior pedicle triangular flap is planned to be transposed intranasally, as a Z-plasty to the intranasal raw area. (j–l) With a double-hook on the muscle layer, the lateral labial elements are dissected off the maxilla in the supraperiosteal plane. This permits greater advancement of the cheek than is possible using subperiosteal dissection. Important muscular bundles are obtained to perform a functional nasal and labial muscle reconstruction. (m–o) The mucosal incisions on the underside of the lateral elements are extended distally, on the anterior side of the gingivolabial sulcus. In cases presenting with a wide alveolar gap, a second inferiorly based flap can be planned to repair the alveolar gingiva and nasal floor to prevent oronasal fistula. (p–r) The mucosal plane closure is completed. The muscular nasal floor repair will be achieved through the tunnel, using a 'U' suture. (s–t) Narrowing of the interalar width observed through the skin is a way to check the correct reposition of the nasal muscles. An interdomal suture, to project and narrow the nasal tip, is performed. Final view of the simultaneous lip and nose reconstruction.

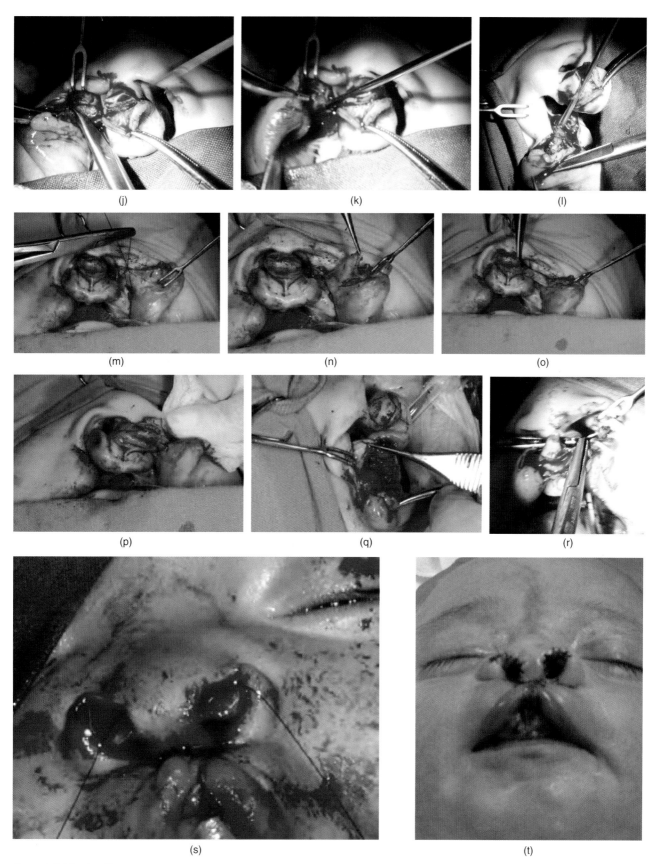

Figure 10.3 (*Continued*)

Muscular nasal floor reconstruction is accomplished using a 'U' stitch, tacking the nasal muscle bundles from both sides through the collumelar tunnel, at the nasal spine level.

The 'C' flap on each side of the columellar base is trimmed to 3 mm in length. The alar bases are advanced, rotated endonasally, and sutured side-to-end to the 'C' flaps to reconstruct the nasal floor.

A back-cut is made at the distal end of the sulcal incision, and the sulcus is closed while the labial flap is pulled mesially with a double hook. The lateral labial mucosal lining forms the anterior wall of the central gingivolabial sulcus.

The orbicular bundles are secured, from superior to inferior, to the periostium of the premaxilla, on both sides of the prolabial flap.

Construction of the median tubercle begins with the insertion of a fine chromic suture to join the white-roll–vermilion flaps at the midline; this is placed about 3 mm medially from the tattooed lateral Cupid's bow point. Excess vermilion-mucosa is trimmed from each flap and the junction aligned to form the median raphe. The tip of the philtral flap is inset into the handle of Cupid's bow and skin closure is completed using 6-0 atraumatic nylon (Mulliken, 1985). See Figure 10.3.

Results

See Figures 10.4 to 10.17.

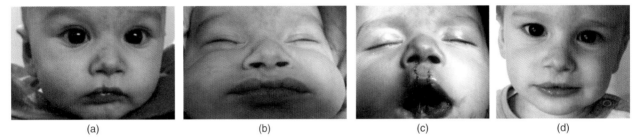

(a) (b) (c) (d)

Figure 10.4 (a–d) Pre and postop frontal and inferior views of an asymmetrical incomplete bilateral cleft lip resolution, with muscular reconstruction of the nasal floor and without touching the nose.

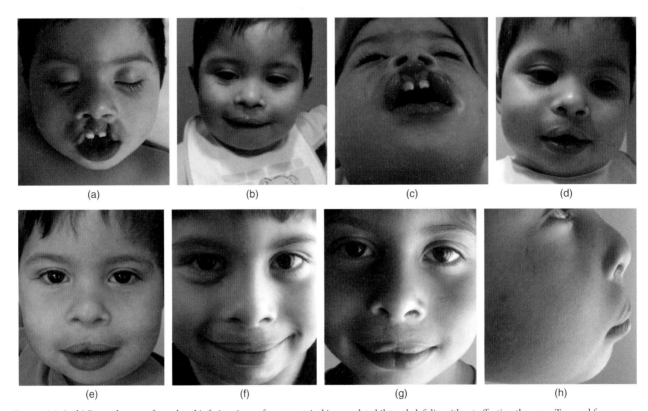

(a) (b) (c) (d)

(e) (f) (g) (h)

Figure 10.5 (a–h) Pre and postop frontal and inferior views of a symmetrical incomplete bilateral cleft lip without affecting the nose. Two and four year follow-up.

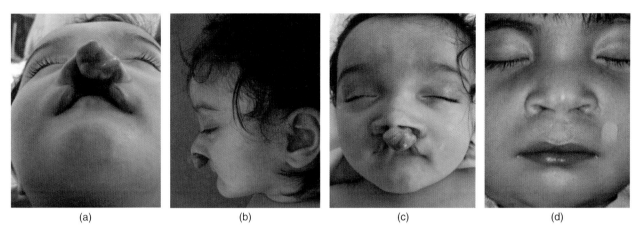

Figure 10.6 (a–d) Pre and postop views of a severe bilateral complete case without presurgical orthopedic. The selected procedure was a two-stage reconstruction. Lips first and nose in a second step, with a good looking philtrum reconstruction.

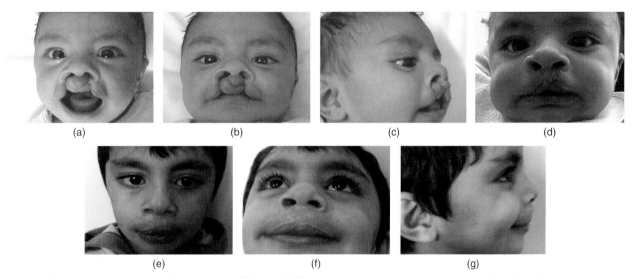

Figure 10.7 (a–g) Pre and postop views of an asymmetrical bilateral cleft lip with previous DPNR technique treatment. The selected procedure was a one-stage reconstruction without touching the nose. Four year follow-up.

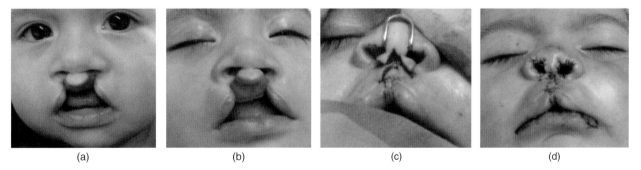

Figure 10.8 (a–d) Pre, intra, and post views of a symmetrical incomplete bilateral cleft lip with a very depressed nose and short lip. An island prolabial flap was performed using both lateral labial flaps to cover the drawn area and elongate the lip. The lateral prolabial flaps were rotated and employed to repair the nasal floor. Rim incisions were utilized to elongate collumela and project the tip of the nose.

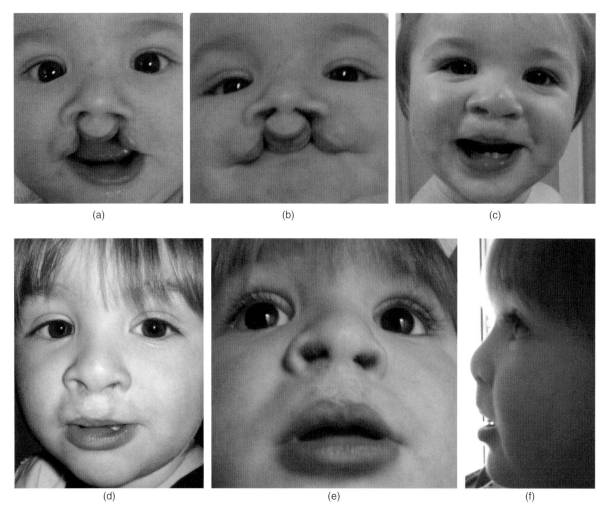

Figure 10.9 (a–f) Pre and post views of a symmetrical complete bilateral cleft lip without presurgical orthopedic. A simultaneous lip and nose reconstruction with bilateral rim incisions was performed. Three year follow-up. This case will probably need a second minimal nose revision.

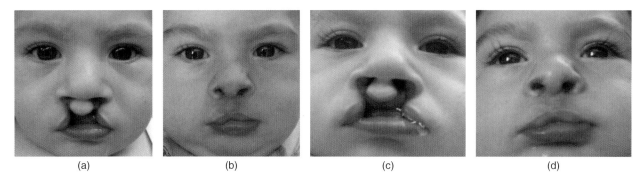

Figure 10.10 (a–d) Pre and post views of a symmetrical complete bilateral cleft lip with previous DPNR technique treatment. Although bilateral rim incisions were utilized at the moment of the simultaneous lip and nose reconstruction, the nose is natural looking and we don't expect mayor changes with growth.

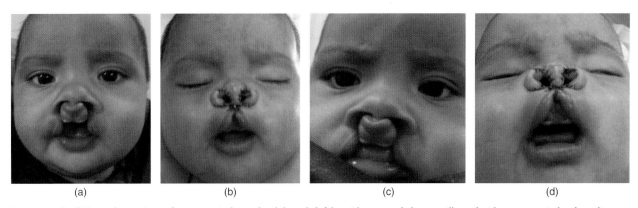

Figure 10.11 (a–d) Pre and post views of a symmetrical complete bilateral cleft lip with a protruded premaxilla, and without presurgical orthopedic. Simultaneous lip and nose reconstruction was performed. The oral plate must necessarily be used from the first postop day. The aim is to guide muscular action to obtain premaxillary retrusion and avoid descent.

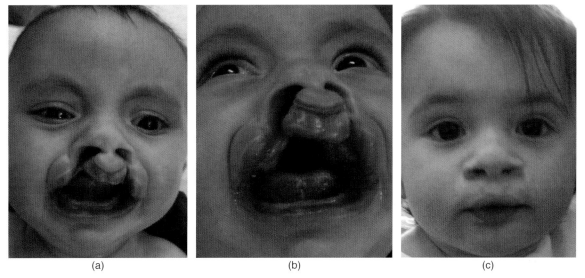

Figure 10.12 (a–c) Preop and one year postop views of a bilateral complete cleft lip with a protruded premaxilla. The DPNR technique although utilized was insufficient to produce complete correction of the nasoalveolar distortion. Simultaneous lip and nose reconstruction was performed and the oral plate was utilized from the first postop day.

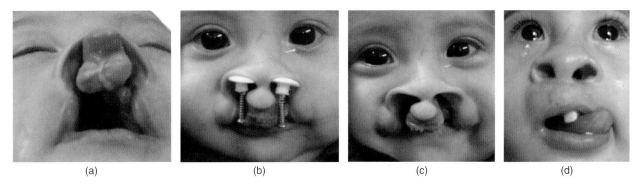

Figure 10.13 (a–d) Pre and postop views of an asymmetrical, with protruded premaxilla, bilateral complete cleft lip. The DPNR technique was effective in ameliorating distortions making the one-step procedure easier.

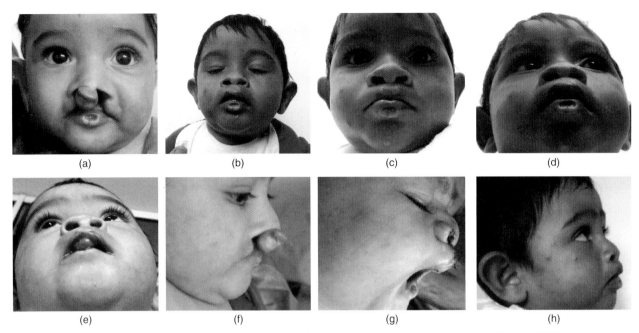

Figure 10.14 (a–h) Pre and one year postop views of an asymmetrical, with protruded premaxilla, bilateral complete cleft lip. The DPNR technique was optimum to correct all distortions. The surgical one-step reconstruction was less aggressive as a result with an increased aesthetic result.

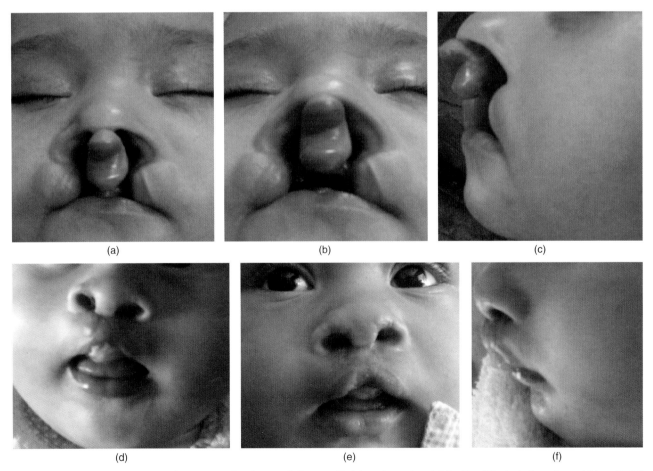

Figure 10.15 (a–i) Pre and post views of a symmetrical, with protruded premaxilla, bilateral complete cleft lip. The difficulty is the petite prolabium. DPNR technique was extremely useful to solve this case in a one-stage procedure. The post op oral plate was effective in guiding the premaxilla to the right position. Six month postop views show a hypertrophic scar as an immediate complication that we expect to solve with massage and compression.

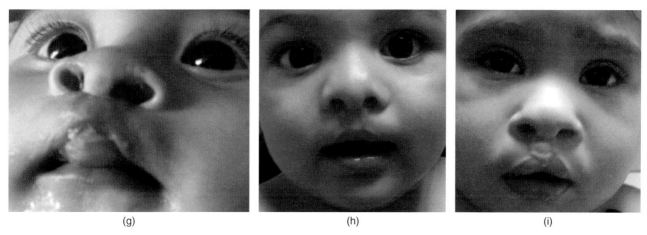

(g) (h) (i)

Figure 10.15 (*Continued*)

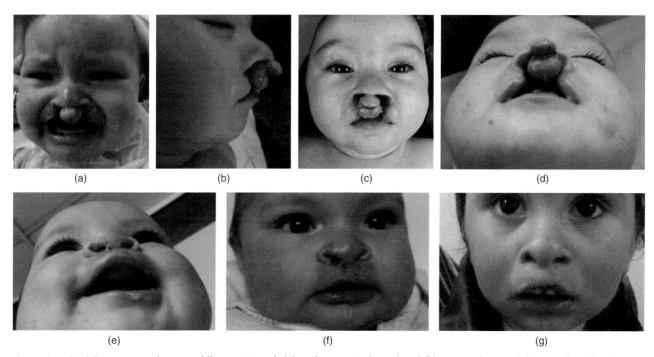

(a) (b) (c) (d)

(e) (f) (g)

Figure 10.16 (a–g) Pre, postop, and two year follow-up views of a bilateral symmetrical complete cleft lip case, with protruded premaxilla. Although one-step reconstruction can be performed any time, it is recommended to wait until 6 months for effective treatment. If not, increased technical difficulties and complications must be expected.

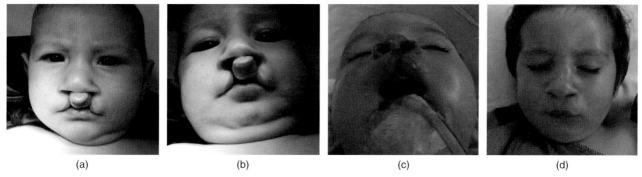

(a) (b) (c) (d)

Figure 10.17 (a–d) For non-severe cases, simultaneous lip and nose repair can be done from 3 months old.

Discussion

Surgeons seem to accept that a repaired bilateral cleft lip will be more noticeable than a repaired unilateral cleft lip (Millard, 1977; Khosla *et al.*, 2012).

Our logic regarding surgical reconstruction changed when we understood the concept that the prolabium is embryologically lip tissue, and thus should stay in the lip; and also that multistage procedures to create a columella are not necessary (McComb, 1975; Mulliken, 2000).

The columella is shortened due to the lateral pull of the alar cartilages and alar base due to the malalignment of the prolabium and the lateral maxillary segments. This displaces the true soft triangle and columella, which flattens the nasal tip and shortens the columellar height.

Primary correction commenced with the onset of the concept that the columella is in the nose (McComb, 1990; Mulliken, 1992).

The alar cartilages and nasal soft tissue envelope can be sculpted, which will rotate the skin of the alar rim medially and add length to the columella. This can be achieved by presurgical remodeling or surgical maneuvers at the time of the primary repair.

Preoperative dentofacial orthopedics is key to set the stage for synchronous bilateral nasolabial closure. Dentofacial orthopedics (active or passive) is not always available or considered necessary in many centers. Therefore, older techniques continue to be practiced: (i) Staged repair: first, closure on one side of the lip (usually the more severely involved) and then, the other side. (ii) Preliminary labial adhesion, either bilateral or one side first. (ii) The third common strategy is to undertake simultaneous bilateral labial repair over the protuberant premaxilla. This method makes it difficult to: (i) primarily correct the nasal deformity, and (ii) design the philtral flap of appropriate dimensions in anticipation of growth. Most of these procedures present early or late complications.

Immediate

Dehiscence occurs more commonly with bilateral lips than unilateral ones, probably due to the stretch of the repair over the protruded premaxilla in patients without presurgical orthodontics. Even mild trauma, like the banging of the head of the child against the shoulder of the parent, may cause disruption of the repair.

With the onset of surgical techniques bringing the lateral orbicularis oris muscles together in the midline after raising the prolabial skin flap, rarely there can be a loss of the prolabium, and even entire premaxilla, due to vascular compromise.

When there is good presurgical alignment of the premaxilla with both the lateral maxillary segments, an adequate advancement of the lateral lip elements from both sides is easier and there is no central vermillion deficiency ("whistle deformity"). The lateral turned down flaps are used to form the central vermillion after turning down the prolabial mucosa.

Gradual

If healing is successful, the philtrum is likely to overgrow to become too wide or abnormally shaped.

If there is much tension, hypertrophic scars can present.

Retrusion and descent of the premaxilla can present if there is no postsurgical orthodontic control and the oral plate is not utilized.

Sequels

A lip that is too tight can occur when too much of the lateral lip elements is discarded, often due to repeated lip advancements to correct central vermillion deficiencies. The best reconstruction available in this instance is a central shield-shaped Abbe flap as recommended by Millard. See Figures 10.18 to 10.24.

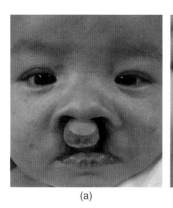 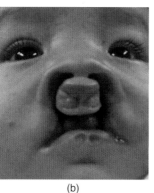 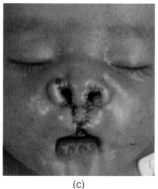 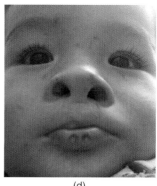

(a) (b) (c) (d)

Figure 10.18 (a–d) Central vermillion deficiency ("whistle deformity") is one of the most common complications.

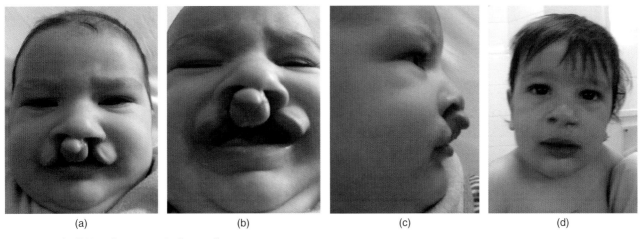

Figure 10.19 (a–d) Nostril asymmetry is also very frequent.

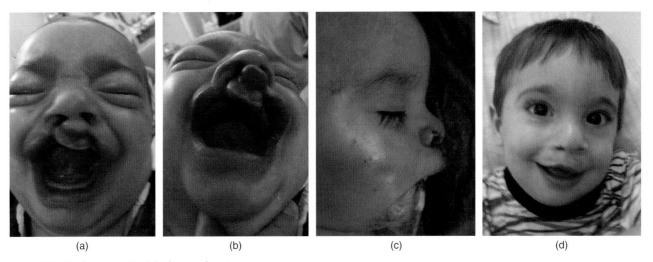

Figure 10.20 (a–d) Asymmetrical alar base implantation.

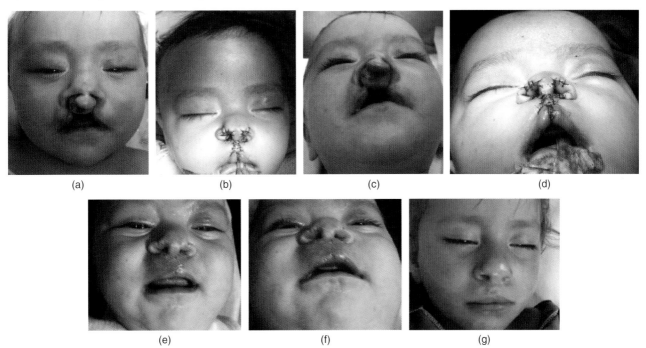

Figure 10.21 (a–g) Although the final result looks great, the DPNR technique gives us the possibility of avoiding surgical nasal repositioning, decreasing surgical aggression and preventing growth alterations.

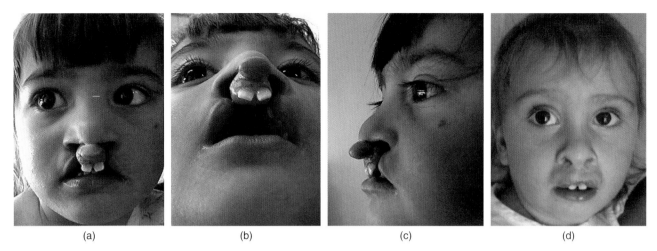

(a)   (b)   (c)   (d)

Figure 10.22 (a–d) Unfortunately we still see older patients who have not received any treatment. We feel the complete simultaneous repair described works very well in these cases.

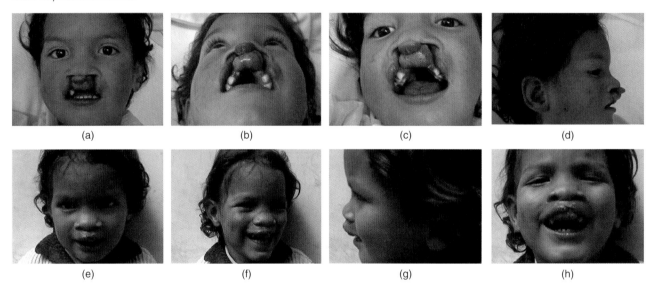

(a)   (b)   (c)   (d)

(e)   (f)   (g)   (h)

Figure 10.23 (a–h) Having a good looking result is not enough; avoiding growth and speech alterations is our commitment, but implementing the early protocol and having a totally rehabilitated child at the age of entering elementary school is our major goal.

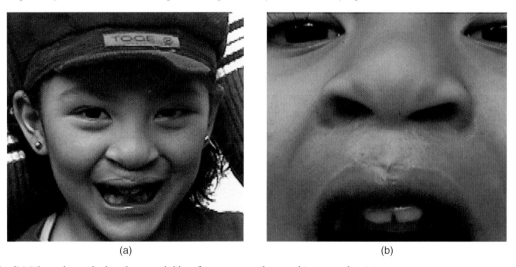

(a)   (b)

Figure 10.24 (a–d) With good growth, the other sequels like a flat nose are easily treated in a second revision.

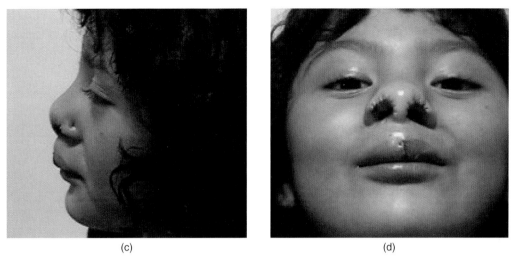

(c)   (d)

Figure 10.24 (*Continued*)

Follow-ups

See Figures 10.25 to 10.29.

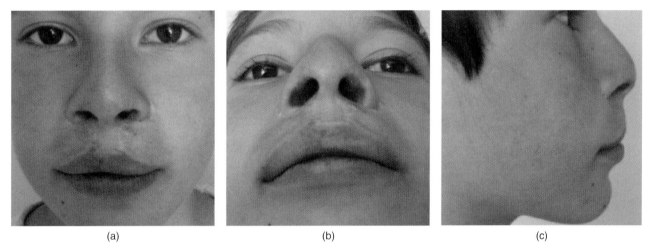

(a)   (b)   (c)

Figure 10.25 (a–c) Frontal, inferior, and lateral views in a 7-year-old patient.

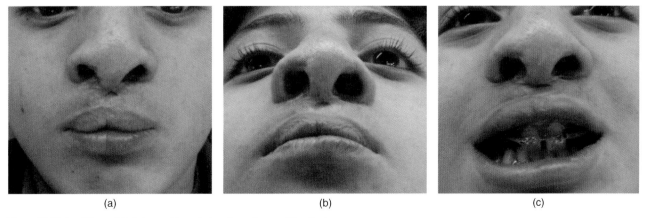

(a)   (b)   (c)

Figure 10.26 (a–c) Frontal, inferior, and lateral views in an 8-year-old patient.

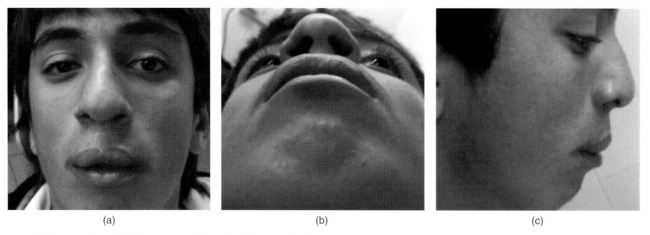

Figure 10.27 (a–c) Frontal, inferior, and lateral views in a 10-year-old patient.

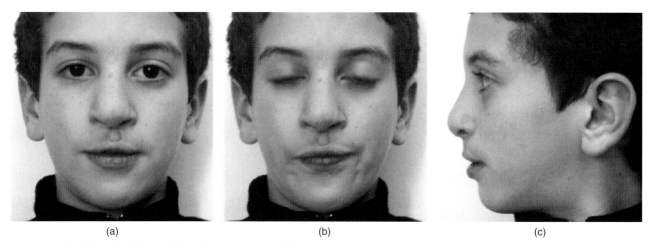

Figure 10.28 (a–c) Frontal, inferior, and lateral views in a 12-year-old patient.

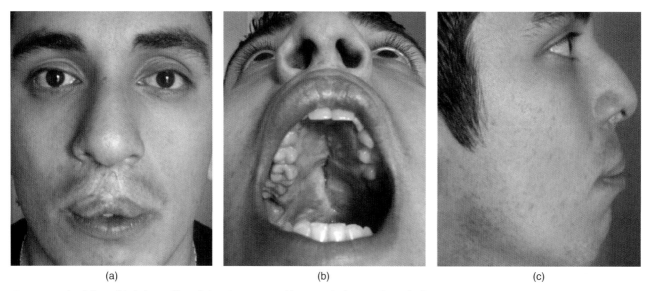

Figure 10.29 (a–g) Frontal, inferior, and lateral views in a 20-year-old patient. Oral views after orthodontic treatment.

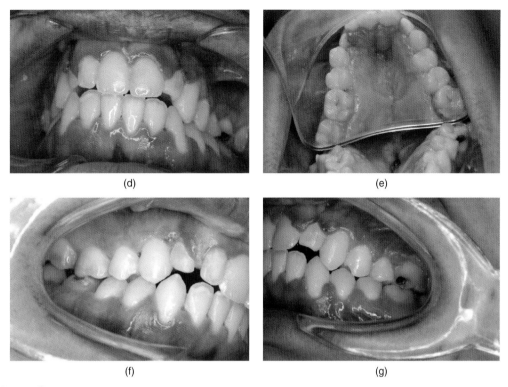

(d)   (e)

(f)   (g)

Figure 10.29 *(Continued)*

Conclusions

The advent of presurgical orthopedics and primary rhino-plasty techniques has made secondary columellar lengthening procedures obsolete. We agree that secondary columellar lengthening procedures are suboptimal and should be avoided. A child born with bilateral cleft lip should not have to suffer because of an ill-conceived and poorly executed primary repair. The operative principles for synchronous nasolabial correction are established. The techniques are within the repertoire of any well-trained and careful surgeon who is genuinely focused on the care of these children. Philtral columns and dimple are the only labial features that seem to be just beyond the surgeon's craft (Mulliken *et al.*, 2003; McComb, 2009).

For too long there has been misplaced emphasis on protocols that are based on the traditional concept of trying to minimize inhibition of midfacial growth. Indeed, some degree of maxillary retrusion is an unavoidable consequence of closure of the lip and palate. First priorities are nasolabial appearance and speech. Midfacial hypoplasia and underbite are entirely correctable after completion of facial growth (Kohout *et al.*, 1998).

Some type of dentofacial orthopedic manipulation is necessary to permit proper philtral design, nasal correction, and alveolar closure (Millard & Latham, 1990). If dentofacial orthopedics fails or if the child presents too late for an appliance to work, consider premaxillary ostectomy and set-back, either at the time of nasolabial repair (in infancy) or synchronously with palatal closure (in late infancy or early childhood).

The surgeon must correct the bilateral lip and nasal deformity in three dimensions while making alterations based on anticipated changes in the fourth dimension. This understanding is only gained by documenting the changing nasolabial features in children with repaired bilateral cleft lip and nasal deformity. Photography is essential and tabulation of revision-rate is useful; however, the future is in computerized three-dimensional photogrammetry (Rogers *et al.*, 2014).

References

Cutting, C. B. (2006) Bilateral cleft lip repair. In: Mathes, S. J. (ed.) *Plastic Surgery*, 2nd edn. Philadelphia, PA: Saunders, p. 235.

Farkas, L. G. and Lindsay, W. K. (1971) Morphology of the adult face following repair of bilateral cleft lip and palate in childhood. *Plast Reconstr Surg* **47**:24–32.

Farkas, L. G., Posnick, J. C., Hreczko, T. M., *et al.* (1992) Growth patterns of the nasolabial region: A morphometric study. *Cleft Palate-Craniofac J* **29**:318–324.

Khosla, R. K., McGregor, J., Kelley, P. K., *et al.* (2012) Contemporary concepts for the bilateral cleft lip and nasal repair. *Semin Plast Surg* **26**(**4**):156–163.

Kohout, M. P., Monasterio Aljaro, L., Farkas, L. G., *et al.* (1998) Photogrammetric comparison of two methods for synchronous repair of bilateral cleft lip and nasal deformity. *Plast Reconstr Surg* **102**:139–149.

McComb, H. (1975) Primary repair of the bilateral cleft lip nose. *Br J Plast Surg* **28**(**4**):262–267.

McComb, H. (1990) Primary repair of the bilateral cleft lip nose: A 15-year review and a new treatment plan. *Plast Reconstr Surg* **86**:882–890.

McComb, H. K. (2009) Primary repair of the bilateral cleft lip nose: A long-term follow-up. *Plast Reconstr Surg* **124**(5):1610–1615.

Millard, D. R., Jr. (1977) *Cleft Craft. The Evolution of its Surgery*. Vol **2**: Bilateral and rare deformities. Boston, MA: Little Brown, pp. 681–710.

Millard, D. R., Jr. and Latham, R. A. (1990) Improved primary surgical and dental treatment of clefts. *Plast Reconstr Surg* **86**:856–71.

Mulliken, J. B. (1985) Principles and techniques of bilateral complete cleft lip repair. *Plast Reconstr Surg* **75**:477–486.

Mulliken, J. B. (1992) Correction of the bilateral cleft lip nasal deformity: Evolution of a surgical concept. *Cleft Palate Craniofac J* **29**:540–545.

Mulliken, J. B. (1995) Bilateral complete cleft lip and nasal deformity: An anthropometric analysis of staged to synchronous repair. *Plast Reconstr Surg* **96**:9–23.

Mulliken, J. B. (2000) Repair of bilateral complete cleft lip and nasal deformity – State of the art. *Cleft Palate Craniofac J* **37**:342–347.

Mulliken, J. B. (2001) Primary repair of bilateral cleft lip and nasal deformity. *Plast Reconstr Surg* **108**:181–194.

Mulliken, J. B., Burvin, R., and Farkas, L. G. (2001) Repair of bilateral complete cleft lip: Intraoperative nasolabial anthropometry. *Plast Reconstr Surg* **107**:307–314.

Mulliken, J. B., Wu, J. K., and Padwa, B. L. (2003) Repair of bilateral cleft lip: Review, revisions, and reflections. *J Craniofac Surg* **14**:609–620.

Mulliken, J. B. (2004) The changing faces of children with cleft lip and palate. *N Eng J Med* **351**:743–737.

Mulliken, J. B. (2009) Repair of bilateral cleft lip and its variants. *Indian J Plast Surg* **42**(Suppl):S79–90.

Mulliken, J. B. and Kim, D. C. (2013) Repair of bilateral incomplete cleft lip: Techniques and outcomes. *Plast Reconstr Surg* **132**(4):923–932.

Rogers, C. R., Meara, J. G., and Mulliken, J. B. (2014) The philtrum in cleft lip: Review of anatomy and techniques for construction. *J Craniofac Surg* **25**(1):9–13.

CHAPTER 11
Cleft palate repair

Ricardo D. Bennun[1] and Luis Monasterio Aljaro[2]
[1] Asociacion PIEL, Maimonides University and National University of Buenos Aires, Argentina
[2] Fundacion Gantz, Santiago de Chile

Introduction

Surgical techniques for cleft lip and palate are continuously evolving, even more so the techniques for cleft palate repair. The techniques, their variations, the outcome and rehabilitation procedures are very well described in the available literature (Schweckendiek & Doz, 1978; Wallace, 1987; Leow & Lo, 2008; Agrawal, 2009).

Cleft palate affects almost every function of the face except vision. Today a child born with cleft palate with or without cleft lip should not be considered as unfortunate because surgical repair has reached a highly satisfactory level. However, for an average cleft surgeon, palatoplasty remains an enigma.

Basically there are three groups of palatoplasty techniques. One is for hard palate repair, the second for soft palate repair, and the third based on the surgical schedule. Hard palate repair techniques are Veau–Wardill–Kilner V-Y, von Langenbeck, two-flap, alveolar extension palatoplasty, vomer flap, raw area free palatoplasty, and so on. The soft palate techniques are intravelar veloplasty, double opposing Z-plasty, radical muscle dissection, primary pharyngeal flap, and so on. And the protocol based techniques are Schweckendiek's, Malek's, whole in one, modified schedule with palatoplasty before lip repair, and so on.

Conventional methods of cleft lip repair deprive the anterior (buccolingual) alveolar mucoperiosteum of blood supply from the facial–internal maxillary arcade. Six months later, at palatoplasty, lingual incisions permanently isolate the lingual mucoperiosteum from its blood supply: the greater palatine artery. The osteogenic alveolar mucoperiosteum is thus converted from a richly supplied boundary zone between the two angiosomes into an isolated tissue dependent on osseus backflow. Cleft-sided growth disturbance is considered from this perspective. Subperiosteal techniques that preserve the blood supply to this tissue are considered in a sequential plan of cleft management (Carstens, 1999) (Figures 11.1–11.3).

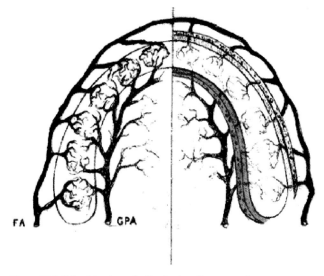

Figure 11.1 Palate blood supply distribution. The two angiosomes description.

Preoperative considerations

Schedule of palatoplasty

The majority accept 6 to 12 months as the optimum age for palatoplasty. Ideally, the development of babbling should be considered as an indicator of the best time to reconstruct the palate. The author advocates palate repair after lip/nose repair, and selects between 8 to 12 months as the ideal period for a complete hard and soft reconstruction.

Endotracheal tube

Being an intraoral surgery, the endotracheal tube (ETT) is an important factor to be considered in palate repair. The ETT has to be placed orally. The tongue blade of the mouth gag retracts the ETT and is placed against the tongue; therefore there is a risk

Cleft Lip and Palate Management: A Comprehensive Atlas, First Edition. Edited by Ricardo D. Bennun, Julia F. Harfin, George K. B. Sándor, and David Genecov.
© 2016 John Wiley & Sons, Inc. Published 2016 by John Wiley & Sons, Inc.

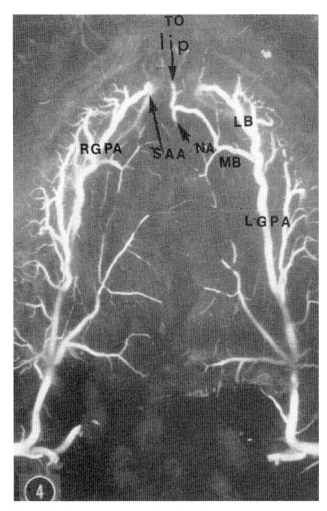

Figure 11.2 Contrasted arteriography of the palate.

of ETT compression between the gag and the mandible (Jaeger, 1999). The use of a preformed RAE tube (Ring, Adair, Elwin tube) facilitates the placement of the palate mouth gag without this risk.

Mouth gag

Basically, there are two types of palate mouth gags commonly in use. Kilner–Dott and Dingman mouth gags. The Dingman gag is a little large and relatively heavy but the inbuilt cheek retractors help in intraoral exposure.

Haemostatic infiltration

Lidocaine Clohidrate 2% with Epinephrine 1:50.000 and a carpule syringe are used for infiltration of the palate 5–7 min before the surgery. Use of a smaller syringe makes the infiltration and hydro-dissection easier in the hard palate region.

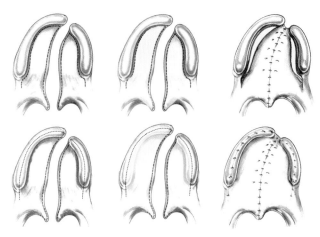

Figure 11.3 The conventional approach and the modifications proposed by Carstens.

Objectives of the cleft palate repair

There are three major objectives of a cleft palate operation, all of these are inter-related:
- To produce anatomical closure of the defect.
- To create an apparatus for development and production of normal speech.
- To minimize the maxillary growth disturbances and dento-alveolar deformities.

Principles of the ideal palatoplasty
- Closure of the defect.
- Correction of the abnormal position of the muscles of the soft palate.
- Reconstruction of the muscle sling.
- Retro-positioning of the soft palate to allow the anterior part of the soft palate to come in contact with the posterior pharyngeal wall during speech.
- Minimal or no raw area should be left on the nasal side or the oral surface.
- Tension-free suturing.
- Two-layer closure in the hard palate region and a three-layer closure of the soft palate.

Surgical technique

An incision of the mucosa along the cleft borders is performed; a subperiosteal dissection around the palatal bone is done to create two mucoperiosteal flaps that will allow us the complete closure of the nasal floor including the anterior palatal portion.

A careful dissection of the levator palati following its liberation from the posterior border of the hard palate is accomplished, until it becomes a compact bundle to be sutured to its corresponding muscle on the opposite side.

By means of lateral compensatory incisions, a scissor separation of both muscular planes is accomplished and the superior constrictor is freed from the pterygoid plate, without needing to break the hamulus, allowing all these muscles to be medially displaced and attached to the palatal flap to meet their components from the opposite side.

Before closure of the nasal mucosal plane, a trimming suture of the deep muscular plane is performed.

One or two alveolar extending palatal flaps are planned according to whether the clinical case is unilateral or bilateral complete. In cases of secondary cleft palatal, a minimal incision variant can be utilized.

In unilateral complete cases the selected flap to be elevated using Carstens' approach is located at the affected side.

Subperiosteal detaching of the palatal plane and a complete muscular dissection of the normal side is performed in a conservative way, avoiding the anterior portion of the alveolar extended incision.

When the cleft is extremely wide, the soft palate is extremely short, or the patient is an adult, a primary pharyngeal flap could be indicated.

The LVP muscle from children with cleft palate has a different morphology compared to normal adult muscle. The differences may be related to different stages in the maturation of the muscles, changes in functional demands with growth and age, or a consequence of the cleft. The lack of contractile tissue in some of the cleft biopsies offers one possible explanation for persistent postsurgical velopharyngeal insufficiency in some patients, despite a successful surgical repair (Lindman *et al.*, 2001) (Figure 11.4).

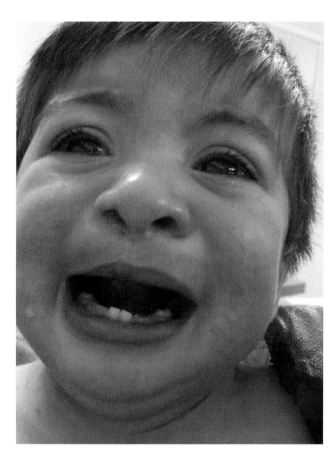

Figure 11.4a One-year-old patient with unilateral complete cleft lip and palate.

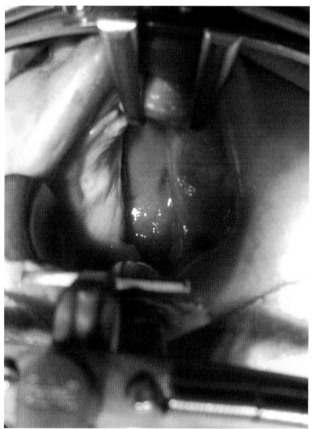

Figure 11.4b Intra oral view of a cleft palate with the alveolar cleft segments correctly approximated.

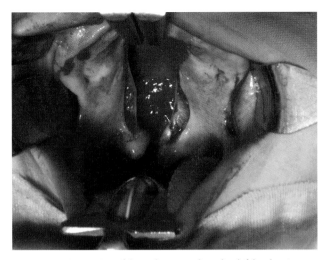

Figure 11.4c An incision of the oral mucosa along the cleft borders is performed.

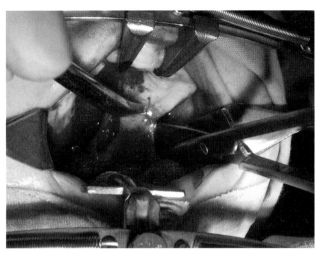

Figure 11.4d A scissor separation of both muscular planes is accomplished.

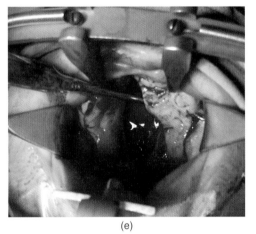

(e)

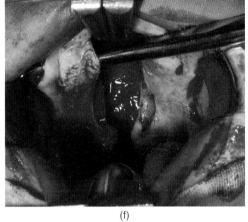

(f)

Figure 11.4e–f A subperiostal dissection of both palatal sides and around de palatal bone is done.

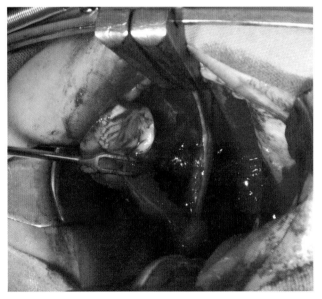

Figure 11.4g Liberation of the levator palati from the posterior border of the hard palate is accomplished.

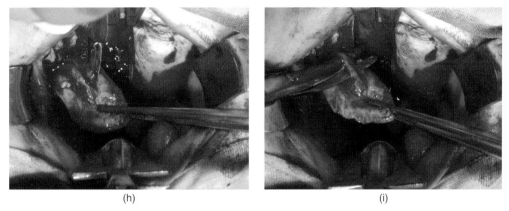

(h)   (i)

Figure 11.4h–i The palatal flap over the cleft side is using an alveolar extension incision. The palatal artery is totally liberated.

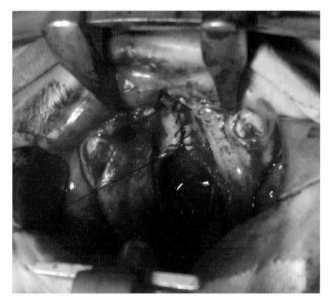

Figure 11.4j A nasal plane closure of the hard and soft palate is completed.

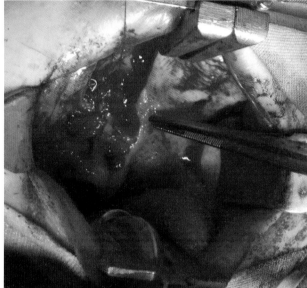

Figure 11.4k To guaranty a satisfactory contact of the anterior wall with pharynx a trimming suture of the deep muscular plane is accomplished.

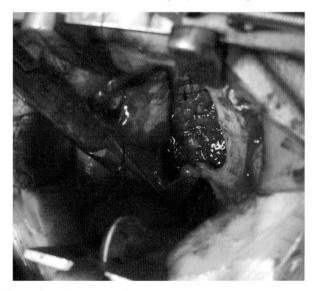

Figure 11.4l A traction suture facilitate the correct uvula reconstruction.

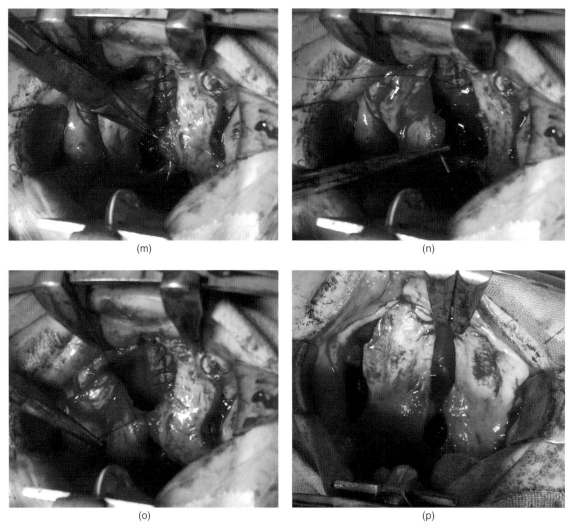

(m)

(n)

(o)

(p)

Figure 11.4m–p A careful dissection of the levator palati, until it becomes a compact bundle, is accomplished and sutured to its corresponding muscle on the opposite side.

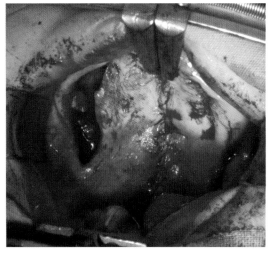

Figure 11.4q The flap results enough to complete the closure of the anterior palatal portion.

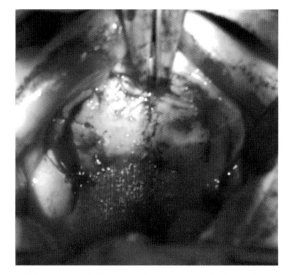

Figure 11.4r At the end of surgery minimal raw area is observed.

Basics of postoperative management

Feeding
Postoperative oral fluid is given as soon as the child regains full consciousness. Early oral feeding pacifies the child, allowing early dismissal.

Postoperative analgesia
In our hospital, paracetamol suppository and oral suspension are used with satisfactory results.

Results

See Figures 11.5–11.8.

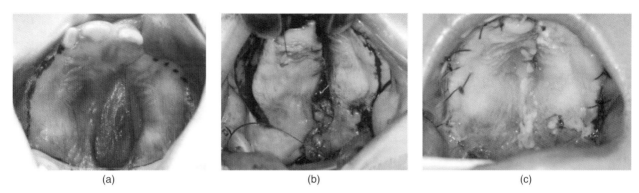

(a)   (b)   (c)

Figure 11.5 (a–c) The Carstens' variant was employed in a unilateral complete case. The normal palate side was selected to be transposed. This procedure was performed by Dr. Monasterio Aljaro.

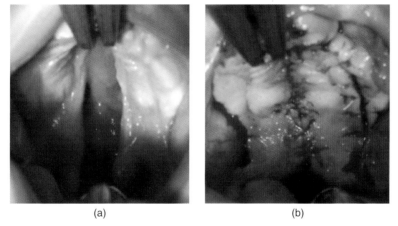

(a)   (b)

Figure 11.6 (a–b) The Carstens' procedure was used in a complete unilateral case. The cleft palate side was selected to be transposed.

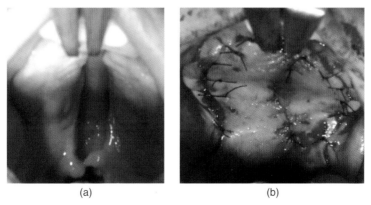

(a)   (b)

Figure 11.7 (a–b) The Carstens' reconstruction was performed in a bilateral complete case. Two muco-periosteal flaps were used to complete the reconstructive surgery.

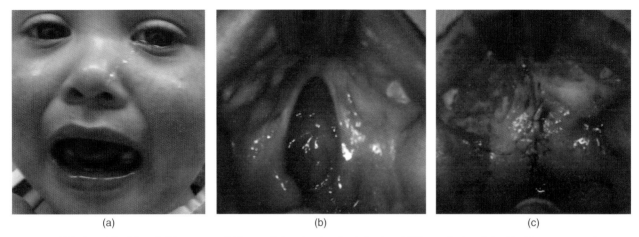

(a)   (b)   (c)

Figure 11.8 (a) Patient with a Pierre Robin sequence. (b) Intraoral view showing the cleft palate. (c) The result of a minimal incision reconstructive procedure.

Complications

Common complications of any palate surgery are as follows:

Immediate complications: hemorrhage, respiratory obstruction, hanging palate, dehiscence of the repair, oronasal fistula formation.

Late complications: bifid uvula, velopharyngeal incompetence, abnormal speech, maxillary hypoplasia, dental malpositioning and malalignment, otitis media.

Hemorrhage

Intraoperative bleeding is not usual in the majority of patients. Use of Lidocaine with Epinephrine solution and a careful dissection by plane reduces the blood loss. Use of bipolar coagulation proves quite useful in achieving hemostasis. Bleeding is more commonly seen in adults and secondary cases.

Respiratory obstruction

Postoperative pulse oximetry is mandatory for all palatoplasty patients until the child is fully awake and is able to maintain O_2 saturation with natural air without any support. If the child is sedated and there is tongue fall, the resulting respiratory problem poses a considerable risk. In high-risk patients with cleft palate with micrognathia or syndromic cleft, it is safer to apply a tongue suture during the postoperative period for 12–24 hours.

Oronasal fistula

The oronasal fistula itself is a major subject for discussion. The incidence varies from less than 2% to over 40% in different publications. Common sites are the junction between the hard and the soft palate and the anterior palate region. However, any part of the palatal repair may have breakdown resulting in oronasal fistula. Most new variations and additional procedures are aimed at reducing the incidence of fistula formation. The fistula may be significant or insignificant. This depends upon the site and the dimension. Every significant fistula requires repair at an appropriate time.

Discussion

Until a few years ago this author used Veau–Wardill–Kilner palatoplasty as the usual repair method in our protocol. In this technique a V-Y procedure is performed, the whole mucoperiosteal flap and the soft palate are retroposed, and the palate lengthened. This procedure leaves an extensive raw area anteriorly and laterally along the alveolar margin with exposed bare membranous bone. The raw area heals with secondary intention. This causes shortening of the palate and can result in velopharyngeal incompetence. Contraction of wounds following surgery can be the first link in a causal chain leading eventually to secondary skeletal deformities (Olin et al., 1974; Moore et al., 1988).

To increase lengthening of the soft palate, a horizontal back-cut in the nasal lining at the junction of hard and soft palate was described (Dorrance & Bransfield, 1946). This procedure also leaves a large raw area on the nasal surface which is left open. This may contract after healing with secondary intention and may undo the palatal lengthening. Since there is single-layer repair in the region of the back-cut, the incidence of palatal fistula is high.

Because of these drawbacks, pushback and V-Y techniques have fallen into disrepute and are now less commonly used.

It is a well-established fact that unrepaired cleft patients have a better maxillary relationship and development. Early and aggressive palatal surgical intervention causes maxillary hypoplasia. For this reason many surgeons used to perform palate repair in two stages. The soft palate repaired early and the hard palate closed later. At the time of introduction of this protocol the soft palate was repaired along with the lip at around 4–6 months of age and the hard palate was repaired at the age of 10–12 years. This indication was later reduced to 4–5 years (Lehman *et al.*, 1990; Lindsay & Witzel, 1990). This delay significantly reduced the cleft width in the hard palate region and was easy to close without the need for extensive dissection. This protocol probably reduced the maxillary hypoplasia but the speech result was compromised.

Vomerine mucoperiosteal tissue is very versatile. Most surgeons utilize the vomer flap only for repair of the cleft anteriorly in the hard palate region and the alveolar region. The vomer flap in this region is invariably used as a superiorly based turnover flap. This tissue has been revisited and has been extensively used for covering palatal defects (Lee *et al.*, 2001). Many varieties of vomer flaps have been described for use in unilateral and bilateral cleft palates for nasal lining and oral mucosa resurfacing (Bumsted, 1981).

In the functional anatomy of the soft palate as applied to wind playing, seven muscles of the soft palate involved in the velopharyngeal closure mechanism are described. These are the tensor veli palatini, levator veli palatini, palatopharyngeus, palatoglossus, musculus uvulae, superior pharyngeal constrictor, and salpingopharyngeus. These muscles contribute to either a palatal or a pharyngeal component of velopharyngeal closure (Evans *et al.*, 2010).

A double reverse Z-plasty for the oral and nasal surfaces of the soft palate was introduced (Furlow, 1986). The cleft margin forms the central limb. The muscle is incorporated into the posteriorly based triangular flap on the left side for ease of dissection. The hard palate region is closed by making an incision along the cleft margin, elevating the mucoperiosteum from the medial side and taking advantage of the high arch. The cleft is closed in two layers without making a lateral incision; with the use of the lateral relaxing incision only when necessary.

On transposition of the triangles there is an effective lengthening of the soft palate, the suture line is horizontal, and there is good overlap of the levator muscle. Many surgeons claim to have better speech outcome with the Furlow repair technique. However, studies have not proved this objectively. The major objection to this technique is the non-anatomic placement of the muscle.

The raw area left over the nasal surface after pushback has always been a matter of concern. A buccal myomucosal flap was used to take care of this raw area created after pushback surgery (Mukherji, 1969) and bilateral buccal mucosal flaps simultaneously for covering the oral and nasal surfaces. This technique has been re-popularized for covering the defect created after the back-cut at the junction between hard and soft palate (Jackson *et al.*, 2004).

Primary pharyngeal flap is only indicated to improve the speech in children with a very wide cleft palate and in adult patients with a short soft palate. Patient postop disadvantages after a pharyngeal flap surgery can be sleep apnea and hyponasality (Stark *et al.*, 1969; Senders & Fung, 2009).

Braithwaite in 1968 was the first to describe the dissection of the levator palati from the posterior border of the hard palate, nasal and oral mucosa and posterior repositioning (Braithwaite & Maurice, 1968). He described an independent reconstruction of the levator sling suturing of both sides of the muscle. Since then intravelar veloplasty has evolved considerably and many surgeons have modified the surgical details to achieve better anatomical muscle sling reconstruction. A radical muscle dissection under a microscope (Sommerlad, 2003) and a transection of the tensor palati keeping its function intact, with the hook of the hamulus, were described (Cutting *et al.*, 1995).

To ensure optimal function of the nasopharyngeal sphincter, adequate exposure, mobilization, and coaptation of the muscles must be carried out (Schweckendiek, 1966; Markus *et al.*, 1993). The muscles concerned in this closure are two slings of the levator palati and palatopharyngeous muscles and the palatopharyngeal sphincter of Whillis. No doubt the nasopharyngeal closure is partly a sphincteric action brought about by contraction of the upper fibers of the superior constrictor muscle which Whillis showed has some fibers inserted into the palatal aponeurosis and which he called the palatopharyngeal sphincter (Whillis, 1930).

Michael Carstens has recently described alveolar extension palatoplasty (AEP). In this technique the entire gingivoperiosteal tissue is incorporated into the mucoperiosteal palatal flap. This is expected to lengthen and widen the flap to cover the larger defect. Carstens claims that this procedure is more favorable to protect both angiosomes. This is expected to reduce maxillary hypoplasia.

In unilateral cases we only move one flap, and in this case our selection is the cleft-side. Our feeling is that covering the gap without making any incision on the normal side makes our reconstructive procedure less aggressive. In this way, the normal side development can be the support for a favorable growth of the affected side.

For soft palate cleft repair our choice is a minimal incisions procedure, but we only recommend this technique to experienced surgeons.

Uvula reconstruction is usually not given enough emphasis; however, parents and patients while assessing cleft palate repair watch the formation of the uvula. Hence the uvula should be repaired with great care in two layers.

Follow-ups

See Figures 11.9 and 11.10.

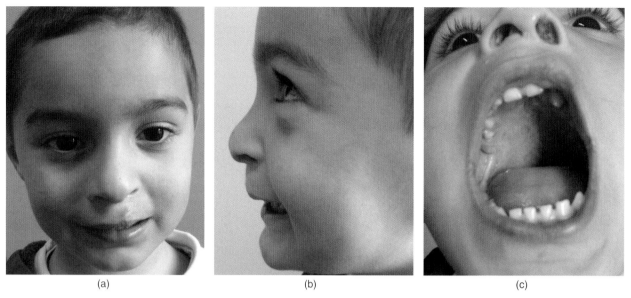

(a)   (b)   (c)

Figure 11.9 (a–c) Frontal, lateral, and intraoral views in a six-years-old patient. Follow up after a Carstens' procedure. No scars retraction, no anterior fistulas or dental arch alterations are observed.

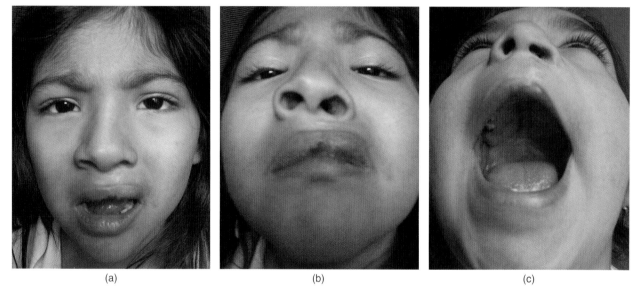

(a)   (b)   (c)

Figure 11.10 (a–c) Frontal, inferior, and intraoral views in an eight-years-old patient. Follow up after a Carstens' procedure.

Conclusion

Cleft palate surgery has seen major refinements over the past 20–30 years. Attempts to create a normal anatomy have improved the overall outcome of surgery. A team approach has decreased the morbidity and secondary deformities caused by the cleft. The current trend of early palate repair, early assessment with improved instrumentation, early evaluation of velopharyngeal function, and the development of procedures for achieving better bony alignment should result in more predictable end results in terms of speech and maxillofacial growth following cleft palate repair.

We have incorporated Carstens' principles in cleft palate repair for six years, following with the two-plane muscular reconstruction of the soft palate. To date we have operated on 84 cases. Following these patients we have noted anticipated dental eruption. The anterior and lateral closure was more comfortable, with almost no raw area. The immediate benefit is that the baby can take from the first day a complete diet including milk and derivatives. As we noted, for good scar evolution we abandoned the use of postop palatal plates with the objective of making scar compression and contention. Although we need prolonged follow-ups, anterior fistulas, skeletal alterations, and VPI rates seem to be progressively decreasing.

References

Agrawal, K. (2009) Cleft palate repair and variations. *Indian J Plast Surg* **42** Suppl:S102–109.

Braithwaite, F. and Maurice, D. G. (1968) The importance of the Levator Palatini muscle in cleft palate closure. *Br J Plast Surg* **21**:60–62.

Bumsted, R. M. (1981) Two-layer closure of a wide palatal cleft. *Cleft Palate J* **18**:110–5.

Carstens, M. H. (1999) Sequential cleft management with the sliding sulcus technique and alveolar extension palatoplasty. *J Craniofac Surg* **10**(6):503–518.

Cutting, C., Rosenbaum, J., and Rovati, L. (1995) The technique of muscle repair in the soft palate. *Op Tech Plast Surg* **2**:215–222.

Dorrance, G. M. and Bransfield, J. W. (1946) The pushback operation for repair of cleft palate. *Plast Reconstr Surg.* **1**:145.

Evans, A., Ackermann, B., and Driscoll, T. (2010) Functional anatomy of the soft palate applied to wind playing. *Med Probl Perform Art* **25**(4):183–189.

Furlow, L. T., Jr. (1986) Cleft palate repair by double opposing Z-plasty. *Plast Reconstr Surg* **78**:724–738.

Jackson, I T., Moreira-Gonzalez, A. A., Rogers, A., *et al.* (2004) The buccal flap a useful technique in cleft palate repair? *Cleft Palate Craniofac J* **41**:144–151.

Jaeger, J. M. and Durbin, C. G., Jr. (1999) Special purpose endotracheal tubes. *Respir Care* **44**:661–683.

Lee, S. I., Lee, H. S., and Hwang, K. (2001) Reconstruction of palatal defect using mucoperiosteal hinge flap and pushback palatoplasty. *J Craniofac Surg* **12**:561–563.

Lehman, J. A., Jr., Douglas, B. K., Ho, W. C., *et al.* (1990) One-stage closure of the entire primary palate. *Plast Reconstr Surg* **86**: 675–681.

Leow, A. M. and Lo, L. J. (2008) Palatoplasty: Evolution and controversies. *Chang Gung Med J* **31**(4):335–345.

Lindman, R., Paulin, G., and Stål, P. S. (2001) Morphological characterization of the levator veli palatini muscle in children born with cleft palates. *Cleft Palate Craniofac J* **38**(5):438–448.

Lindsay, W. K., Witzel, M. A. (1990) Cleft palate repair: Von Langenbeck Technique. In: Bardach, J. and Morris, H. L. (eds) *Multidisciplinary Management of Cleft Lip and Palate*. Philadephia: Saunders, p. 303.

Markus, A. F., Smith, W. P., and Delaire, J. (1993) Primary closure of cleft palate: A functional approach. *Br J Oral Maxillofac Surg* **31**:71–77.

Moore, M. D., Lawrence, W. T., Ptak, J. J., *et al.* (1988) Complications of primary palatoplasty: A twenty-one-year review. *Cleft Palate J* **25**:156–162.

Mukerji, M. M. (1969) Cheek flap for short palates. *Cleft Palate J* **6**:415–420.

Olin, W., Jr., Morris. J., Geil, J., *et al.* (1974): Contraction of mucoperiosteal wounds after palate surgery in beagle pups. *J Dent Res* **53**(special issue):149(Abstr. 378).

Schweckendiek, W. (1966) Primary veloplasty. In: Schuchardt, K. (ed.) *Treatment of Patients with Clefts of Lip, Alveolus and Palate*. Stuttgart: Thieme.

Schweckendiek, W. and Doz, P. (1978) Primary veloplasty: Long term results without maxillary deformity – a 25 year report. *Cleft Palate J* **15**:268–274.

Senders, C. W. and Fung, M. (2009) Factors influencing palatoplasty and pharyngeal flap surgery. *Arch Otolaryngol Head Neck Surg* May;**117**(5):542–545.

Sommerlad, B. C. (2003) A technique for cleft palate repair. *Plast Reconstr Surg* **112**:1542–1548.

Stark, R. B., Dehaan, C. R., Frileck, S. P., *et al.* (1969) Primary pharyngeal flap. *Cleft Palate J* **6**:381–383.

Wallace, A. F. (1987) A history of the repair of cleft lip and palate in Britain before World War II. *Ann Plast Surg* **19**:266–275.

Whillis, J. (1930) A Note on the muscles of the palate and the superior constrictor. *J Anat* Oct;**65**(Pt **1**):92–95.

PART 3

Orthodontic treatment

Correction of transverse problems in cleft patients using the Maimonides protocol

Julia F. Harfin
Maimonides University, Argentina

Esthetics and improvement of their smile are two of the most important factors for cleft lip and palate patients, and the orthodontist plays a very important role not only in straightening teeth but also in improving the patient's smile.

Due to genetic and environmental processes, failure of fusion between the palatal process and the medial nasal process causes different types of orofacial clefts.

The incidence of hypodontia in children with various types of clefts, inside and outside the cleft region, and the possible association between the cleft and the side of the missing teeth were studied by Shapira *et al.* (2000).

They found a statistically significant difference when they compared cleft with non-cleft patients. Some theories include genetic and environmental factors during teeth development. This congenital absence of permanent teeth has important clinical implications for the treatment and retention plan since there is a close relationship among the number of teeth, the width of the palate, and the facial profile.

A congenitally missing permanent maxillary lateral incisor on the cleft-side is commonly found, with or without a supernumerary tooth in the cleft region.

The constricted palatal morphology is created in part by the width and size of the cleft and may be worsened by primary lip and palate surgery repair performed during childhood (Yang *et al.*, 2012).

The higher prevalence of posterior cross-bite among cleft palate patients has been widely reported and its correction has to be done prematurely in order to compensate for restrained growth.

It is advisable to perform rapid maxillary expansion in growing patients as soon as possible. Successfully separating the midpalatal suture in cleft palate patients can be achieved after or before a bone grafting procedure, but the younger the patient,

the better the result that can be achieved. However, the real challenge is to determine the best protocol to avoid relapse, especially in the transverse dimension.

The type of the scar plays an important role in the stability of the maxillary dental arch width after orthodontic treatment in patients with cleft lip and palate. Similar results have been obtained in growing and non-growing patients with or without a secondary bone graft. Fixed appliance therapy is preferred over a removable appliance for normalization of the position and inclination of the teeth, since better control is achieved with a huge improvement of dental function and esthetics.

A fixed retention wire between the anterior teeth is highly advisable in conjunction with a removable appliance to maintain the arch width obtained. Unfortunately there aren't any special types of brackets or wires to treat all these patients, though new alloys are very useful. The help of a speech therapist is invaluable during and after the orthodontic treatment.

A 9-year old patient was referred for orthodontic treatment. Her chief complaint was the unesthetic appearance of the anterior teeth. She had a unilateral cleft lip and palate with a visible cross-bite on the same side (Figure 12.1). Her smile was asymmetric and the midline was not coincident.

The patient had a convex profile with protrusive lips and she did not like smiling (Figure 12.2).

The front and occlusal photographs confirmed the lack of eruption of the lateral incisors and the midline deviation. Also, there was a significant maxillary arch constriction on the cleft-side in concordance with the palatal scar (Figure 12.3).

There was also significant crowding on the mandibular arch with the Class I molar on the right side and Class II molar on the left side (Figure 12.4). The temporary upper molars were in cross-bite position.

Cleft Lip and Palate Management: A Comprehensive Atlas, First Edition. Edited by Ricardo D. Bennun, Julia F. Harfin, George K. B. Sándor, and David Genecov.
© 2016 John Wiley & Sons, Inc. Published 2016 by John Wiley & Sons, Inc.

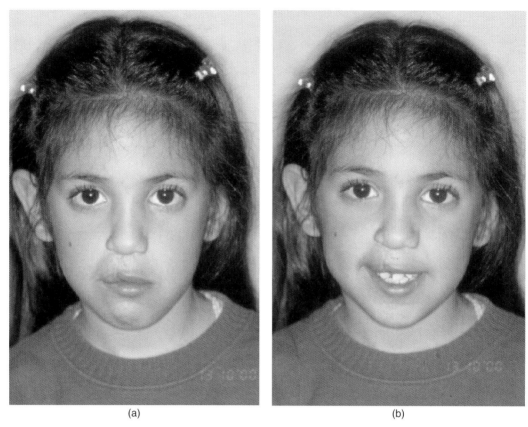

Figure 12.1 (a) Pre-treatment front and (b) smile photographs.

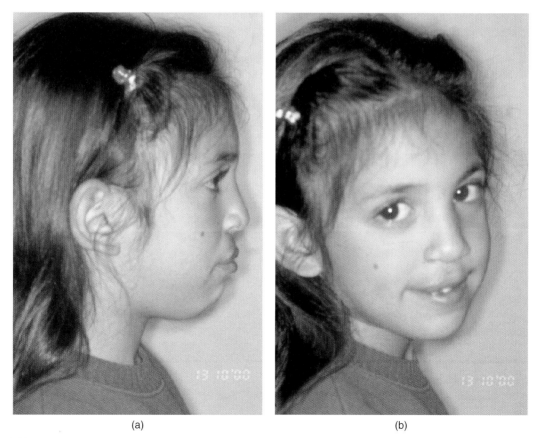

Figure 12.2 (a, b) Pre-treatment lateral photographs.

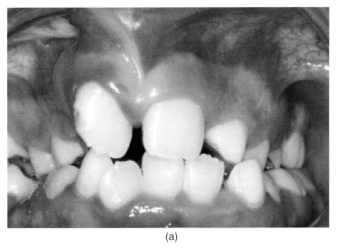
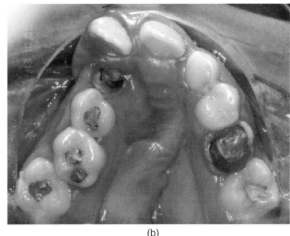

(a)   (b)

Figure 12.3 (a) Front and (b) occlusal photographs at the beginning of treatment.

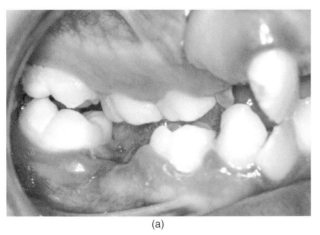
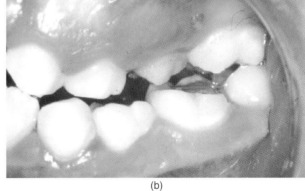

(a)   (b)

Figure 12.4 (a) Right and (b) left photographs from the first visit.

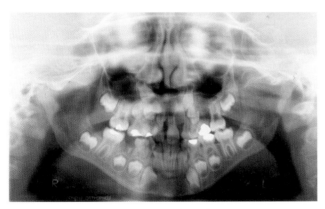

Figure 12.5 Pre-treatment panoramic radiograph.

The panoramic radiograph confirmed the different stages of development of the upper and lower permanent teeth (Figure 12.5). The upper right lateral incisor was absent.

Cephalometric analysis showed that the patient had a severe dolico-phacial pattern with a small and retruded mandible (Figure 12.6a). The constriction of the right upper arch was clearly visible in the occlusal radiograph (Figure 12.6b).

The treatment objectives for the patient were to:
(1) align and level the arches,
(2) normalize overjet and overbite,
(3) improve the transverse dimension,
(4) normalize the occlusal plane,
(5) improve oral health,
(6) improve the smile,
(7) long-term retention.

A fixed rapid maxillary expander with two long mesial arms was placed to improve the width of the maxillary arch. Only one activation a day was recommended in order to preserve the soft palate scar tissue (Figure 12.7). A six-month retention period was advised after completion of the expansion.

Pre-programmed brackets were used to begin the alignment with a Ni-Ti 0.016" arch. An open coil spring was placed to correct the upper midline and to recover space from the right upper canine (Figure 12.8). After the expansion, the right upper canine began its eruption behind the central incisors.

More space was achieved after five months with the open coil spring in place. The right upper canine migrated slowly towards

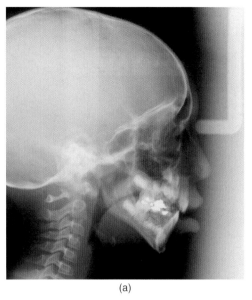

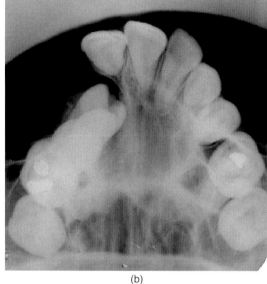

Figure 12.6 Pre-treatment (a) lateral and (b) occlusal radiographs.

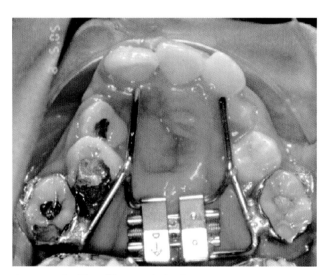

Figure 12.7 Rapid maxillar expander in place.

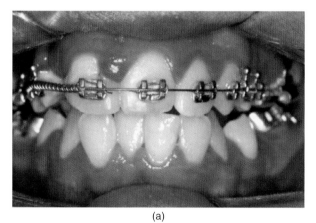

(a)

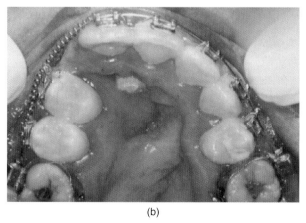

(b)

Figure 12.8 (a, b) Pre-programmed brackets with a Ni-Ti coil spring to begin alignment.

to the newly achieved space without any orthodontic intervention (Figure 12.9).

In the lateral views, alignment of the upper arch was observed with an inactive open coil spring to maintain the canine space (Figure 12.10). Extraction of the lower first bicuspids was indicated. Oral hygiene was fairly good.

Pre-programmed brackets on the lower arch were bonded in order to complete the alignment and leveling. The improvement in the position of the upper right canine was evident (Figure 12.11)

The use of a multistrand arch is recommended to maintain the correct torque and inclination of the upper incisors. To improve smile esthetics, it was necessary to bond the upper right lateral incisor bracket on the upper right canine. Reinforcement of oral hygiene is advisable (Figure 12.12).

The alignment and leveling of the upper and lower arch was almost achieved five months later. The upper right canine was recontoured as a lateral incisor and the first upper bicuspid as a cuspid (Figure 12.13).

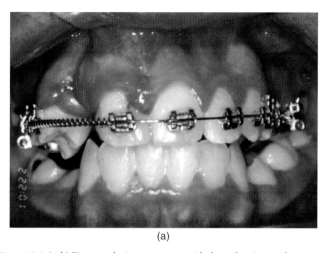
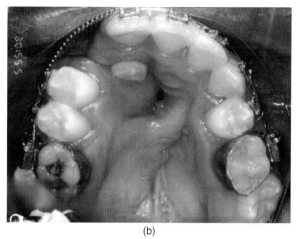

(a)   (b)

Figure 12.9 (a, b) Five months into treatment with the coil spring in place.

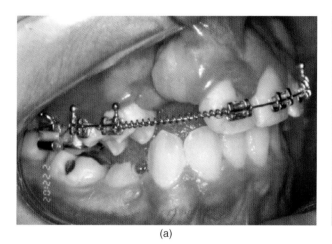
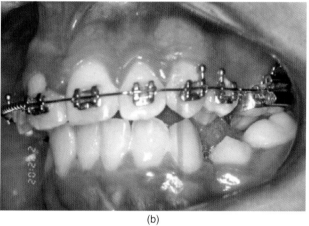

(a)   (b)

Figure 12.10 (a, b) Lateral views at this stage of treatment. Space for the upper right canine was achieved.

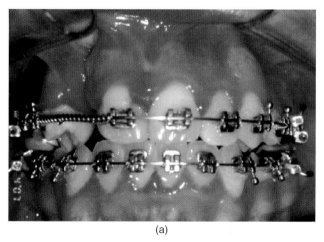
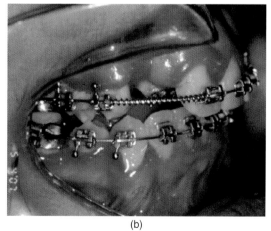

(a)   (b)

Figure 12.11 (a, b) The same type of brackets were bonded on the lower arch.

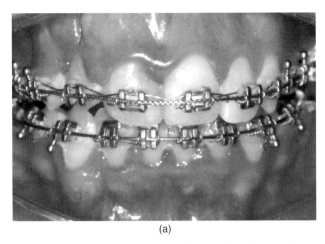 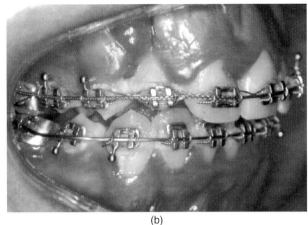

(a)   (b)

Figure 12.12 (a) Front and (b) right lateral photographs at this stage of treatment.

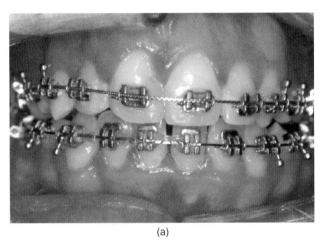 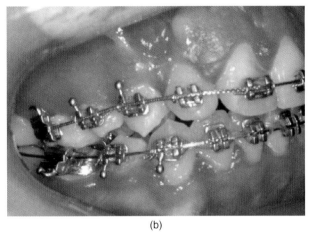

(a)   (b)

Figure 12.13 (a, b) The recontouring of the upper right canine as a lateral incisor is clearly visible.

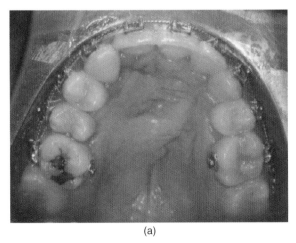 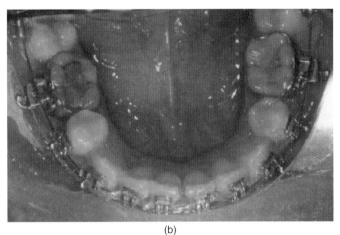

(a)   (b)

Figure 12.14 (a, b) All the extraction spaces are totally closed.

After analyzing the upper and lower arch, it was possible to confirm that all the extraction spaces were closed (Figure 12.14).

The results at the end of the treatment clearly demonstrate the normalization of the upper arch that was achieved, with normal overjet and overbite (Figure 12.15).

The results were evident when panoramic and lateral radiographs at the end of the orthodontic treatment were examined (Figure 12.16).

Final smile photographs confirmed the huge improvement of her smile, and consequently her self-esteem, obtained solely

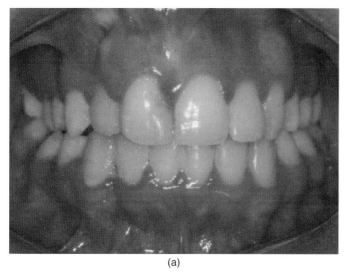

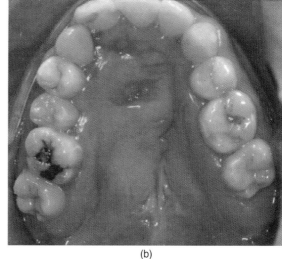

Figure 12.15 (a) Front and (b) occlusal photographs at the end of the treatment.

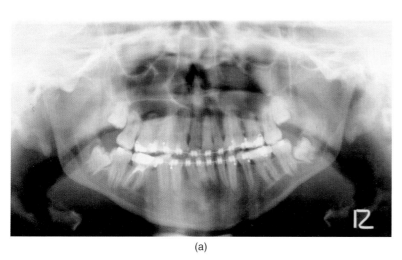

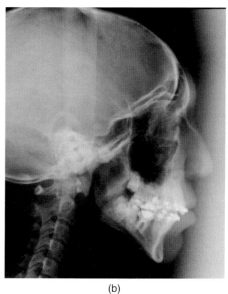

Figure 12.16 (a) Panoramic and (b) lateral radiograph at the end of the orthodontic treatment.

through an orthodontic procedure and without any new surgery (Figure 12.17).

The changes in the transversal width and shape of the maxillary arch when pre- and post-orthodontic treatment photos are compared clearly demonstrate the normalization and correction of the lateral cross-bite and how the soft tissues accompanied this expansion (Figure 12.18).

Removable or fixed expanders can be used, but fixed appliances are normally more controllable and are easy to activate. A long-term retention period is recommended in order to maintain the results.

Ishikawa *et al.* (1998) indicated that the dental arch form in cleft patients is determined by the location and type of scar tissues. Also the degree of relapse has a close relationship with the type of scar and tension of the soft tissues (Nicholson & Plint, 1989).

The following 12-year old patient is another example of the use of this protocol. At the beginning of the treatment, the use of a hyrax-type appliance was highly advisable. As always, the activation was once a day in order to protect the palate soft tissues (Figure 12.19).

The upper left canine began its eruption during the expansion process.

After the RME was completed, brackets on the upper arch were bonded to complete the alignment and leveling of the arches. Space for a future implant to replace the upper left lateral incisor was achieved with the help of an open Ni-Ti coil spring. Also a

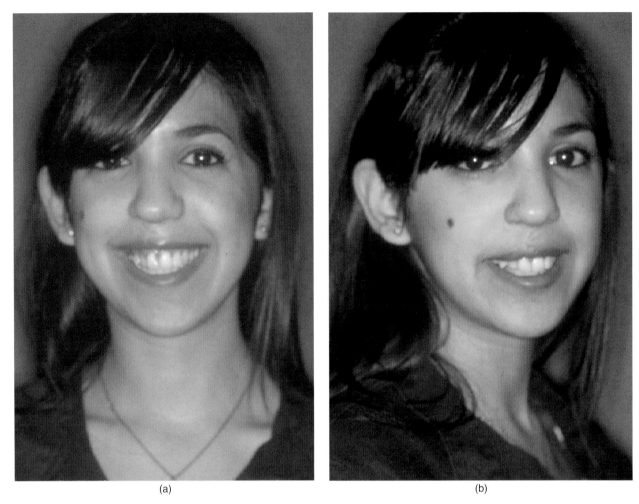

(a)   (b)

Figure 12.17 (a) Front and (b) smile post-treatment photographs.

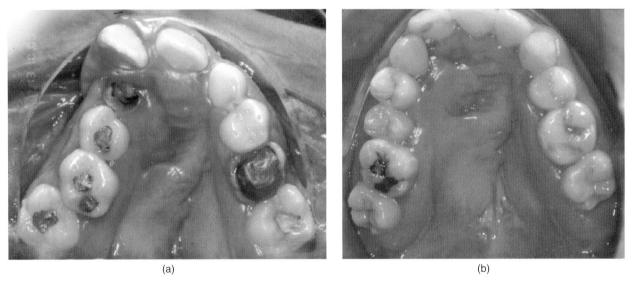

(a)   (b)

Figure 12.18 (a) Pre- and (b) post-treatment occlusal photographs.

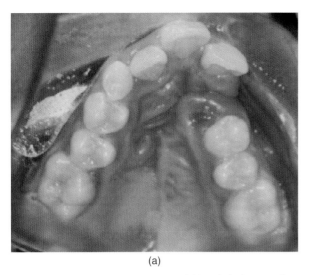

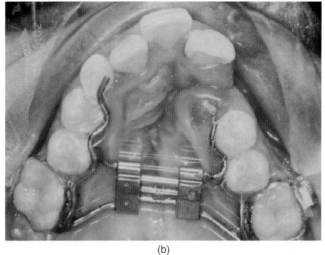

(a)   (b)

Figure 12.19 (a) Occlusal pre-treatment and (b) with the hyrax appliance in place.

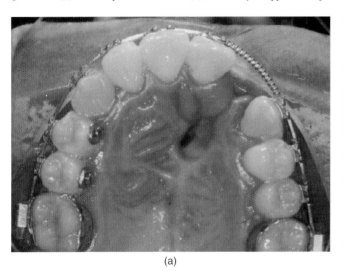

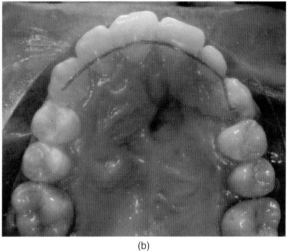

(a)   (b)

Figure 12.20 (a, b) During alignment and with the retention wire in place.

Table 12.1 Protocol results.

	Pre	Post	2 years post
Intercanine width	24.8/2.4	30.4/2.6	29.4/2.3
Inter 1st molar width	49.2/3.7	53.2/3.4	51.9/2.1

fixed retention wire was recommended until the patient was 18 years old (Figure 12.20).

After analyzing 22 patients (9 girls and 13 boys) between 9 and 18 years of age with unilateral cleft lip and palate that were treated with RME, the following results were achieved (Table 12.1). No major differences were found in either sex.

The expansion was greater in the anterior area than in the molar area. The relapse that was observed was in direct relation to the type and length of the retention appliance that was used. It is important to remember that the palatal scar plays an important role during the retention period and, because of this, permanent retention was recommended.

Conclusions

The orthodontist plays an important role within the multi and interdisciplinary cleft team from the child's birth. Patients with cleft palate can be treated satisfactorily solely with orthodontic appliances and without orthognatic procedures (Shultes *et al.*, 2000). Few studies have been conducted to evaluate the post-treatment stability of dental arch widths in patients with unilateral or bilateral cleft lip and palate after orthodontic treatment and retention.

There are some issues to take into account:

(1) the inward forces generated by lip and cheek pressure,
(2) the tension produced by the scar tissue,

(3) the cleft's width and size,

(4) the age of the patient.

It is very important to pay attention to the size of the scar and its location as the causative factor for relapse tendency. The negative effect of the scar in relation to relapse of the incisor lateral position after the orthodontic treatment is something to bear in mind.

An important study was published in order to investigate the relapse tendency in the maxillary dental arch width according to the different types of maxillary arch form (Al-Gunaid *et al.*, 2008). The authors concluded that significant differences in the relapse of interpremolar and intermolar widths were recognized between patients with collapse of the minor or both segments, when compared to patients with symmetrical arch form. However, the real issue is how to prevent relapse of the maxillary expansion. Individualized long-term protocols have to be developed for each patient with a four to six month control during the first five years and a yearly control afterwards. There is no one special appliance that can cater for all patients. The post-orthodontic phase of treatment is fundamental and patients should be made aware of its importance. Longitudinal follow-up studies are necessary.

References

Al-Gunaid, T., Asahito, T., Yamaki, M., *et al.* (2008) Relapse tendency in maxillary arch width in unilateral cleft lip and palate patients with different maxillary arch forms. *Cleft Palate Craniof J* **45**:278–283.

Ishikawa, H., Nakamura, S., Misaki, K., *et al.* (1998) Scar tissue distribution on palates and its relation to maxillary dental arch form. *Cleft Palate Craniofac J* **35**:313–319.

Nicholson, P. T. and Plint, D. A. (1989) A long-term study of rapid maxilllary expansion and bone grafting in cleft and palate patients. *Eur J Orthod* **11**:186–192.

Shapira, Y., Lubit, E., and Kuftinek, M. (2000) Hypodontia in children with various types of cleft. *Angle Orthodontist* **70**:16–21.

Shultes, G., Gaggl, A., and Kärcher, H. (2000) A comparison of growth impairment and orthodontic results in adult patients with clefts of palate and unilateral clefts of lip, palate and alveolus. *Brit J Oral Max Surg* **38**:26–32.

Yang, C. J., Pan, X. G., Qian, Y. F., and Wang, G. M. (2012) Impact of rapid maxillary expansion in unilateral cleft lip and palate patients after secondary alveolar bone grafting: Review and case report. *Oral Surg Oral Med Oral Pathol Oral Radiol* **114**:25–30.

CHAPTER 13

Changes in arch dimension after orthodontic treatment in cleft palate patients

Julia F. Harfin

Maimonides University, Argentina

Dental abnormalities are commonly seen in patients with palatal clefts. Often at least one tooth is missing, irregularities in shape and size are present, and the teeth on both sides of the cleft can be more affected with hypoplasia.

The frequency of missing teeth in the maxilla in and outside the cleft area is higher in patients with cleft lip and palate when compared to normal patients. The absence of one or more teeth in the permanent dentition near the cleft area is frequently observed. The permanent lateral incisor is affected the most. It is possible that some damage to the germs of the permanent teeth may occur during hard palate surgery (Lekkas *et al.*, 2000). The new surgery protocol tends to avoid this problem.

The presence of periodontal problems in teeth close to the cleft areas was reported by Brägger and Almeida (Brägger *et al.*, 1990; de Almeida *et al.*, 2007, 2009). They reported that in individuals with clefts the prevalence of recession was 10 times higher than that in the same teeth in individuals without cleft. But in patients with high control of their oral hygiene there is no reason to expect more prevalence and severity of periodontal pockets and gingival inflammation than in other areas of the same patient. There are no major differences regarding gender and age. The timing and sequencing of the treatment is also very important.

The transverse dental and skeletal relationship is one of the main considerations to take into account when the treatment plan is designed, since anterior and lateral cross-bite occurs in more than 70% of repaired cleft lip and palate patients (Li & Lin, 2007). Upper arch crowding, absent teeth, and posterior cross-bite are very common in growing and non-growing patients with repaired uni- or bilateral cleft lip and palate. The need for maxillary expansion in many patients with labial and palatal clefts has been recognized in nearly all the

publications related to orthodontic treatment over the past 60 years (Nicholson & Plint, 1989).

Orthodontic upper arch expansion using RME (rapid maxillary expansion) or a quad-helix (slow dental expansion) is normally carried out to correct the compression of the palate present in almost all of these patients. Due to social and economic circumstances, many of these patients were not treated during their childhood and adolescence. As a result of this, a significant compression of the maxilla is present (Figures 13.1 and 13.2).

In order to avoid or diminish this compression, a new surgical protocol was designed. Unfortunately there is no specific cephalogram nor specially designed bracket to treat this type of patient.

Orthodontics plays an important role in the normalization of the maxillary transverse deficiency during childhood, adolescence or adulthood. Maxillary transverse expansion is one of the best options to correct a narrow or collapsed upper jaw. The ideal time is before the total eruption of the permanent teeth but it is possible to achieve good results in non-growing patients too. A strict weekly control is necessary to avoid any dental side-effects such as bone recessions on the labial side.

In young patients, the normalization of the transverse dimension allows a better coordination of the upper and lower arches. A slight and controlled overexpansion is also indicated. The results vary among appositional bone on the alveolar process, buccal tipping of bicuspids and molars, or a combination of both.

Correction of the anterior and posterior cross-bite is recommended as soon as possible in order to achieve a better intermaxillary relationship, improve esthetics and reduce functional disturbances. The width of the cleft and/or the scar are determinants when choosing the best treatment plan for these particular patients.

Cleft Lip and Palate Management: A Comprehensive Atlas, First Edition. Edited by Ricardo D. Bennun, Julia F. Harfin, George K. B. Sándor, and David Genecov.
© 2016 John Wiley & Sons, Inc. Published 2016 by John Wiley & Sons, Inc.

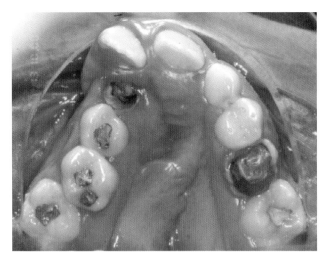

Figure 13.1 A 17-year-old woman.

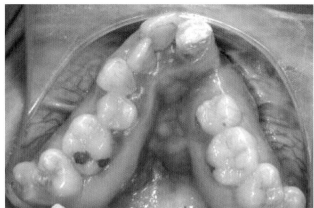

Figure 13.2 A 37-year-old woman.

It is necessary to control the relapse that could occur to some extent after the orthodontic treatment as a consequence of the constriction of the scar tissues in the palate in combination with high pressure from the facial muscles. Nicholson and Plint (1989) reported interdental width relapse in more than 50% of patients treated with only RME and no difference between bone graft and non graft patients. Dental arch transverse stability is normally reached when overexpansion with good lateral posterior occlusion is achieved after orthodontic treatment and in conjunction with a long-term retention plan.

The following patients demonstrate how a significant improvement can be achieved. When RME is used, only one turn a day to activate the appliance is suggested instead of twice a day, in order to protect the constricted palatal soft tissue.

The 39-year-old patient in Figure 13.3 is a clear example. He was looking for some orthodontic and/or prosthetic treatment to improve his smile and avoid orthognatic surgery. He had received primary lip repair and palatoplasty, but he could not remember when the surgery had been performed. The upper right lateral incisor was absent and an important palatal cross-bite on the same side was present in concordance with the deviation of the midline. Mesiorotation of the first right molar was also evident (Figure 13.3). The direction and type of the scar is clearly visible.

The Class III molar on the right side and Class II molar on the left side were present. The upper right lateral incisor was missing and the right premolars were in cross-bite position (Figure 13.4).

The panoramic radiograph confirmed the absence of the lateral incisor and the size of the cleft. An important cavity on the left first molar is also present. The right upper second molar and all the third molars had been extracted (Figure 13.5a). Cephalometric analysis indicated a dolichofacial patient (VERT -1.16) with a retruded mandible (−14.9 mm according to McNamara *et al.*, 2003) (Figure 13.5b).

The treatment objectives were to:
(**1**) align and level the arches,
(**2**) normalize the dental midlines,

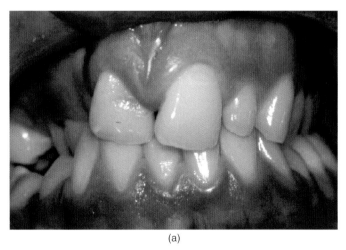

(a)

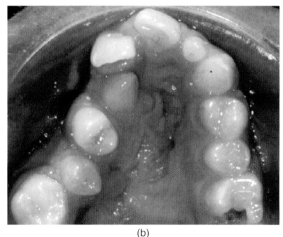

(b)

Figure 13.3 (a) Front and (b) occlusal pre-treatment photographs.

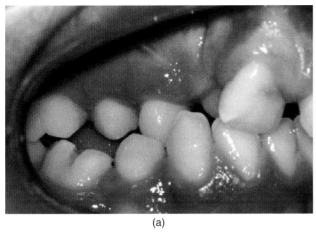 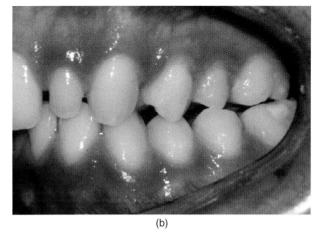

(a)   (b)

Figure 13.4 (a) Right and (b) left sides before treatment.

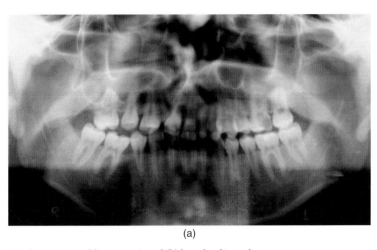 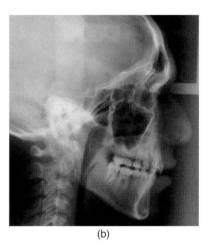

(a)   (b)

Figure 13.5 Pre-treatment (a) panoramic and (b) lateral radiographs.

(3) correct the right cross-bite,

(4) open the upper right lateral space for prosthesis replacement,

(5) improve periodontal health,

(6) improve smile esthetic,

(7) long-term retention plan.

Even though he was a non-growing patient, a rapid-maxillary expander was placed to improve the maxillary arch. One day activation for 21 days was suggested and then pre-programmed brackets with a round Ni-Ti-Cu arch wire (0,014″) were placed (Figure 13.6).

After six months the rapid-maxillary expander was removed and, keeping in mind the normalization of the midline, an open coil spring between the upper right canine and the central incisor was placed (Figure 13.7). Changes in the arch form and size are noticeable.

Once the midline correction had been achieved, the next step was to obtain adequate space to replace the upper lateral incisor. A plastic tooth with a conventional bracket was ligated to the arch and then an open Ni-Ti coil spring was placed mesial to the first bicuspid to normalize the position the right canine (Figure 13.8).

For esthetic and functional reasons, a provisional fixed prosthesis was placed the same day the brackets were removed (Figure 13.9).

The comparison between the buccal front photograph pre- and post-treatment confirmed the significant improvement in his smile and dental occlusion. The treatment objectives were fully achieved. Now, the gingival line was parallel to the occlusal plane and the midlines were coincident (Figure 13.10).

When pre and post-intraoral maxillary occlusal photos were compared, an important and effective change was confirmed. The inter bicuspid and intercanine width were clearly improved (Figure 13.11). To maintain the results a removable plaque was recommended for long-term use, for 20 hours a day. This is the only method that will avoid relapse due to disfunctional muscular activity. This protocol appears to be extremely useful in growing and non-growing cleft palate patients.

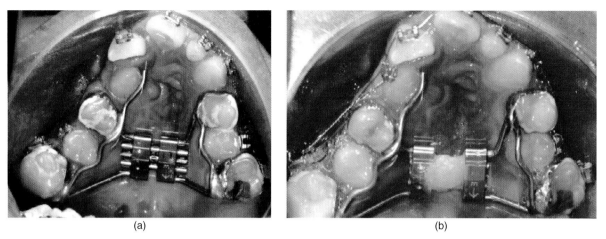

Figure 13.6 RME (a) 3 and (b) 21 days after activation period and with pre-programmed brackets in place.

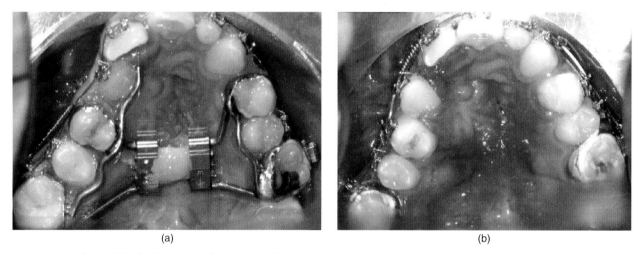

Figure 13.7 (a) Before and (b) after the removal of the rapid-maxillary expander.

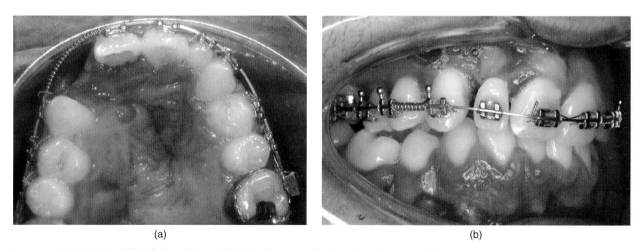

Figure 13.8 (a) Occlusal and (b) right lateral view with Ni-Ti coil spring and a plastic lateral incisor in place.

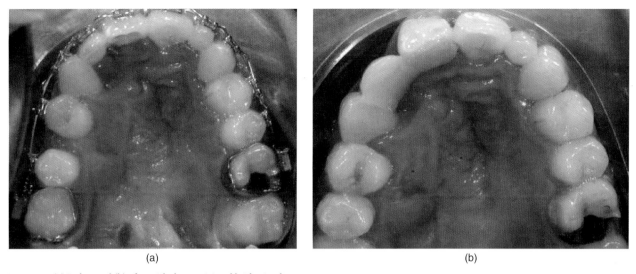

Figure 13.9 (a) Before and (b) after with the provisional bridge in place.

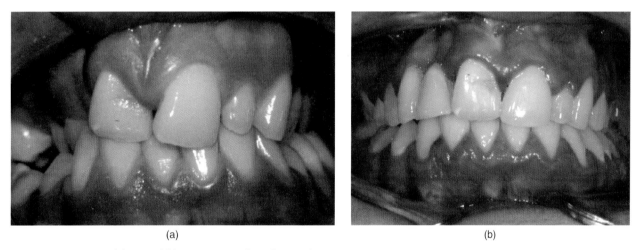

Figure 13.10 Comparison (a) pre- and (b) post-treatment front photographs.

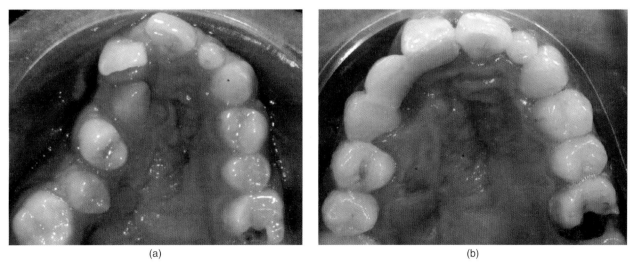

Figure 13.11 Comparison maxillary arch (a) pre- and (b) post-treatment.

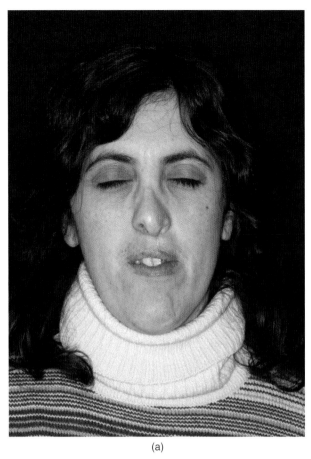
(a)

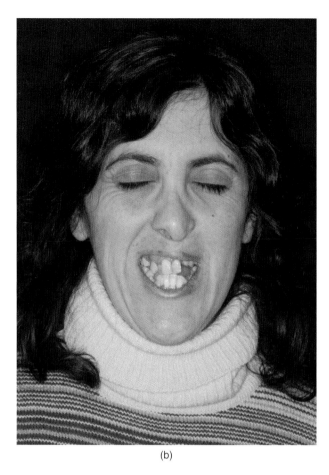
(b)

Figure 13.12 Pre-treatment (a) front and (b) smile photographs.

For esthetic and functional reasons, a provisional fixed prosthesis was placed the same day the brackets were removed (Figure 13.9).

The next patient was a very challenging case. She came to the Orthodontic Department seeking a second opinion. She was very unhappy with her smile. The first dentist had suggested the extraction of the upper central and lateral incisors and also the canines, replacing them with implants. Due to economic circumstance she refused the idea. The second dentist recommended the same extractions and a removable prosthesis to replace them.

The facial photographs show a non-esthetic smile and an asymmetric face. The nose was deviated to the right and the chin to the left. To that date, she had received eight different surgeries to repair the lip, palate, and nose (Figure 13.12).

After analyzing the front dental photographs, important crowding and malocclusion were confirmed. The midlines were not coincident and a lateral compression was evident on both sides. In the lower arch there was a clear lack of space for the lower canines. The result was an important facial and dental asymmetry. She also complained about difficulties in eating and swallowing. It was difficult to move the mandible to achieve centric relation due to significant maxilla–mandibular discrepancy. No temporomandibular clicks or pain were present (Figure 13.13).

The right lateral view showed a remarkable Class III canine and the absence of the right second molar. On the left side a significant cleft between the first left bicuspid and the central incisor was visible. The upper left lateral incisor and canine were absent (Figure 13.14). Additionally, a severe Curve of Spee was present.

The triangular shape of the maxilla was the result of the type of cleft palate surgery and lack of functional activity. Two upper bicuspids were extracted when she was an adolescent (Figure 13.15a) as well as the second right lower molar. The lower arch had 10 mm discrepancy (Figure 13.15b).

The panoramic Rx confirmed the absence of the left lateral, canine, and first bicuspid, the upper right bicuspid and the second right lower molar. The canine's root was positioned very high and horizontally (Figure 13.16a) and the lower left third molar was mesio-inclined. The asymmetry was confirmed in the lateral Rx and also the significant anterior openbite (Figure 13.16b). Cephalometric analysis indicated a severe dolichofacial pattern (VERT-2.23) with an increased lower facial height (61°).

The patient's treatment objectives were to:
(1) align and level the arches,
(2) normalize the overjet and overbite,
(3) improve the occlusal plane,
(4) improve smile esthetics,
(5) maintain periodontal health,

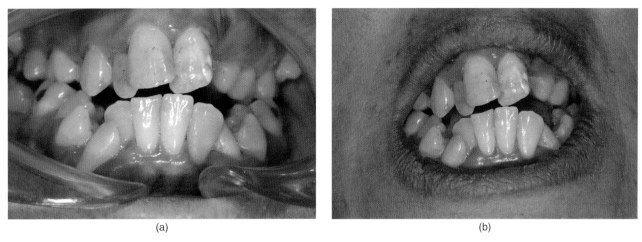

Figure 13.13 Pre-treatment (a) front and (b) smile dental photographs.

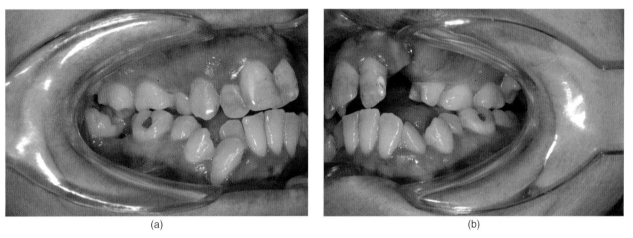

Figure 13.14 (a) Right and (b) left side at the initial phase. The upper left cleft and lack of space are evident.

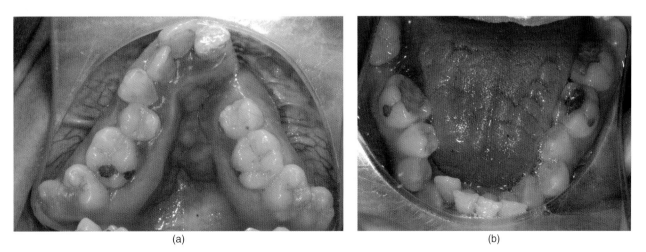

Figure 13.15 Pre-treatment (a) upper and (b) lower arches. The triangular shape of the maxillary arch is very interesting.

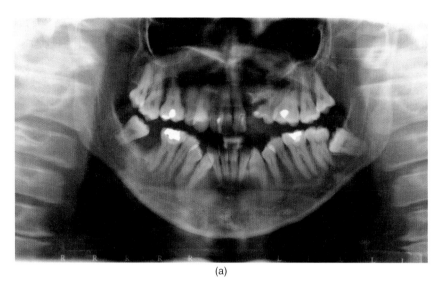

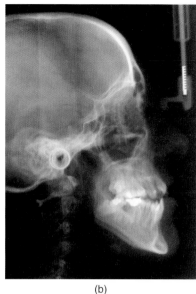

(a)

(b)

Figure 13.16 Pre-treatment (a) panoramic and (b) lateral radiograph.

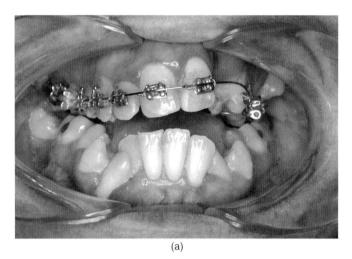

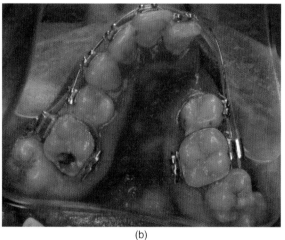

(a)

(b)

Figure 13.17 (a, b) Pre-programmed brackets with 0.016″ Ni-Ti-Cu archwire to begin alignment.

(6) open up space for the absent left lateral incisor and canine,
(7) long-term retention.

The treatment plan was proposed according to the malocclusion, the bone structure, and the amount of periodontal support.

To improve periodontal health, monthly oral hygiene instruction including scaling and root planning was highly recommended.

To begin the alignment and leveling of the upper arch, pre-programmed 0.022″ metal brackets were placed in conjunction with a 0.016″ Ni-Ti-Cu archwire. Activation took place every 6 weeks (Figure 13.17).

Eight months later the upper arch was almost normal. Bands were placed on the second molars in conjunction with a Ni-Ti open coil that was placed on the left side aiming for enough space to replace the absent teeth. At this time brackets on

the lower arch were bonded for initial alignment and leveling (Figure 13.18).

Extraction of the lower right first premolar was decided upon to compensate the previous extraction of the upper first bicuspids. In order to facilitate the extraction a bracket was bonded on the lower first right bicuspid three months before the extraction. This method is very useful in order to loosen the bicuspid and facilitate the extraction process, avoiding root and/or bone fractures (Figure 13.19).

The process of closing the extraction space began two weeks later. For esthetic reasons a plastic lateral incisor and canine with brackets were added to the upper archwire. This procedure boosted her self-esteem to such a degree that she decided to begin studying to become a dental hygienist (Figure 13.20).

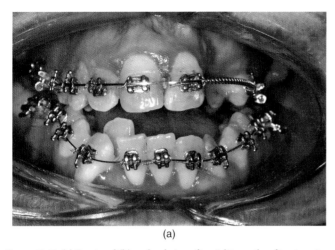
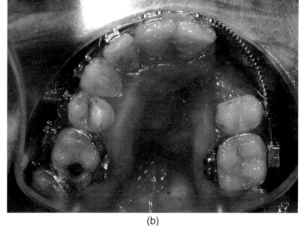

Figure 13.18 (a) Front and (b) occlusal view after eight months of treatment.

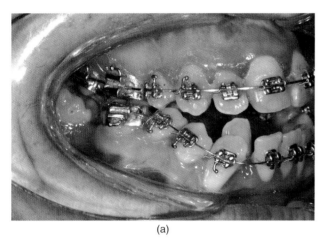
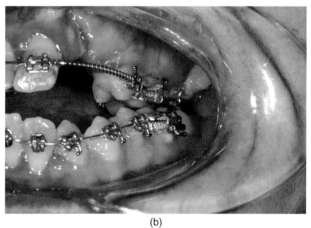

Figure 13.19 (a) Right and (b) left lateral view after eight months of treatment.

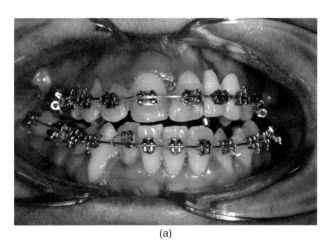
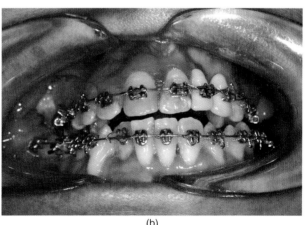

Figure 13.20 (a, b) Frontal photographs after 16 months in treatment with plastic teeth in place to enhance esthetics.

Tubes on the second molars were added in order to help normalization of the occlusal plane. The Class I canine on the right side was almost correct (Figure 13.21). Oral hygiene was fairly good.

Experience has demonstrated that it is important to maintain the last archwire for at least three to four months to prevent any type of relapse, particularly on the left side. The relapse on the scar zone of soft tissue is difficult to predict. On the

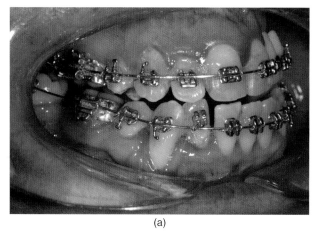

(a)   (b)

Figure 13.21 (a, b) The right and left canines are nearly in place.

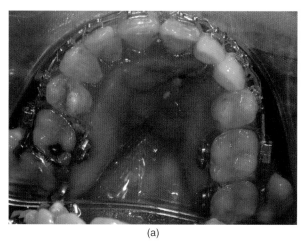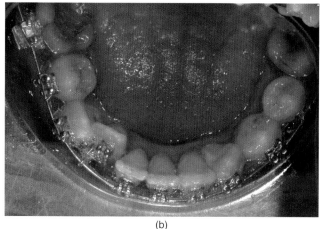

(a)   (b)

Figure 13.22 (a) Upper and (b) lower arcades after 23 months in treatment.

lower arch, the space from the first bicuspid extraction was totally closed and the lateral incisor moved into its place (Figure 13.22).

The patient decided to finish the treatment as her husband got a new job in another province. Figure 13.23 shows the results after two years of treatment. A provisional fixed prosthesis was cemented the same day the brackets were debonded. To maintain the treatment results, a removable upper and lower retainer was recommended indefinitely (Figure 13.23). The midlines were normalized and the overjet and overbite were improved.

The post-treatment facial photographs demonstrate the results that were achieved with just an orthodontic procedure. Not only were the upper and lower teeth aligned, but the improvement of the soft tissues was remarkable. She promised us she would continue her studies in her new location (Figure 13.24).

The panoramic Rx and the lateral radiograph at the end of the treatment were coincident with the clinical results. No signs of bone or root resorption were present (Figure 13.25).

This is a clear example of the results that can be achieved when the teeth are moved with very slow and gradual forces. When low load deflection arches are used, the teeth are moved with the bone, while when strong forces are used, the teeth are moved through the bone. Comparison of the pre and post-treatment maxillary arch confirms this hypothesis (Figure 13.26).

Comparison of the pre and post-treatment panoramic radiographs shows the complete normalization of the Curve of Spee (Figure 13.27).

Analyzing the front photographs before and after treatment demonstrates not only that the smile improved but also the patient's attitude towards life. Now when she smiles she feels more confident and her eyes are a clear reflection of this attitude (Figure 13.28). The positive effect of the orthodontic treatment on her appearance and self-esteem is remarkable and easy to see.

The real challenge is how to maintain the results. It is important to control the new arch form and its width since the lateral musculature tends to return to the original shape.

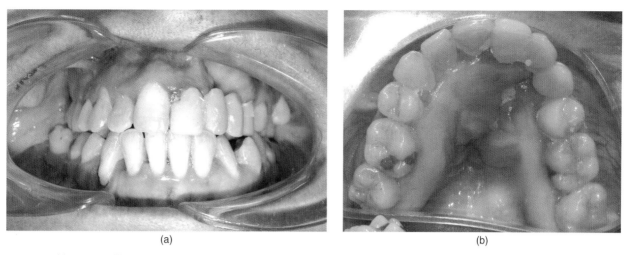

Figure 13.23 (a) Front and (b) occlusal photographs at the end of the treatment with a temporary bridge in place.

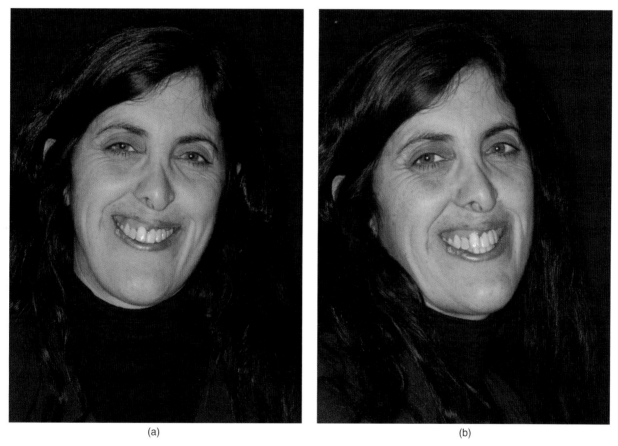

Figure 13.24 (a, b) Final smile photographs.

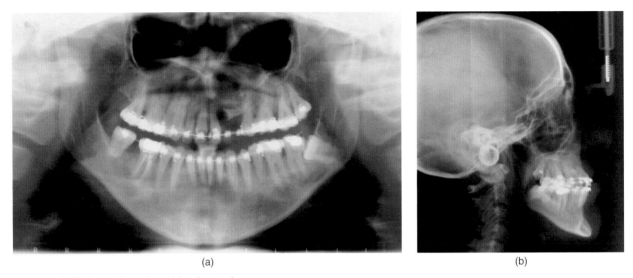

Figure 13.25 (a, b) Final radiographs with brackets in place.

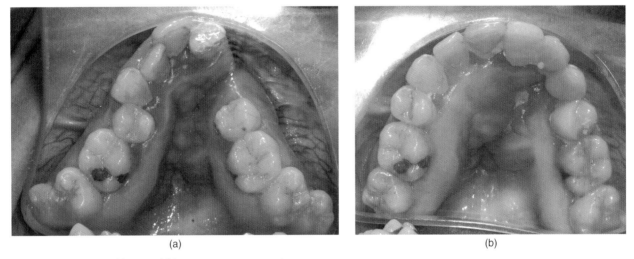

Figure 13.26 Comparison (a) pre- and (b) post-treatment upper arch.

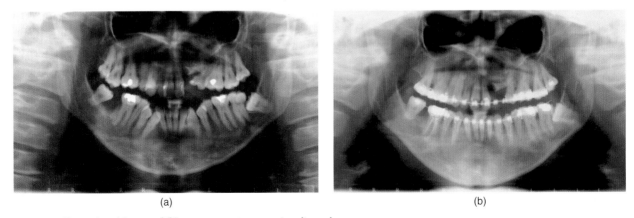

Figure 13.27 Comparison (a) pre- and (b) post-treatment panoramic radiographs.

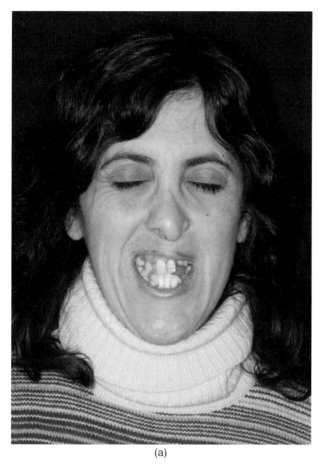 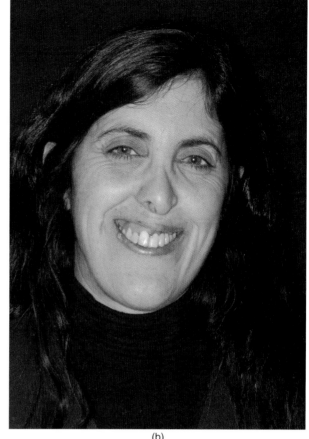

(a) (b)

Figure 13.28 (a) Pre- and (b) post-treatment frontal photographs.

Experience has demonstrated that expansion is less stable at the first bicuspid and cuspid area and for that reason it is recommended to leave the expander in as long as possible. The author recommends the use of a transpalatal bar with lateral arms as a retention appliance for a long period of time.

Normalization of the soft tissues of the face is the "gold standard" in all patients that were born with cleft lip and palate clefts (Sinko *et al.*, 2005; Marcusson *et al.*, 2001; Thomas *et al.*, 1997). Better results have been achieved with the application of this protocol over the last seven years in conjunction with an individualized orthodontic treatment. Designing new surgical procedures in these cleft lip and palate patientsis recommended in order to not alter their facial growth as a consequence of the scars after surgical repair.

Conclusions

The patient's treatment was unconventional but it was successful in significantly improving her masticatory function and smile along with favorable dental and facial esthetics without any orthognatic surgery.

It is possible to achieve the normalization of the transverse dimension only with orthodontic movements without bone-grafting procedures. The secret is to move teeth with very low and continuous forces and in this way the teeth will move with bone to their new position.

The role of the orthodontist in the cleft palate team is very important. He/she has to manage the maxillofacial growth in children and improve the occlusion and prepare the mouth for future prosthetic and reconstructive procedures in the adults.

The maintenance of the corrected transverse dimension is very challenging and along-term control is necessary to keep the palatal width that was achieved, thus the retention plan is one of the most important phases of the treatment plan (Nicholson & Plint, 1989).

Different designs of functional appliances are suggested in order to maintain the results, since it is very difficult to control the muscular activity, particularly on the cleft-side. An acrylic plate in the maxilla to maintain the expansion achieved is recommended.

Comprehensive care from infancy to adult age is essential to achieve esthetic and functional result. The orthodontist has a great responsibility in managing this type of patient, as this deformity also influences ability to find a job, gain social credit, find a spouse, and so on. While men can hide scars or conceal a retruded maxilla with a moustache, a nice and harmonious smile is key for success in our society.

References

Bragger, U., Nyman, S., Lang, N. P., *et al.* (1990) The significance of alveolar bone in periodontal disease: A long term observation in patients with cleft lip, alveolus and palate. *J Clin Periodont* **17**:370–384.

De Almeida, A. L., Madeira, L. C., Freitas, K. C., *et al.* (2007) Cross-sectional evaluation of the presence of gingival recession in individuals with cleft lip and palate. *J Peridontol* **78**:29–36.

De Almeida, A. L., Gonzalez, M. K., Greghi, S. L., et al. (2009) Are teeth close to the cleft more susceptible to periodontal disease? *Cleft Palate Craniofac J* **46**(**2**):161–165.

Li, W. and Lin, J. (2007) Dental arch width stability after quahelix and edgewise treatment in complete unilateral cleft lip and palate. *Angle Orthod.***77**:1067–1072.

Lekkas, C., Latief, B. S., ter Rahe, S. P. N., and Kuijpers-Jagtman, A. M. (2000) The adult unoperated cleft patient: Absence of maxillary teeth outside the cleft area. *Cleft Palate Craniofac J* **37**(**1**): 17–20.

Marcusson, A., Akerlind, I., and Paulin, G. (2001) Quality of life in adults with repaired complete cleft lip and palate. *Cleft Palate Craniofac J* **38**:379–385.

Marcusson. A., Paulin, G., and Ostrup, L. (2002) Facial appearance in adults who have cleft lip and palate treated in childhood. *Scand J Plast Reconstr Surg Hand Surg* **36**:16–23.

Nicholson, P. T. and Plint, D. A. (1989) A long term study of rapid maxillary expansion and bone grafting in cleft lip and palate patients. *EJO* **11**:186–192.

Sinko, S., Jeagsch, R., Prechtl, V., *et al.* (2005) Evaluation of esthetic, functional and quality-of-life outcome in adult cleft-lip and palate patients. *Cleft Palate Craniofac J* **42**:355–361.

Thomas, P. T., Turner, S. R., Rumsey, N., *et al.* (1997) Satisfaction with facial appearance among subjects affected by a cleft. *Cleft Palate Craniofac J* **34**:226–231.

CHAPTER 14

Real orthodontic treatment in adult cleft patients

Julia F. Harfin

Maimonides University, Argentina

The aim of this chapter is to show the positive soft tissues changes that can be achieved using only orthodontics. With a worldwide incidence of 1/750–1000 live births, facial clefts rank as the second most frequent congenital malformation. Facial esthetics is a very important aspect of an individual's general perception of life (Richman *et al.*, 1985; Persson *et al.*, 2002). Treating these patients is a real challenge from a biomechanical, functional, and esthetic point of view since they may have scars on the lip, nasal deformity, missing teeth, poor occlusion in a retruded maxilla, or a combination of all of these that have to be taken into account when determining the treatment objectives. Cleft lip and palate patients may also have a less attractive facial appearance, more speech problems, and in general more psychological problems. Management of labial–alveolar–palatal clefts requires an interdisciplinary rather than a multidisciplinary team (Chuo *et al.*, 2008).

As has been described and demonstrated, the ideal time to perform lip and nose surgical reconstruction is between 2–6 months of age or at a minimum of 10 pounds of weight and it is advisable to complete the closure of the palate before 12 months of age. However, in many cases economic constraints delay treatment time and patients come to the clinic when they are adults, looking for a way to improve their esthetic and functional conditions. Some come with previous surgeries and others without.

Patients' expectations concerning the results of the treatment have increased over the years and the importance of psychological aspects on health-related quality of life is undeniable.

Strict plaque control with regular application of fluoride solutions is recommended to avoid periodontal tissue destruction and formation of carious lesions (Bragger *et al.*, 1992).

Rx and cephalometric studies are similar to those performed on normal patients, however the results must be individualized to each patient. There are no specific brackets to treat these patients but pre-programmed brackets are recommended. It is advisable to use low load deflexion wires, especially near the cleft. The activation period should be further apart: every 4 to 8 weeks. Since the arch shape and the size of the maxillary dental arch are influenced by palatal muscle strain and scar retraction after several different surgeries, an individualized long-term retention plan is inevitable (Yang *et al.*, 2012).

The means of achieving good orthodontic results in patients who cannot afford additional orthognatic surgery will be demonstrated. Dental and skeletal post-treatment long-term stability is a fundamental point in the treatment of cleft-palate patients and the following three patients clearly illustrate these concepts.

Patient 1

This patient is a clear example of the results that can be achieved considering the previous statements. She was sent to the Orthodontics Department at Maimonides University, for a second opinion, after two years of treatment in another hospital. Her main concern was the lack of alignment in the maxilla and her uneven smile. She had been told that with orthodontic treatment only her smile could not be improved since she was 32 years old. She also presented with pain at the temporomandibular joints, more evident on the right side.

The front photograph showed an asymmetric face. The left side was longer than the right one. The height of the eyes, the ears and the upper lip gave evidence of this asymmetry, and this was more evident when she smiled (Figure 14.1).

A retruded upper lip was confirmed on the lateral photograph as well as an open nasolabial angle (Figure 14.2).

Cleft Lip and Palate Management: A Comprehensive Atlas, First Edition. Edited by Ricardo D. Bennun, Julia F. Harfin, George K. B. Sándor, and David Genecov.
© 2016 John Wiley & Sons, Inc. Published 2016 by John Wiley & Sons, Inc.

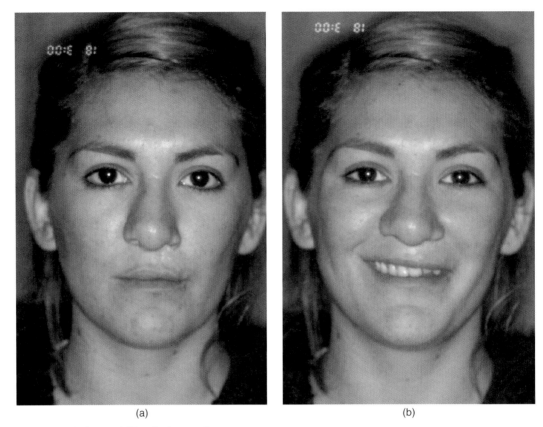

Figure 14.1 Pre-treatment (a) front and (b) smile photographs.

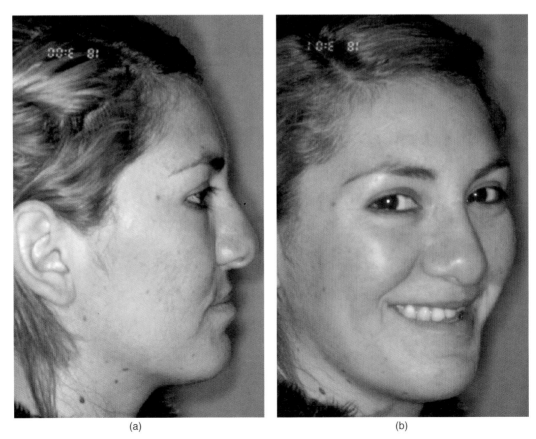

Figure 14.2 (a) Profile and (b) smile profile pre-treatment photographs.

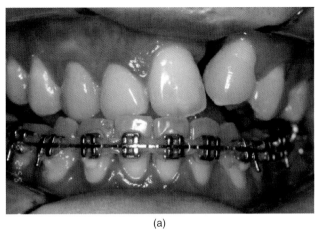
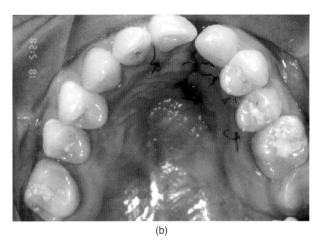

(a) (b)

Figure 14.3 (a) Front and (b) upper occlusal pre-treatment photographs.

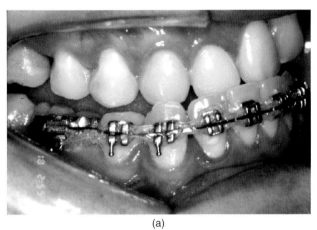
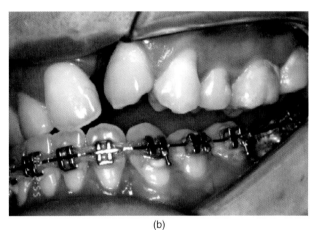

(a) (b)

Figure 14.4 Pre-treatment (a) right and (b) left sides.

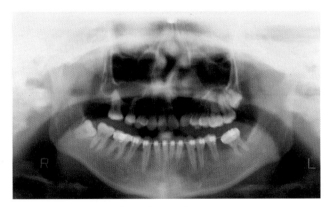

Figure 14.5 Panoramic radiograph at the first appointment.

When the front photograph was analyzed, the absence of the left central and lateral incisor was confirmed (Figure 14.3). The midlines were not coincident and all the teeth of the right side were clearly displaced to the left. There was no visible space to replace the upper left central and lateral incisors, and at the same time overjet and overbite were diminished. One month earlier she had received a palatal surgery and some sutures were still in place. In the first appointment she came with brackets on the lower arch and an edge-to-edge bite in the anterior region. Oral hygiene was good.

The first upper right molar and the first lower left molar had been extracted five years earlier. Negative overbite and overjet in conjunction with an important lateral openbite were present (Figure 14.4). The cleft on the left side was totally visible.

The absence of the upper central and lateral left incisors, the first upper right molar and the first lower left molar were confirmed in the panoramic Rx (Figure 14.5). The lower right third molar and the upper left third molar had not erupted at the time. No root resorption was noticeable.

Treatment objectives

After studying her radiographs, photographs, and models, it was decided that the ideal treatment would be a new orthodontic treatment in combination with an orthognatic surgery to improve facial, functional and dental esthetics.

As a result of economic and personal problems the patient refused another surgery, and an orthodontic treatment with all its limitations was proposed.

The objectives were to:

(1) align and level the arches,
(2) correct the midline,
(3) normalize the overjet and overbite,
(4) achieve a Class I canine and molar,
(5) improve the nasolabial angle,
(6) improve the smile,
(7) replace the absent teeth,
(8) long-term retention.

Pre-programmed brackets were used in the upper arch with a Ni-Ti open coil spring (Figure 14.6) with the objective of opening up space for the incisors that were absent. At this point, no bracket on the upper left canine was recommended.

The first phase for alignment and leveling was performed with a round Ni-Ti-Cu archwire in conjunction with a Ni-Ti open coil

spring activated every four weeks, as can be observed in the lateral photographs (Figure 14.7).

It is highly recommended to use a low load deflexion arch with a continuous force. Three months later, some space was open (Figure 14.8) and there were some changes in the position of the upper right central incisor.

Seven months later almost the whole space required to replace the upper left central incisor was achieved. A central incisor plastic tooth with a bracket was added to improve the anterior esthetic (Figure 14.9). At the same time a button was placed on the mesial side of the canine to improve its position.

Four months after the last photograph, the canine was nearly in the right position but a little more space was necessary to replace the upper left lateral incisor. The midlines were almost coincident. Some stripping in the lower anterior region was performed to normalize lower incisor position (Figure 14.10). Overjet and overbite were improved.

Similar results were observed on the lateral views. A 0.016″ × 0.016″ SS arch with a continuous elastic was used in the lower

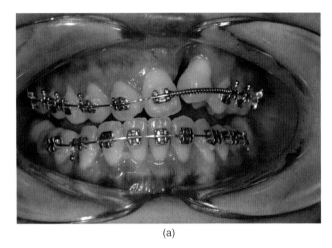
(a)

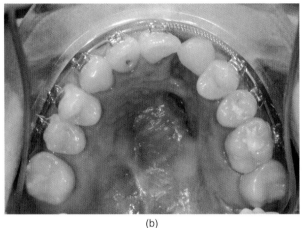
(b)

Figure 14.6 (a) Front and (b) occlusal photographs with a Ni-Ti coil spring in place.

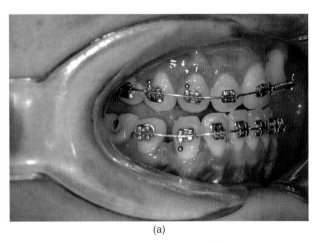
(a)

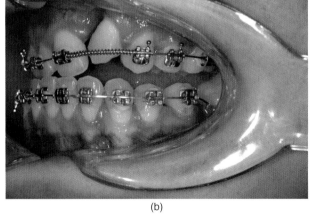
(b)

Figure 14.7 (a, b) Lateral views at the beginning of the treatment.

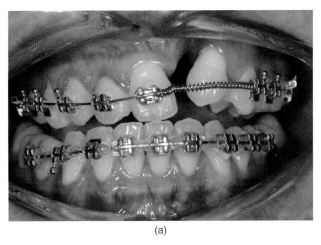
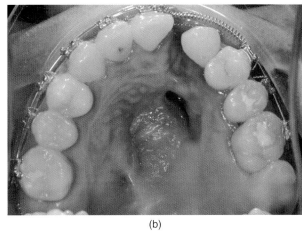

(a)   (b)

Figure 14.8 (a) Front and (b) occlusal view after three months of treatment.

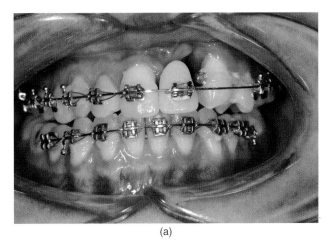
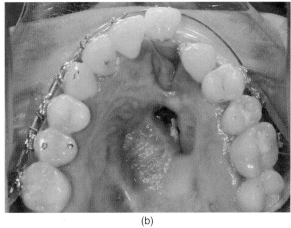

(a)   (b)

Figure 14.9 Front and occlusal photographs after seven months in treatment with a plastic central incisor in place to enhance esthetics.

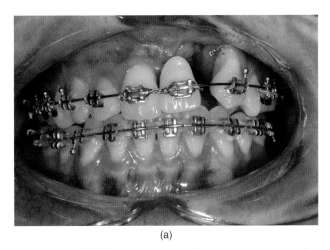
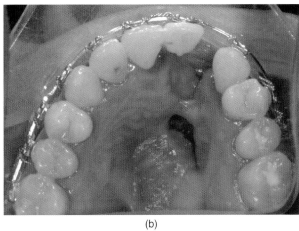

(a)   (b)

Figure 14.10 (a, b) Midlines are almost coincident and overjet and overbite are improved.

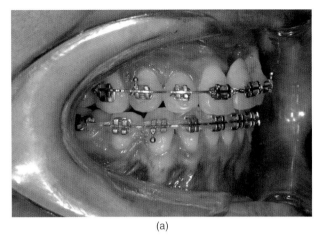

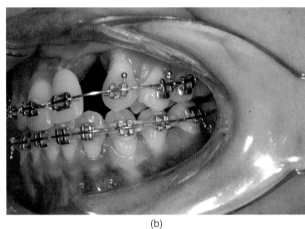

(a)
(b)

Figure 14.11 (a, b) Lateral views at this stage of treatment.

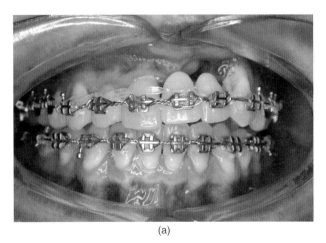

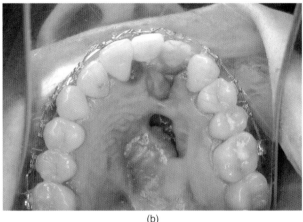

(a)
(b)

Figure 14.12 (a) Frontal and (b) occlusal photographs with the central and lateral plastic incisors in place.

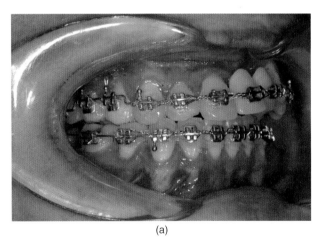

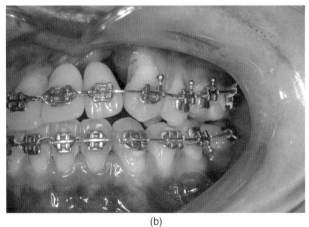

(a)
(b)

Figure 14.13 (a) Right and (b) left sides with SS archwires with compensatory bends in place.

arch and a 0.016″ × 0.022″ SS in the upper arch (Figure 14.11). A Class I canine on the right side was achieved. Oral hygiene was normal.

When space for the upper left lateral incisor was obtained, another plastic incisor with a bracket was placed with an elastic up to the right second bicuspid, in order to maintain the midline (Figure 14.12).

The Class I molar and canine on the right side were completely normal (Figure 14.13) but there was a little difference on the left side. A few bends in the archwire were required to improve

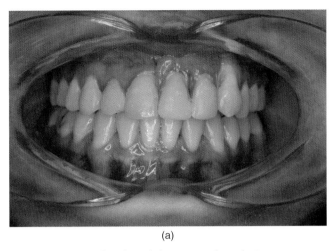

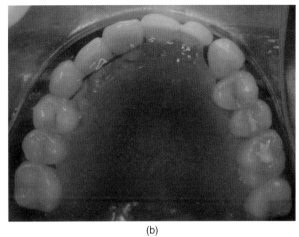

Figure 14.14 (a, b) Final results with the provisional prosthesis.

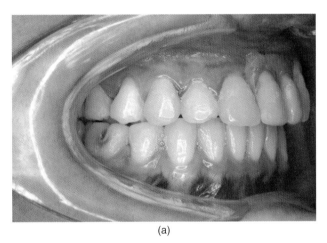

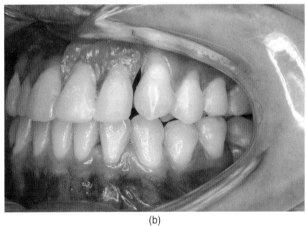

Figure 14.15 (a, b) Lateral views at the end of the treatment.

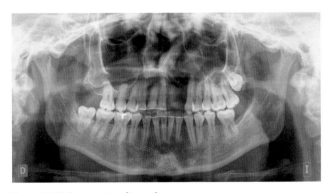

Figure 14.16 Panoramic radiograph post-treatment.

occlusion. Some periodontal attachment was lost on the canine's mesial side because of the proximity of the cleft.

The front and occlusal photograph at the end of the treatment confirmed the excellent results that were obtained (Figure 14.14). The absent incisors on the left side were replaced with a provisionary plastic prosthesis until the patient could afford the final one. To maintain the results, a fixed retention wire was placed on the upper right side.

Similar results were observed on the lateral views (Figure 14.15). The gingival tissues were completely normal and the gingival line was parallel to the occlusal plane. Overjet and overbite were within normal values.

The final panaromic Rx confirmed the clinical results (Figure 14.16). In the left anterior region there was enough space for future implants and good parallelism among the roots was present. All the space of the lower left first molar was closed and no signs of root resorption were visible.

The final front photographs show the unexpected results that were obtained. The improvement of the visible scar is clearly noticeable and the smile reflects a happy woman (Figure 14.17).

An important improvement of the profile was confirmed. The nasolabial angle and the upper lip were almost normal (Figure 14.18).

Comparison of the pre- and post-treatment profile photographs is remarkable. Not only the thickness and position of

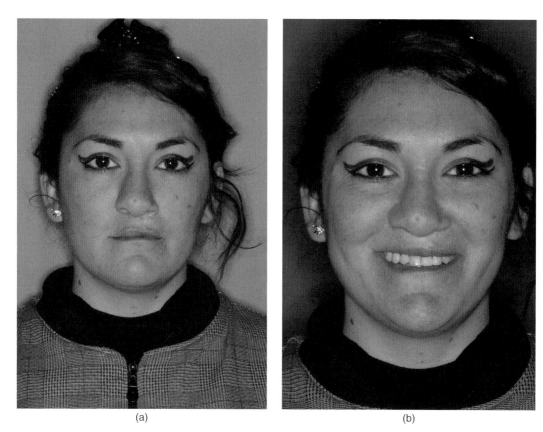

Figure 14.17 (a, b) Final front photographs.

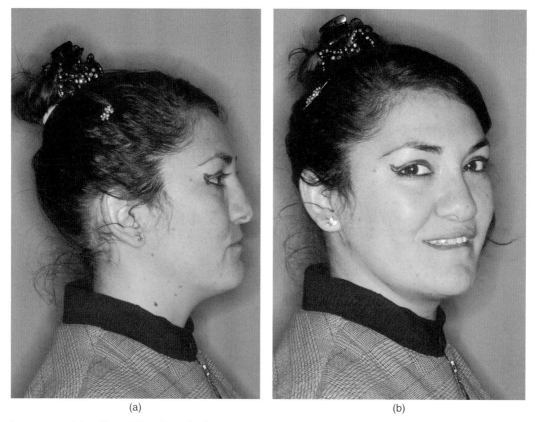

Figure 14.18 Post-treatment (a) profile and (b) smile profile photographs.

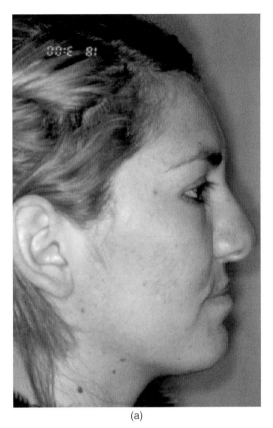

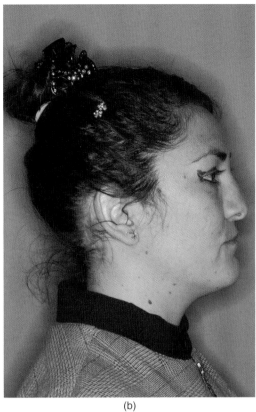

(a)   (b)

Figure 14.19 Comparison (a) pre- and (b) post-treatment profile.

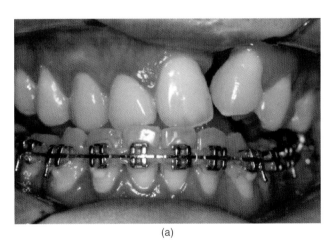

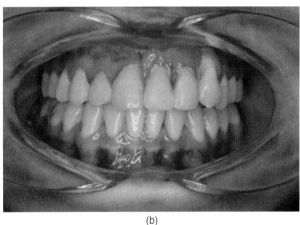

(a)   (b)

Figure 14.20 The benefits of the orthodontic treatment were remarkable when the (a) pre- and (b) post-treatment front photographs were compared.

the upper lip but also the nasolabial angle were really improved (Figure 14.19).

The comparison of the photographs from the first visit and at the end of the orthodontic treatment with the provisional removable prosthesis in place confirms that is possible to recover the occlusion in this type of patient solely with orthodontics (Figure 14.20). The occlusal plane is parallel to the gingival line. The gingival tissues, the midline, overjet, and overbite are completely normalized.

The same results were observed when the maxillary occlusal photographs were analyzed. Despite the age of the patient, the changes in the upper arch shape and width were clearly visible (Figure 14.21).

Excellent results were confirmed when the pre and post-treatment front photographs were compared (Figure 14.22). There is an important improvement not only of the smile but also of the position of the upper lip.

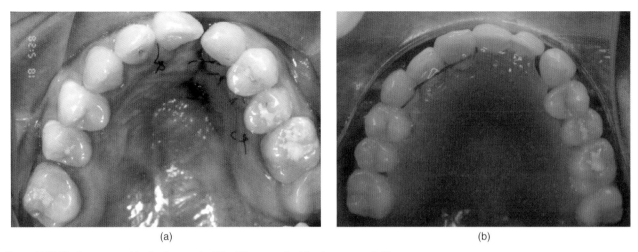

(a)   (b)

Figure 14.21 The improvement in the shape and width of the upper dental arch was remarkable.

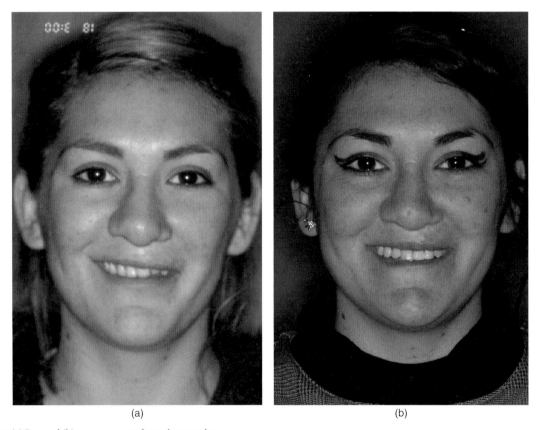

(a)   (b)

Figure 14.22 (a) Pre- and (b) post-treatment front photographs.

Three years later the results were even better. The soft tissues were more relaxed (Figure 14.23) and the smile line continues stable. The patient's smile and eyes were the best evidence of her happiness.

The front dental and occlusal upper photographs confirmed the stability of the results (Figure 14.24). It is important to highlight good oral hygiene. For economic reasons she continued using the same removable prosthesis.

Similar results were observed on the right and left sides (Figure 14.25). The occlusion was improved and no temporomandibular symptoms were present.

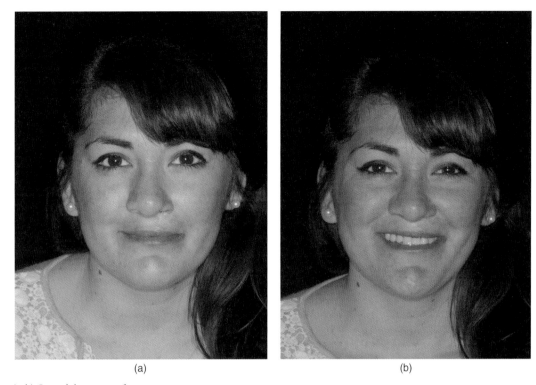

Figure 14.23 (a, b) Control three years after treatment.

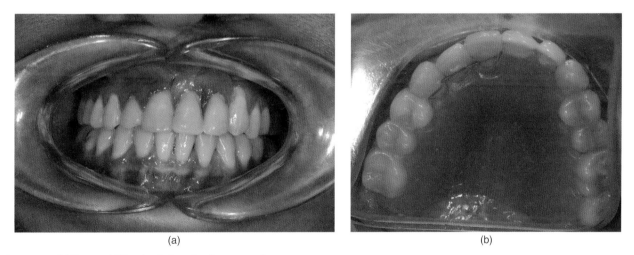

Figure 14.24 (a) Front and (b) occlusal view after three years of treatment.

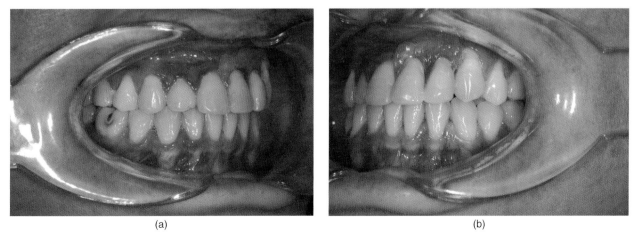

Figure 14.25 (a, b) Control three years post-treatment.

Patient 2

This is a 28-year-old patient who was sent to the Orthodontic Department to improve the position of the upper canines before the design of a new prosthesis. It was a very challenging situation as he had lost the premaxilla during the first months of life. No temporomandibular symptoms were present. He had an unesthetic smile and some scars were clearly visible on the upper lip (Figure 14.26).

A convex profile with protrusion of the lower lip can be observed on the lateral photograph. The nasolabial angle was almost normal (Figure 14.27).

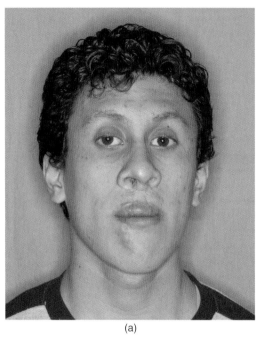
(a)

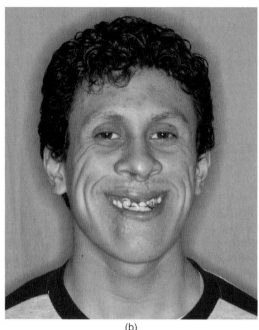
(b)

Figure 14.26 Pre-treatment (a) front and (b) smile photographs.

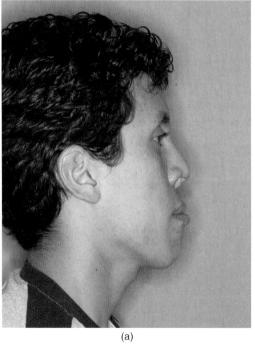
(a)

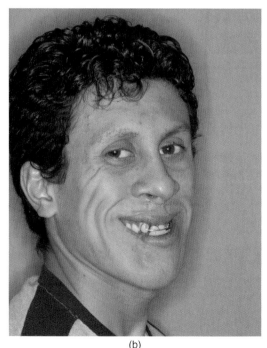
(b)

Figure 14.27 Pre-treatment (a) lateral and (b) smile photographs.

The following front photographs show the anterior region with and without the removable prosthesis. The absence of the premaxilla and the central and lateral incisors could be acknowledged (Figure 14.28).

Also see the lateral views with the removable appliances in place. The previous dentist covered the occlusal surfaces with an acrylic plate (Figure 14.29).

The upper occlusal photograph showed a triangular shape and confirmed the lack of space for the replacement of the upper incisors. The upper arch collapse was evident. In the lower arch, significant crowding was visible (Figure 14.30).

The panoramic rx confirmed the mesioinclination of the upper right and left canines and the absence of the premaxilla. The first left lower molar had an endo-perio problem (Figure 14.31).

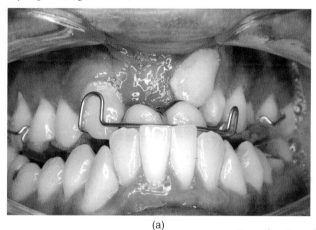

(a)

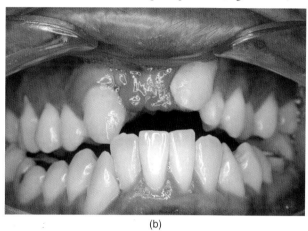

(b)

Figure 14.28 Front view (a) with and (b) without the removable prosthesis in the first appointment.

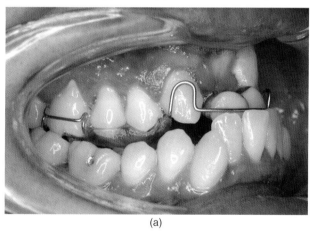

(a)

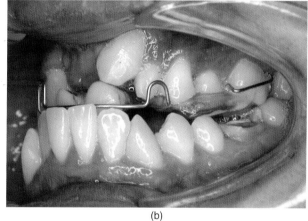

(b)

Figure 14.29 (a, b) Lateral views at the beginning of the treatment.

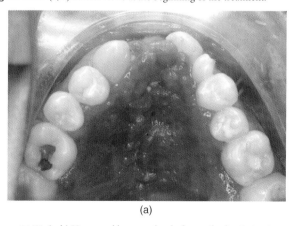

(a)

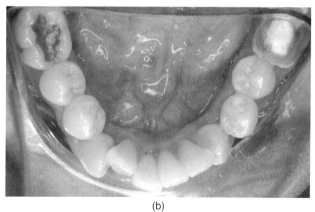

(b)

Figure 14.30 (a, b) Upper and lower arches before orthodontic treatment.

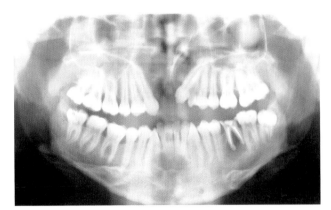

Figure 14.31 Panoramic radiograph pre-treatment. Note the absence of the premaxilla and the inclination of the upper canines.

On the lateral Rx a negative overjet and overbite were confirmed. The length of the mandibular corpus was greater than normal, according Rickett's analysis (Figure 14.32).

The treatment objectives were to:

(1) align and level the arches,
(2) provide enough space to replace the central and lateral upper incisors,
(3) improve dental and facial esthetics,
(4) improve periodontal health.

To achieve these objectives, extraction of the first left lower molar and the first right lower bicuspid was decided upon as well as the temporary upper left canine.

A fixed maxilllary expander was placed in the maxilla in order to improve its shape. For esthetic reasons a plastic central incisor was added. As an adult patient with no more growth expected, only one turn a day was recommended for just four weeks (Figure 14.33).

To align and level the upper arch, preprogrammed brackets were recommended along with a Ni-Ti-Cu 0.018″ wire. A Ni-Ti

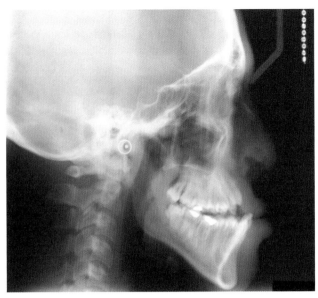

Figure 14.32 The absence of the premaxilla was confirmed on the lateral radiograph.

coil spring was added to help the normalization of the position of the upper right and left canine in order to gain space for a future prosthesis (Figure 14.34).

Four months later, brackets were placed in the lower arch. The extraction of the lower first molar had been done three months earlier and the second bicuspid was distalized with very low and controlled forces. Class III elastics on the left side were suggested (Figure 14.35).

No bracket on the lower right canine was placed until the extraction of the first lower right bicuspid was performed. Class III elastics between the first lower first bicuspid to the first upper left molar were indicated (1/8 medium) with 20 hours per day use (Figure 14.36).

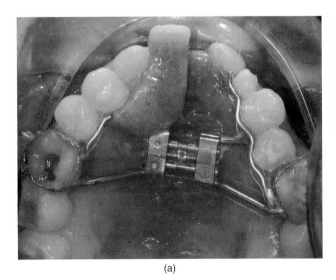

(a)

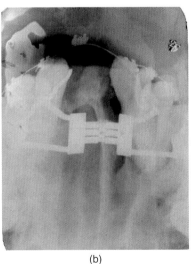

(b)

Figure 14.33 Occlusal (a) photograph and (b) radiograph with the maxillary expander in place.

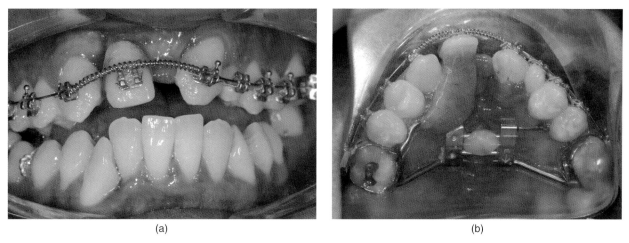

Figure 14.34 (a) Front and (b) occlusal view with the frontal Ni-Ti coil spring in place.

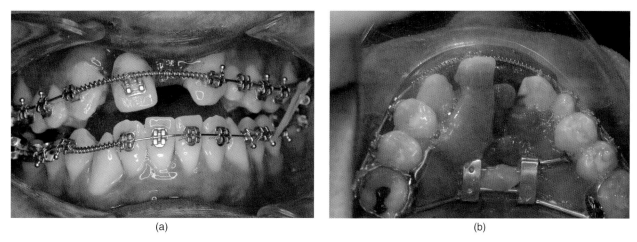

Figure 14.35 (a, b) After four months in treatment, Class III elastics on the left side were recommended.

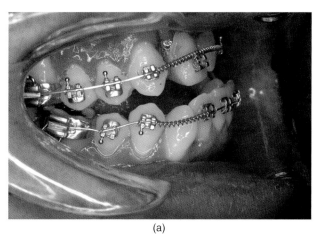
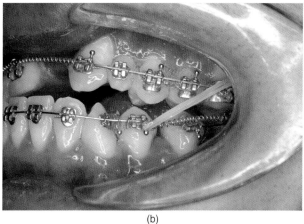

Figure 14.36 (a) Right and (b) left photographs at this stage of treatment.

Five months later the entire space for the replacement of the four incisors was almost complete. The upper arch seemed to be pretty normal (Figure 14.37).

In the lateral views, closing of the extraction spaces was observed. A SS archwire (0.016″ × 0.022″) in the upper and lower arch was recommended in order to improve torque (Figure 14.38).

To improve the lateral occlusion, Class III elastics were recommended (1/8 medium force). The use of two elastics per side for 16–20 hours a day was suggested (Figure 14.39).

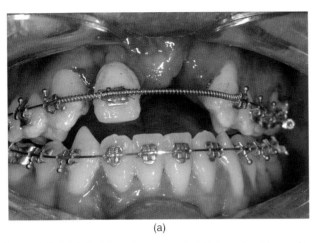
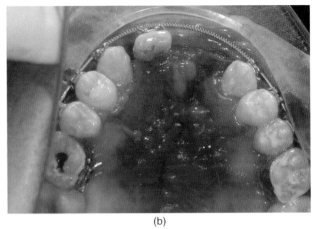

(a)   (b)

Figure 14.37 (a, b) The intercanine space and width have almost been achieved.

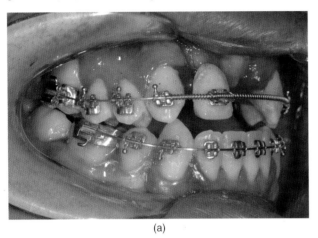
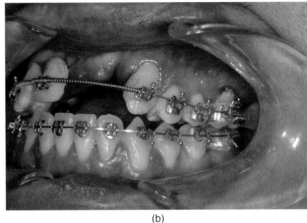

(a)   (b)

Figure 14.38 (a, b) The right and left extraction spaces were totally closed.

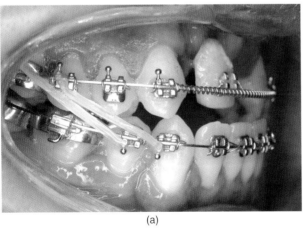
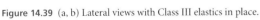
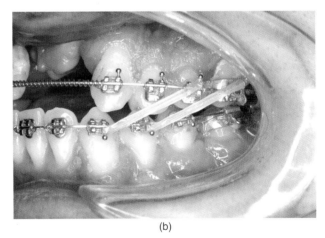

(a)   (b)

Figure 14.39 (a, b) Lateral views with Class III elastics in place.

When the upper arch showed enough space for replacement of the upper incisors, and all the extraction lower spaces were closed, the pre-programmed retention plan was put in place (Figure 14.40).

A removable appliance with the four replacement upper incisors was placed the same day the brackets were removed.

Oral hygiene was fair (Figure 14.41). A standard overjet and overbite were achieved, midlines were normalized and the occlusal plane was almost normal.

At the upper arch the removable prosthesis was in place and a fixed multistrand wire was placed on the lower arch to maintain the position of the anterior teeth (Figure 14.42).

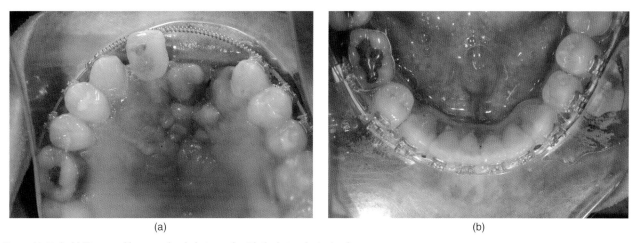

(a)   (b)

Figure 14.40 (a, b) Upper and lower occlusal photograph with the last archwire in place.

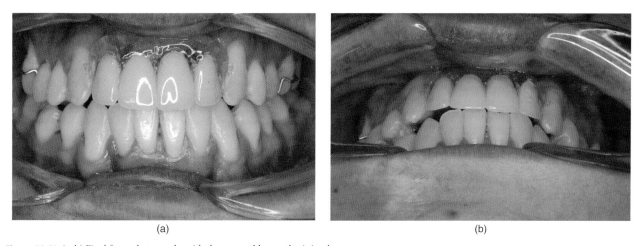

(a)   (b)

Figure 14.41 (a, b) Final front photographs with the removable prosthesis in place.

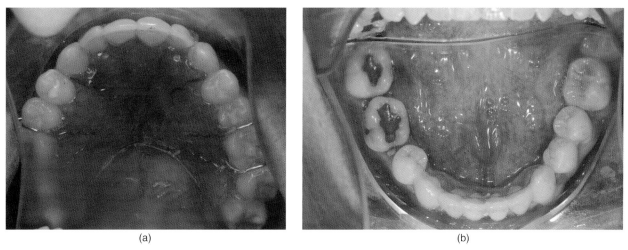

(a)   (b)

Figure 14.42 (a, b) Upper and lower occlusal photographs at the end of the treatment.

The right and left photographs confirmed the results achieved (Figure 14.43).

The improvement of the smile was better than expected not only on the front photographs but also on his profile. The relation between the upper and lower lip improved despite the age of the patient and the lack of premaxilla (Figure 14.44).

The lateral final photographs showed a harmonious profile despite the absence of the premaxilla (Figure 14.45).

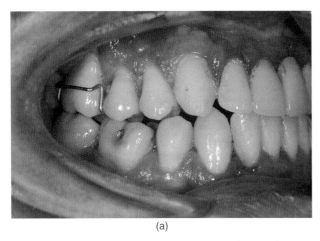

(a)   (b)

Figure 14.43 (a, b) The lateral views with the upper prosthesis in place.

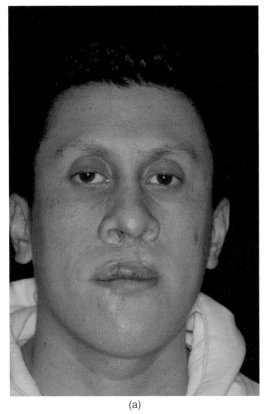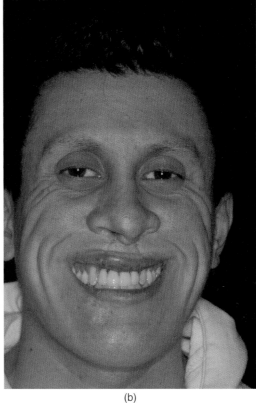

(a)   (b)

Figure 14.44 (a, b) Final front photographs.

The comparison between pre- and post-treatment front oral photographs clearly demonstrate the results that were achieved in relation to the dental alveolar process (Figure 14.46).

The same results were visible when the facial photographs were analyzed. No maxillary distraction osteogenesis was performed using a rigid external distraction device with dentoskeletal anchorage (Akarsu *et al.*, 2012). The boost to his self-esteem allowed him to continue his studies (Figure 14.47).

Despite his age, 28, with no more active growth, the change in the palatal arch was remarkable. The acrylic removable appliance not only replaced the four upper incisors but also acted as a transversal retainer (Figure 14.48). It is widely accepted that maintenance of the palatal transversal dimension is one of the critical points in the treatment of the cleft palate patients.

Despite the absence of the premaxilla in a non-growing patient, normalization of the upper arch form was achieved solely through an orthodontic procedure.

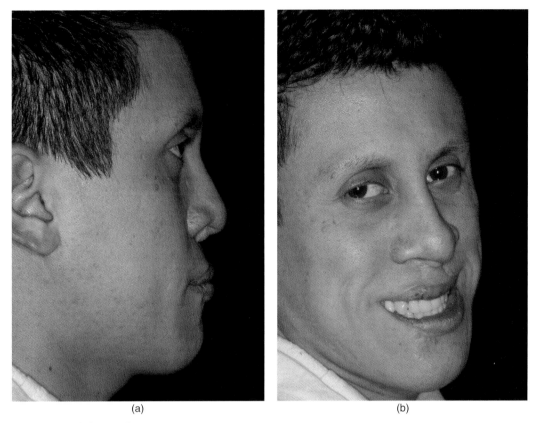

Figure 14.45 (a, b) Final lateral photographs.

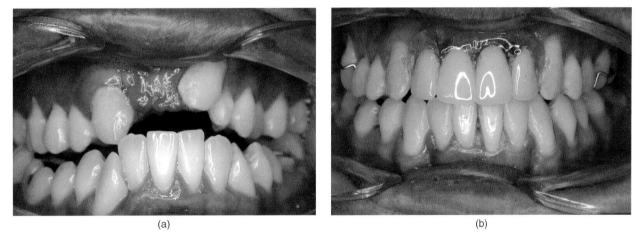

Figure 14.46 Comparison (a) pre- and (b) post-treatment front photographs.

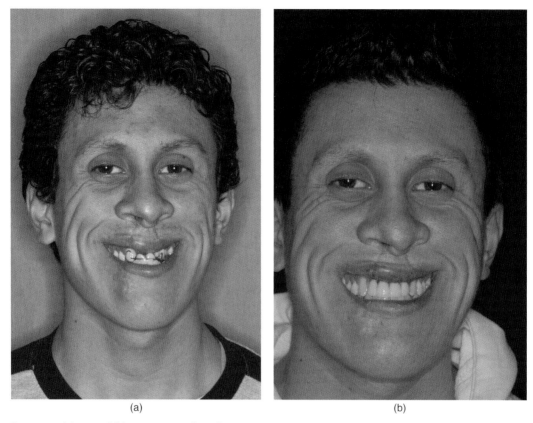

(a)   (b)

Figure 14.47 Comparison (a) pre- and (b) post-treatment front photos.

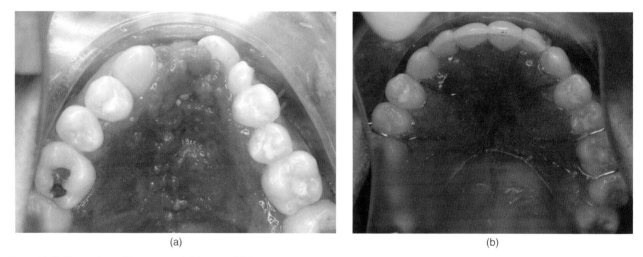

(a)   (b)

Figure 14.48 Comparison of the upper arch (a) pre- and (b) post-treatment.

Patient 3

This patient was sent to the Orthodontic Department in search of another opinion. Her former orthodontist suggested an orthognatic surgery that included a maxillary advancement and retroposition of the mandible. For economic reasons the patient refused the treatment. Other colleagues offered to extract the front teeth and replace them with implants, but she didn't want to lose more teeth. She had an asymmetric face with a concave profile with a short philtrum. The upper lip is clearly retrusive (Figure 14.49).

The front photograph showed an inverted occlusion and the absence of the left upper right lateral incisor. The midlines were almost normal. The upper occlusal photograph confirmed the absence of the left lateral upper incisor, the left 1first upper molar and the first right bicuspid. No open cleft at the palatal area was present (Figure 14.50).

The lateral views confirmed the anterior and posterior cross-bite, the disto-inclination of the right upper canine and the mesio-inclination of the upper left canine (Figure 14.51). Oral hygiene was fairly normal.

The panoramic Rx confirmed the absence of the upper left lateral incisor, the first right bicuspid, the first upper left molar, and the first lower right molar. Upper and lower third molars were present (Figure 14.52).

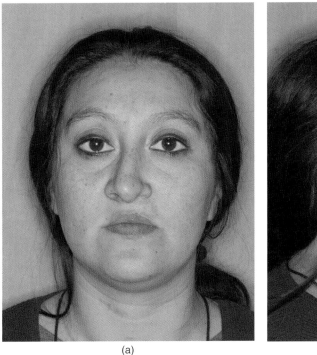
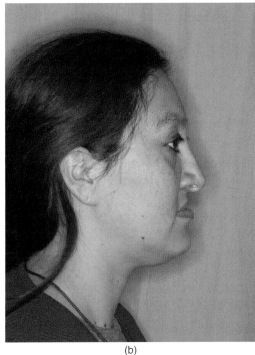

(a)   (b)

Figure 14.49 Pre-treatment (a) front and (b) lateral photograph. The profile is clearly concave with a prognatic chin.

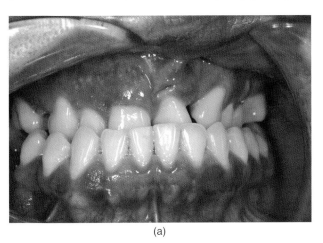
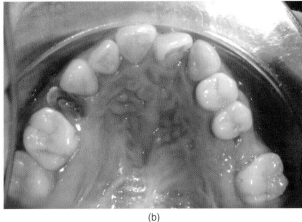

(a)   (b)

Figure 14.50 (a) Front and (b) occlusal view at the beginning of the treatment.

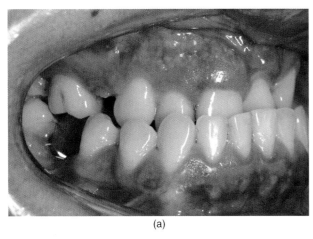
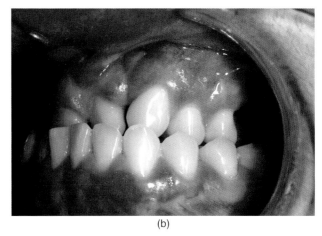

(a)   (b)

Figure 14.51 (a, b) Pre-treatment lateral photographs.

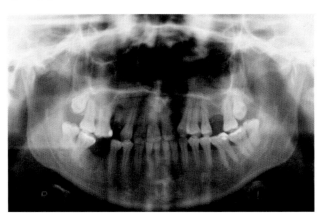

Figure 14.52 Panoramic Rx pre-treatment.

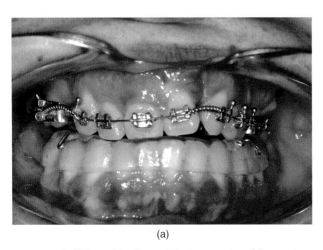
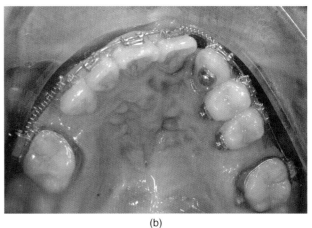

(a)   (b)

Figure 14.53 (a, b) Lower bite plane to help the correction of the negative overbite and a Ni-Ti coil spring to obtain the correct space for the upper lateral incisor.

The treatment objectives were to:

(1) align and level the arches
(2) normalize the overjet and overbite
(3) re-open the space for the upper left lateral incisor and replace the upper right bicuspids,
(4) close the space of the upper first left molar,
(5) improve facial and dental esthetics,
(6) long-term retention

In order to help correct the anterior cross-bite, a plastic bite plane was placed on the lower arch along with pre-programmed 0.022″ brackets with a Ni-Ti-Cu 0.018″ wire and Ni-Ti coil springs (Figure 14.53).

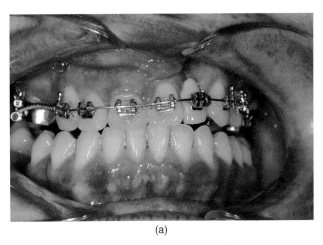
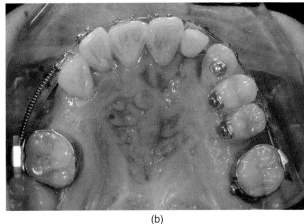

(a)   (b)

Figure 14.54 (a) Front and (b) occlusal photographs after 6 months in treatment.

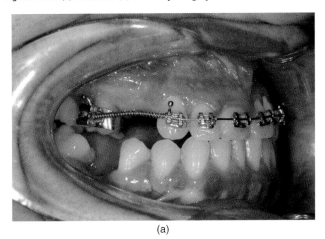
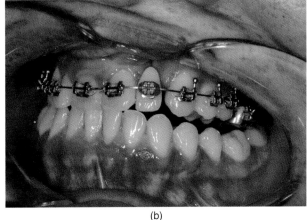

(a)   (b)

Figure 14.55 (a) Right and (b) left photographs with an open coil spring on the right side.

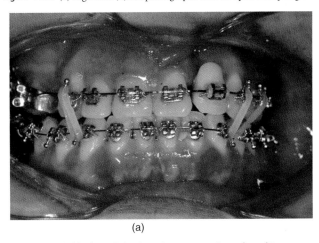
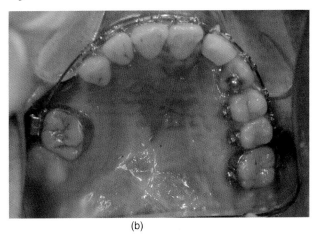

(a)   (b)

Figure 14.56 (a, b) Class III elastics to improve overjet and overbite were recommended.

After 6 months in treatment, the space for the upper left lateral incisor was obtained and the anterior cross-bite was almost corrected. For esthetic reasons a plastic lateral incisor was added to the arch (Figure 14.54).

The lateral photographs showed the progression of the treatment. Low and continuous forces were recommended in conjunction with an open coil spring on the right side (Figure 14.55). Overjet and overbite are improving according to the treatment plan.

In order to improve occlusion, brackets in the lower arch were bonded in conjunction with Class III elastics. The whole space of the absent first upper left molar was closed, and almost normal overjet and overbite were achieved (Figure 14.56).

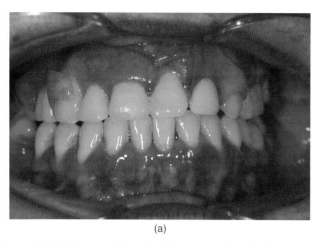

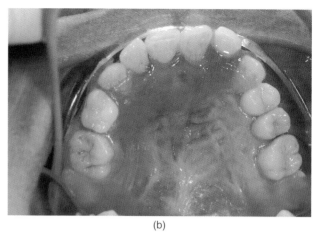

(a)   (b)

Figure 14.57 (a) Front and (b) occlusal photograph at the end of the treatment with the provisional removable prosthesis in place.

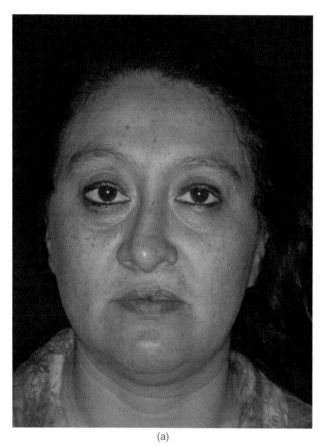

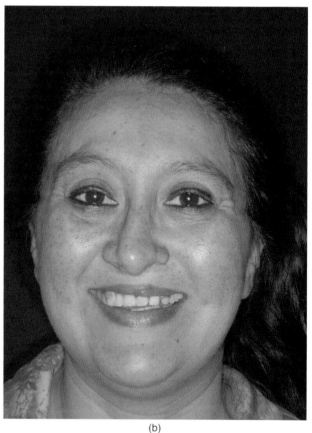

(a)   (b)

Figure 14.58 (a, b) Final smile photographs.

The final front dental photographs confirmed that the objectives were achieved. Overjet and overbite were normalized as well as the curve of Spee. The total treatment time was 25 months and a provisionary plastic removable appliance was placed to replace the absent upper teeth (Figure 14.57).

The smile photographs clearly showed the improvement achieved. The upper lip improvement was noticeable (Figure 14.58).

The comparison between the pre- and post-treatment front photographs clearly demonstrated that the all the dental objectives were achieved, in spite of the fact that she was a non-growing patient (Figure 14.59).

A long-term retention plan is mandatory to maintain the results in surgical and non-surgical patients (Hirano & Suzuki, 2001).

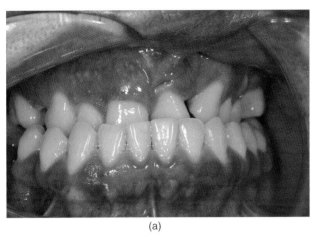 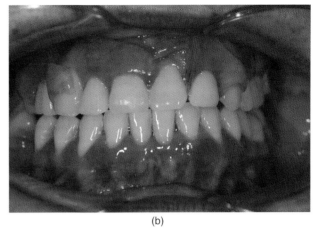

(a)   (b)

Figure 14.59 Comparison (a) pre- and (b) post-treatment. Excellent results were achieved using only orthodontic treatment.

Conclusions

It is well known that facial esthetics is a very important aspect of an individual's general perception of life. Unfortunately, not all the patients have the opportunity to receive multidisciplinary treatment and reach adulthood with severe dental and skeletal deformities (Felemovicius & Monasterio, 2004). As all patients are completely different, it is very difficult to describe a protocol that fits all of them step by step, but there are some characteristics that help the orthodontist decide the best treatment plan.

An efficient plaque control program has to be instituted with regular check-ups and close supervision and regular professional maintenance, especially at the cleft zone, for the entire life of the patient (Gaggl *et al.*, 1999).

When controlled forces are used, no more root resorption is found on the teeth near the cleft.

These three patients clearly demonstrate how, with only slow orthodontic movements, impressive, positive facial and dental changes are possible. Since many do not have the necessary resources for some esthetic and orthognatic surgeries, this protocol encourages orthodontists to treat these challenging patients (Thomas *et al.*, 1997; Sinko *et al.*, 2005).

Changes in the thickness and position of the upper lip are remarkable and they are in concordance with the position of the upper incisors without additional surgeries.

Improvement of their functional outcomes such as biting, chewing, swallowing, and comprehensibility of speech, are also significantly important (Marcusson *et al.*, 2001, 2002).

All the patients recognize that improvement of facial esthetics improves quality of life, especially women because of the importance given to physical attractiveness in our society (Jeffery & Boormann, 2011). After the orthodontic treatment, some of these patients decide to pursue college education in order to progress in life, since self-esteem and social support are highly related to success in life.

New materials and diagnostic tools have contributed significantly to the improvement in orthodontic treatment outcomes in these challenging cleft patients.

An interdisciplinary team is key to achieving positive results.

References

Akarsu, B., Taner, T., Tuncbilek, G., and Mavili, M. (2012) Maxillary protraction in adult cleft lip and palate by a rigid external distraction device with dentoskeletal anchorage. *Eur J Dent* **6**(**2**):206–211.

Bragger, U., Schurch, E., Jr., Salvi, G., *et al.* (1992) Periodontal conditions in adult patients with cleft lip, alveolus and palate. *Cleft Palate Craniofac J* **29**:179–185.

Chuo, B., Seatly, Y., Jeremy, A., *et al.* (2008) The continuing multidisciplinary needs of adult patients with cleft lip and/or palate. *Cleft Palate Craniofac J* **45**:633–638.

Felemovicius, J. and Ortiz Monasterio, F. (2004) Management of the impaired adult cleft patient: The last chance. *Cleft Palate Craniofac J* **41**:550–558.

Gaggl, A., Schultes, G., Karcher, H., and Mossbock, R. (1999) Periodontal disease in patients with cleft palate and patients with unilateral and bilateral clefts of lip, palate and alveolus. *J Periodontol* **70**: 171–178.

Hirano, A. and Suzuki, H. (2001) Factors related to relapse after LeFort I maxillary advancement osteotomy in patients with cleft lip and palate. *Cleft Palate Craniofac J* **38**:1–9.

Jeffery, S. L. and Boormann, J. G. (2011) Patient satisfaction with cleft lip and palate services in a regional centre. *Br J Plast Surg* **54**: 189–191.

Marcusson, A., Akerlind, I., and Paulin, G. (2001) Quality of life in adults with repaired complete cleft lip and palate. *Cleft Palate Craniofac J* **38**: 379–385.

Marcusson, A., Paulin, G., and Ostrup, L. (2002) Facial appearance in adults who have cleft lip and palate treated in childhood. *Scand J Plast Reconstr Surg Hand Surg* **36**:16–23.

Persson, M., Aniansson, G., Becker, M., and Svensson, H. (2002) Self–concept and introversion in adolescents with cleft lip and palate. *Scand J Plast Reconstr Surg Hand Surg* **36**:24–27.

Richman, L. C., Holmes, C. S., and Eliason, M. J. (1985) Adolescents with cleft lip and palate: Self perceptions of appearance and behavior related to personality adjustment. *Cleft Palate J* **22**: 93–96.

Sinko, S., Jeagsch, R., Prechtl, V., *et al.* (2005) Evaluation of Esthetic, Functional and Quality of life outcome in adult cleft-lip and palate patients. *Cleft Palate Craniofac J* **42**:355–361.

Thomas, P. T., Turner, S. R., Rumsey, N., *et al.* (1997) Satisfaction with facial appearance among subjects affected by a cleft. *Cleft Palate Craniofac J* **34**:226–231.

Yang, C. J., Pan, X. G., Qian, Y. F. and Wang, G. M. (2012) Impact of rapid maxillary expansion in unilateral cleft lip and palate patients after secondary alvelolar bone grafting: Review and case report. *Oral Surg Oral Med Oral Pathol Oral Radiol* **114**(**1**):e25–30.

CHAPTER 15

Strengthening surgical/orthodontic interrelationships

Julia F. Harfin[1] and Ricardo D. Bennun[2]

[1] Maimonides University, Argentina
[2] Asociacion PIEL, Maimonides University and National University of Buenos Aires, Argentina

Introduction

Pediatric dentistry provides oral health information that should follow the child with cleft lip and palate from the first day of life until establishment of mixed dentition, craniofacial growth, and dentition development. At present, with the introduction of the Dynamic Presurgical Nasoalveolar Remodeling (DPNR) Technique in our protocol, pediatric dentistry plays a transcendental role in correcting facial distortions previous to surgery, and transforming primary reconstruction in a less aggressive procedure (Monasterio, 2008).

Well-trained surgeons, using fewer incisions and dissections, and respecting blood supply and growth centers, are key to prevent facial growth alterations. Restitution of normal morphology and a correct muscular reconstruction are the ideal complement to complete a proper functional orthopedic treatment (Susami et al., 2006; Moreira et al., 2014).

Orthodontic intervention starts in the mixed dentition, at 8 or 9 years of age. At this stage, rapid maxillary expansion can be performed if necessary. When the permanent dentition is complete, comprehensive orthodontic treatment is initiated, aiming toward tooth alignment and space closure (Fudalej et al., 2011; Freitas et al., 2012; Wiggman et al., 2013). Maxillary permanent canines are commonly moved mesially in order to substitute absent maxillary lateral incisors.

Patient 1

We have selected the present case evolution over 17 years in a bilateral cleft lip and palate patient. This case is a good example of a correct protocol implementation by the interdisciplinary team, and a good response by the patient without leaving his treatment at any time.

After presurgical treatment as a newborn, a one-stage lip and nose reconstruction was performed at the age of 4 months following Mulliken's principles. The complete cleft palate repair was accomplished at the age of 1, using the Veau–Wardill–Kilner procedure. The palatal plate was used for 6 months after surgery.

Periodic controls were every 6 months, with no complications detected. Orthodontic intervention started on time (Garib et al., 2012).

The patient was perfectly happy with the surgical result, and his speech evolution was totally normal. See Figures 15.1 to 15.10.

Cleft Lip and Palate Management: A Comprehensive Atlas, First Edition. Edited by Ricardo D. Bennun, Julia F. Harfin, George K. B. Sándor, and David Genecov.
© 2016 John Wiley & Sons, Inc. Published 2016 by John Wiley & Sons, Inc.

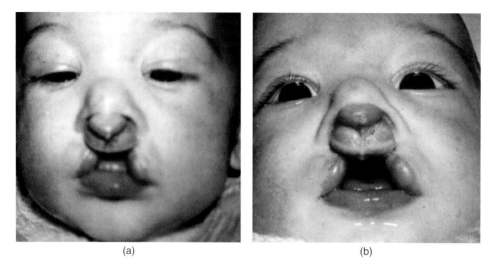

Figure 15.1 Pre-surgical frontal and inferior view.

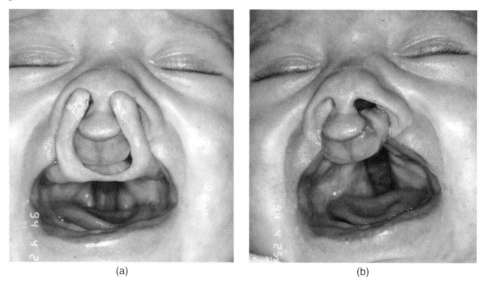

Figure 15.2 (a) Lower view showing presurgical remodelling treatment. (b) Patient ready for lip/nose reconstruction procedure.

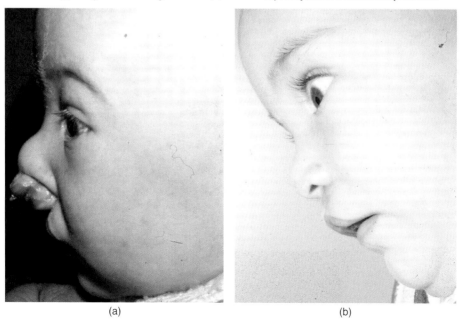

Figure 15.3 Pre- and post-op lateral views.

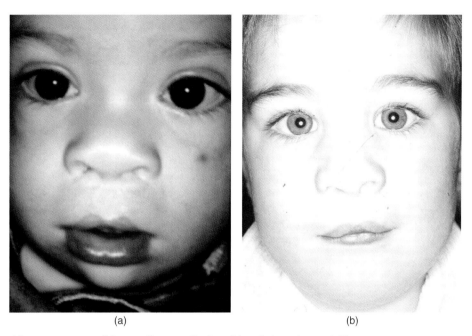

(a)   (b)

Figure 15.4 1 years and 2 years post surgery follow up. The normalization of the soft tissues is remarkable.

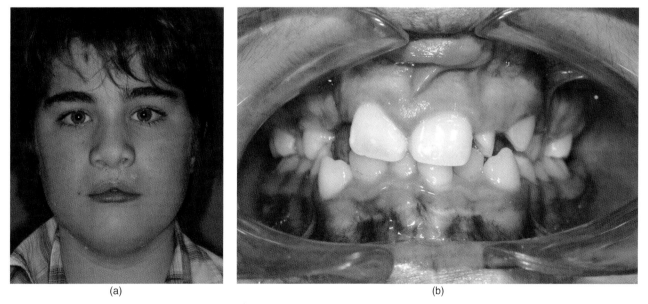

(a)   (b)

Figure 15.5 (a) At 12 years of age the patient began the orthodontic treatment. A little asymmetry is confirmed. (b) A midline deviation was confirmed upon analyzing the dental front photograph.

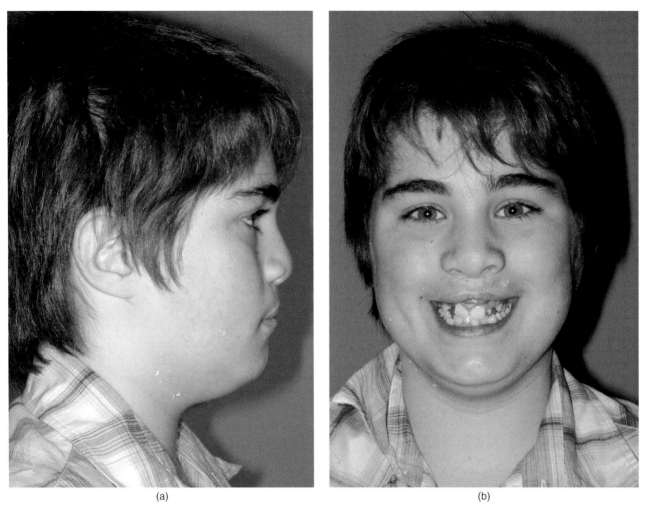

Figure 15.6 (a) At this time he was able to close his lips normally and his profile was a little convex. (b) Dental and facial midlines were not coincident.

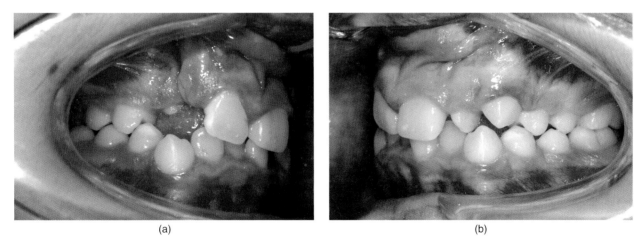

Figure 15.7 (a) Class I molar was confirmed upon analyzing the dental front photograph. (b) Oral hygiene was fairly good.

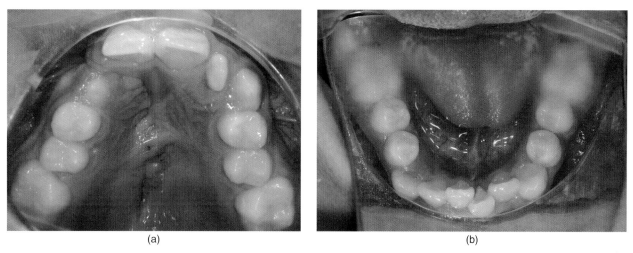

Figure 15.8 (a) There was some compression on the upper arch. The position of the scar was visible. (b) A significant lower anterior crowding was present.

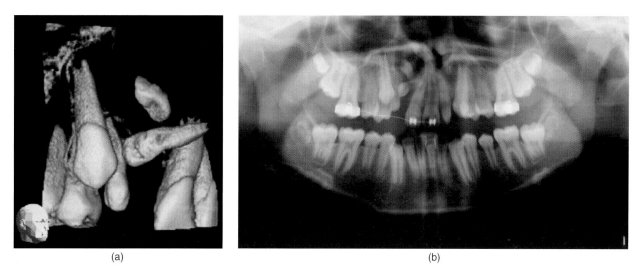

Figure 15.9 (a) The Rx clearly shows the position of the lateral incisor and the presence of a supernumerary tooth on the right side near the cleft. (b) Panoramic radiograph at the beginning of the orthodontic treatment.

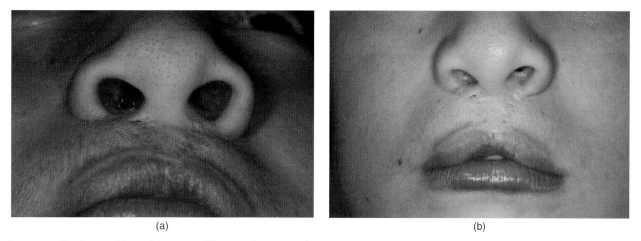

Figure 15.10 The shape and form of the nose and lips were almost normal.

TREATMENT OBJECTIVES

(1) Align and leveling the arches
(2) Maintain Clase 1 molar
(3) Normalize the position of the right upper lateral incisor and canine
(4) Normalize overjet and overbite
(5) Correct midlines
(6) Improve periodontal health
(7) Long term retention

TREATMENT PLAN

(1) Extract the supernumerary tooth
(2) Erupt the right upper lateral incisor and canine
(3) Correct the lower anterior crowding
(4) Maintain Class I molar
(5) Normalize overjet and overbite
(6) Level the Curve of Spee
(7) Fixed upper and lower retention

See Figures 15.11 to 15.17.

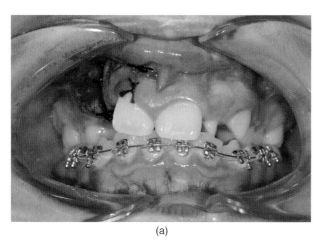
(a)

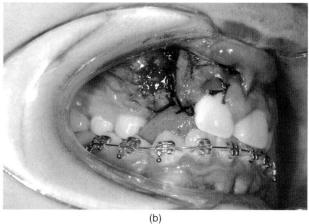
(b)

Figure 15.11 A close flap was performed in order to bond a bracket on the labial surface of the canine.

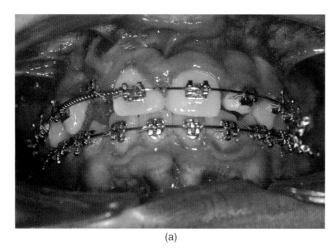
(a)

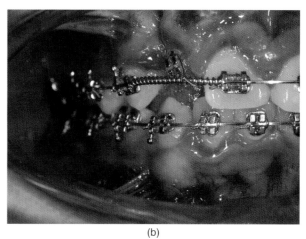
(b)

Figure 15.12 (a) Two weeks after the surgery a low and continuous force was recommended to move the tooth with bone. The ideal activation is every 4–6 weeks. The ideal activation is every 4–6 weeks. Pre-programmed brackets with TMA archwire in the upper arch were used. (b) When the canine was in place, a ligature was placed on the upper right lateral incisor.

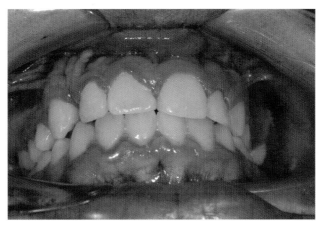

Figure 15.13 At the end of the treatment the objectives were fulfilled. Midlines were corrected.

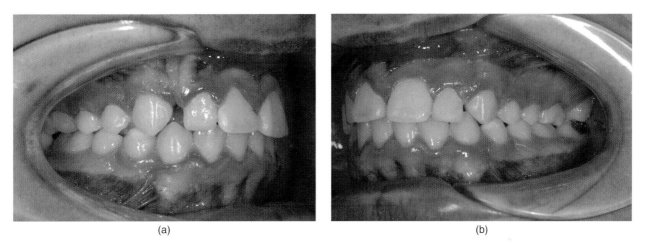

(a) (b)

Figure 15.14 The gingival margins were totally normalized even in the cleft zone. A multidisciplinary team is essential to reach these results.

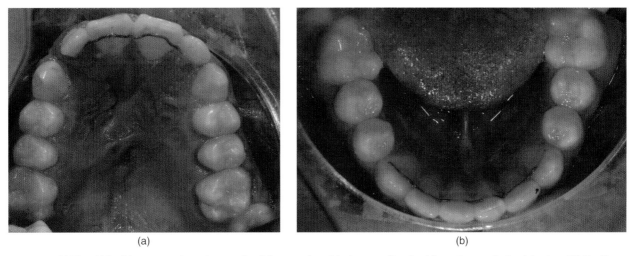

(a) (b)

Figure 15.15 (a) The width of the upper arch was improved and the upper lateral incisor as well as the right canine were in the right place. (b) Significant lower crowding was corrected and a fixed retention wire was bonded from right to left canine.

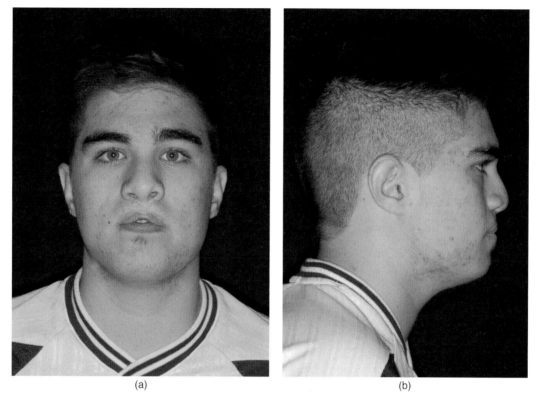

(a)   (b)

Figure 15.16 (a) The final frontal picture confirms the excellent result that was achieved. (b) The lateral view shows a good naso-labial angle and a normal upper lip/lower lip relation.

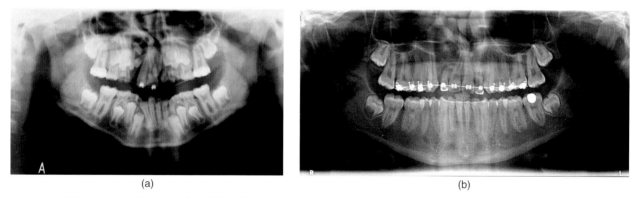

(a)   (b)

Figure 15.17 (a) Impressive results were confirmed when the pre- and post-panoramic radiographs were compared. (b) Some root resorption on the upper right lateral incisor was totally foreseeable.

The orthodontist plays an important role in treating these challenging cases. It is possible to manage the direction of growth patterns, and in this way, to modify them to a certain point in the final outcome.

The possibility to erupt impacted teeth near the cleft is confirmed when low and continuous forces are applied.

Another important goal is to improve the periodontal conditions of the teeth near the cleft in order to obtain a better esthetic and functional occlusion without any secondary bone graft.

Patient 2

The second case is a female patient born 17 years ago with bilateral cleft lip and palate.

At the age of 5 months and after an incomplete presurgical treatment, a one-stage lip reconstruction was performed by the same senior surgeon and using the same technique. The palate was completely repaired by the same surgeon and with the same technique utilized in the former patient, at the age of 1 year old.

A palatal plate was utilized 6 months after surgery.

Periodic controls were every 6 months.

Orthodontic treatment started at 13 years of age when almost all the teeth were erupted. Pre-programmed brackets with the help of Ni-Ti Cu arch wires, are highly recommended in order to normalize the width and shape of the upper arch. No extractions were planned in her lower arch in spite her Class III tendency. Upper and lower fixed retainers were recommended for a long period of time. The patient returned after 3 years for a nose revision. See Figures 15.18 to 15.32.

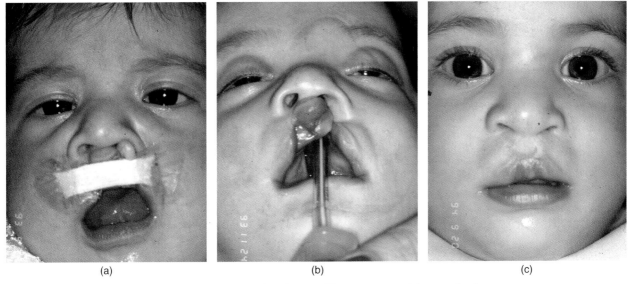

(a)   (b)   (c)

Figure 15.18 (a) Pre-treatment front photograph at 4 months of age. (b) Frontal lower pre-op view. (c) 10 months after surgery.

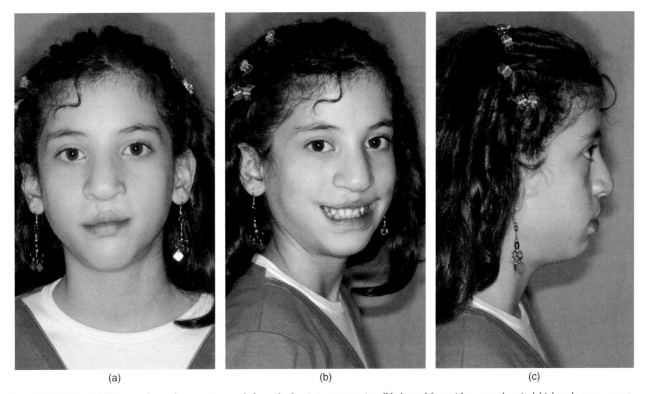

(a)   (b)   (c)

Figure 15.19 Patient at 13 years of age who came in search for orthodontic treatment. A well balanced face with a normal nasio-labial angle, was present with some asymmetry at the middle and lower third.

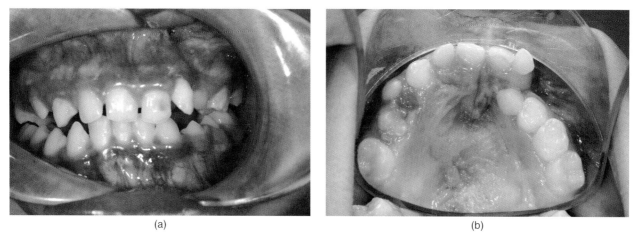

(a)   (b)

Figure 15.20 (a) On the front view, a non-coincident midline was observed in conjunction with the labial position of the left upper lateral incisor. (b) The occlusal photograph confirmed the palatal displacement of the left bicuspid and canine.

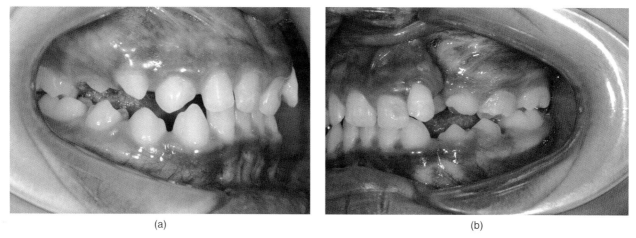

(a)   (b)

Figure 15.21 (a) Significant retroinclination of the upper and lower incisors was present. (b) The cleft was clearly visible distal to the labially displaced upper left lateral incisor.

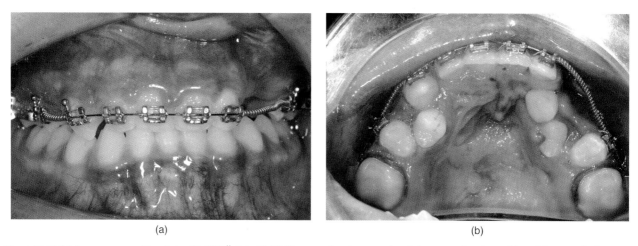

(a)   (b)

Figure 15.22 (a) Pre-programmed brackets with 0.022″ slot with Ni-Ti open coil springs were bonded to normalize the position of the upper incisors. (b) Occlusal view at this time of the treatment. The upper second bicuspids were rotated 180° and in a palatal position.

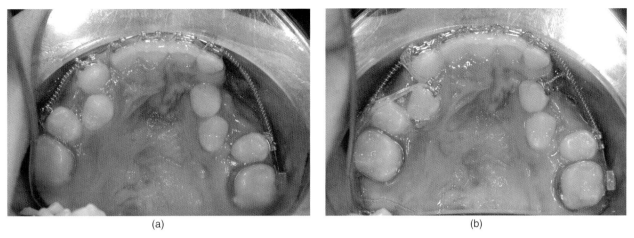

(a)   (b)

Figure 15.23 (a) Two months later with the open Ni-Ti coil spring in place. The upper right second bicuspid was in its position. The scars on the left side were more noticeable than on the right side. (b) Low and continuous forces were used to displace the palatal teeth to their normal position.

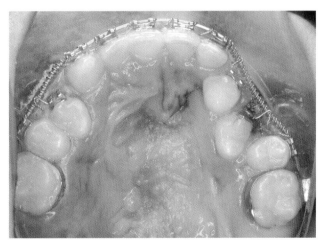

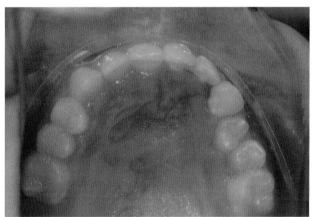

Figure 15.24 This was the situation after 12 months of treatment. The bicuspids and the canine were labially displaced with very low forces.

Figure 15.25 Final occlusal photograph after 22 months of orthodontic treatment.

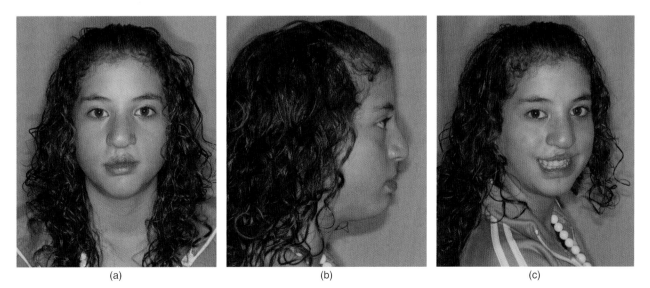

(a)   (b)   (c)

Figure 15.26 Final facial photographs at the end of the treatment. There is considerable improvement not only in the front but also in the profile.

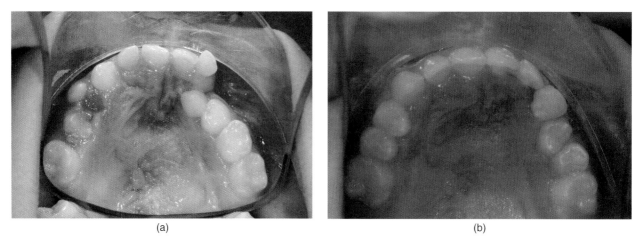

(a)   (b)

Figure 15.27 The comparison of the occlusal upper arch pre- and post-treatment showed the improvement in its width and shape. (a) Early transverse expansion of the maxilla is an effective method for normalizing maxilo-mandibular discrepancies in cleft-palate patients. A fixed and removable appliance is advisable for long term periods in order to avoid relapse in the transversal width, specially on the scar area.

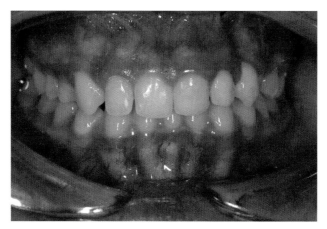

Figure 15.28 The alignment of the teeth was achieved even though the midlines were not completely corrected. The gingival line was normal as well the overjet and overbite.

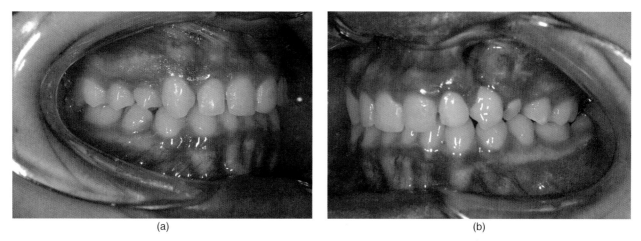

(a)   (b)

Figure 15.29 (a) Lateral views at the end of the orthodontic treatment. Gingival tissues were almost normal and the arches were well coordinated. Long term fixed and removable retainers are advisable.

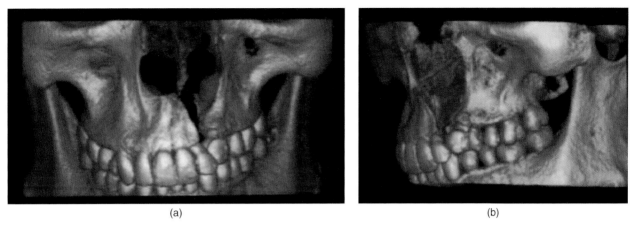

(a)   (b)

Figure 15.30 Front and left side CT scan after the orthodontic treatment.

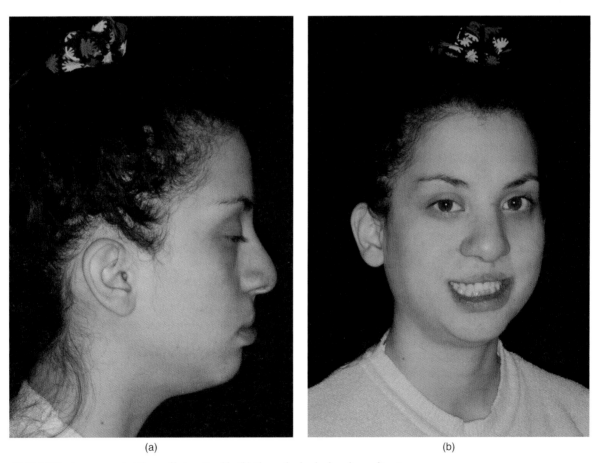

(a)   (b)

Figure 15.31 (a) The improvement at the profile is noticeable. (b) The smile clearly show her melioration.

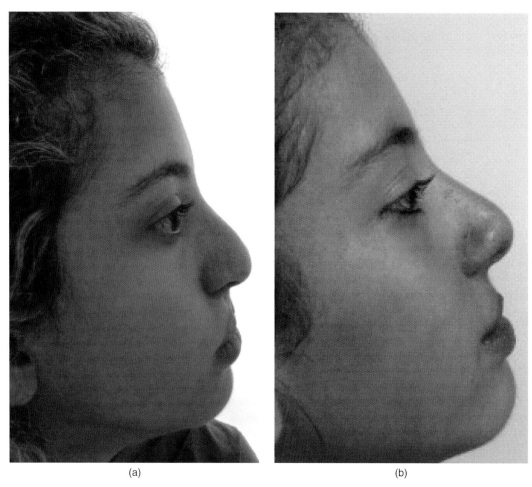

(a)   (b)

Figure 15.32 Pre- and post-nose surgery. The enhancement of the nasio-labial angle is clearly visible.

Post treatment records showed that the treatment objectives were achieved. There is no doubt regarding the importance of presurgical orthopedics.

Dental and facial esthetics can be achieved with an individualized treatment plan in a multidisciplinary team.

Long term control is necessary to maintain dental and soft tissues results. This protocol provides excellent results, both functionally and esthetically.

Surgery of the lip and nose is necessary for patients with cleft lip and palate since a good looking nose is important during one's life, especially in adolescents and young adults.

Successful clinical outcome is dependent on the close communication within the team (pediatrician, oral surgeon, orthodontists, speech pathology, etc.).

Conclusions

The first case presented was solved with only two surgical procedures and the patient has finished his treatment with excellent result. The second one required three surgeries, and orthodontics was completed in one step.

No major facial growth alterations were found in either case. Speech and hearing evolution were totally normal in both cases.

Most surgeons agree that bilateral cleft lip repair is twice as difficult with half of the results. Bearing this point in mind, the author's suggestion would be a change in our paradigm. The aim of halving the difficulty and doubling the results could be achieved by presurgically reducing the distortion.

Patients with unilateral/bilateral cleft lip and palate, and without genetic background, would not necessarily be candidates for alveolar bone graft. Poor midface growth and orthognatic surgery requirement can also be avoided if an adequate surgical procedure and treatment protocol are implemented.

References

Freitas, J. A., Garib, D. G., Oliveira, M., *et al.* (2012) Rehabilitative treatment of cleft lip and palate: Experience of the Hospital for Rehabilitation of Craniofacial Anomalies-USP (HRAC-USP) Part 2: Pediatric dentistry and orthodontics. *J Appl Oral Sci* **20**(**2**):268–281.

Fudalej, P., Katsaros, C., Bongaarts, C., *et al.* (2011) Dental arch relationship in children with complete unilateral cleft lip and palate following one-stage and three-stage surgical protocols. *Clin Oral Investig* **15**(**4**):503–510.

Garib, D. G., Yatabe, M. S., Ozawa, T. O., *et al.* (2012) Alveolar bone morphology in patients with bilateral complete cleft lip and palate in the mixed dentition: cone beam computed tomography evaluation. *Cleft Palate Craniofac J* **49**(**2**):208–214.

Monasterio Aljaro, L. (2008) *Tratamiento Interdisciplinario de las Fisuras Labio Palatinas*. Santiago de Chile: Impresora Optima S.A.

Moreira, I., Suri, S., Ross, B., *et al.* (2014) Soft-tissue profile growth in patients with repaired complete unilateral cleft lip and palate: A cephalometric comparison with normal controls at ages 7, 11, and 18 years. *Am J Orthod Dentofacial Orthop* **145**(**3**):341–358.

Susami, T., Ogihara, Y., Matsuzaki, M., *et al.* (2006) Assessment of dental arch relationships in Japanese patients with unilateral cleft lip and palate. *Cleft Palate Craniofac J* **43**(**1**):96–102.

Wiggman, K., Larson, M., Larson, O., *et al.* (2013) The influence of the initial width of the cleft in patients with unilateral cleft lip and palate related to final treatment outcome in the maxilla at 17 years of age. *Eur J Orthod* **35**(**3**):335–340.

PART 4

Improving results in cleft lip and palate interdisciplinary management

CHAPTER 16

To what extent could dental alveolar osteogenesis be achieved solely with orthodontic treatment in flap patients?

Julia F. Harfin

Maimonides University, Argentina

It is well known that patients with lip and palate clefts have typical characteristics such as deficiency in midface development, orthodontic Class III tendency, abnormal nasolabial angle, oranasal fistulae in some cases, alterations in the number and positions of the lateral incisors, and agenesis or supernumerary teeth.

Treatment alternatives for unilateral or bilateral missing lateral incisors are space closure or opening spaces for their replacement by fixed or removable prosthesis. Implants in the cleft area are often complicated due to the lack of bone and the need for another bone graft.

It is difficult to determine a unique protocol that suits all patients, because they are all different; but the management of implant spaces can help to achieve more esthetic and less invasive results. This method is essentially recommended for large defects or for patients who do not want iliac crest bone graft or other types of grafts.

It is well recognized that orthodontic treatment must be performed to improve the maxilo–mandibular relationship, the facial profile, and the positioning of the cleft alveolar segments. An adequate and individualized diagnosis and treatment plan significantly improves the results with more predictable outcomes. Closing the alveolar bone defect is one of the keys to achieving a better occlusion at the end of the treatment (Iseri et al., 2005).

In seeking alternatives to close important palatal clefts when a secondary bone graft doesn't achieve the expected results, and using the same concepts that periodontists use to improve height and width before implants are placed in patients with reduced bone height, this procedure offers a new alternative. The concept was presented by Dr. Allan Fontanelle more than 20 years ago in patients without clefts, and today it plays an important role in the dental and prosthetic rehabilitation in normal and cleft palate patients. This protocol is highly recommended in all patients no matter their age or width of the cleft as it can help to avoid extra surgeries to solve the deficiency of the buccolingual alveolar width into which teeth can be moved (Yen et al., 2005). As always, monthly oral hygiene instruction including scaling and root planning is highly recommended (Brägger et al., 1985; Teja et al., 1992; de Alemeida et al., 2009).

The following 12-year-old patient is a clear example of this protocol. He was referred by his dentist to the Orthodontic Department to improve his dental occlusion. His cleft lip and palate had been surgically repaired when he was a child. No temporomandibular symptoms were present. The front photograph showed a fairly symmetrical face in conjunction with a functional mandibular deviation to the left side (Figure 16.1).

His profile was straight and the nasal–labial angle presented an open angle. The lateral smile showed malposition of the lateral incisors. The scar on the upper lip is fairly visible (Figure 16.2).

On the dental front photograph, an important overbite on the central incisors was observed. The occlusal view confirmed the double side cleft and a significant palatal cleft that was still open. The deep overbite at the central incisors was nearly 100%. It is important to highlight that the upper lateral incisors were present. The maxillary midline deviated 2 mm to the right (Figure 16.3).

From the lateral view an important deep overbite was confirmed at the incisor area and some openbite was present at the bicuspid area in combination with considerable mobility in the premaxilla (Figure 16.4).

Cleft Lip and Palate Management: A Comprehensive Atlas, First Edition. Edited by Ricardo D. Bennun, Julia F. Harfin, George K. B. Sándor, and David Genecov.
© 2016 John Wiley & Sons, Inc. Published 2016 by John Wiley & Sons, Inc.

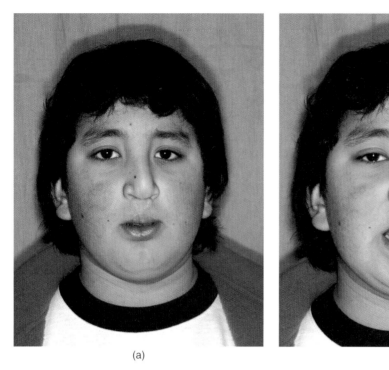

Figure 16.1 (a, b) Front pre-treatment photographs.

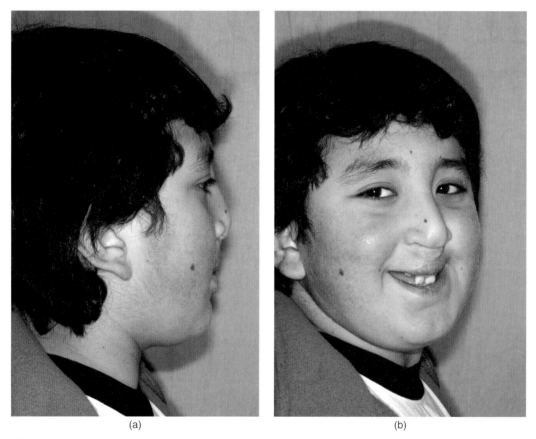

Figure 16.2 (a, b) Lateral pre-treatment photographs.

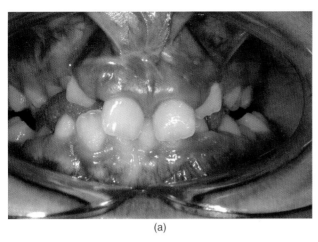
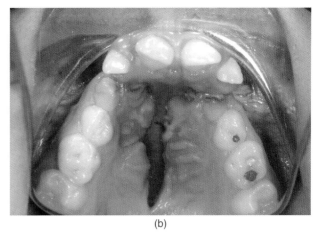

(a)   (b)

Figure 16.3 (a, b) Frontal and upper occlusal buccal pre-treatment photographs.

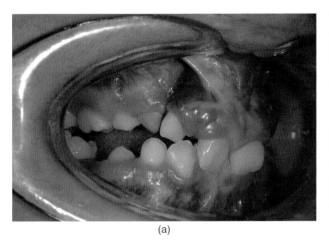
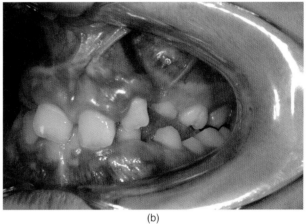

(a)   (b)

Figure 16.4 (a, b) Lateral views at the beginning of treatment.

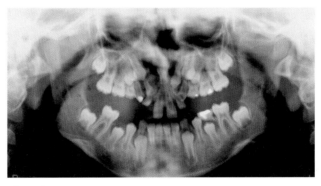

Figure 16.5 Pre-treatment panoramic radiographs.

The panoramic radiograph confirmed the presence of the upper lateral incisors and all the bicuspids and molars were present at different stages of eruption (Figure 16.5).

The lateral and occlusal radiographs confirmed the important deep overbite and clefts (Figure 16.6).

The patient's treatment objectives were to:

(1) align and level the arches,
(2) normalize the overjet and overbite,
(3) achieve a Class I canine and molar,
(4) normalize the dental midline,
(5) replace the missing teeth,
(6) long-term retention.

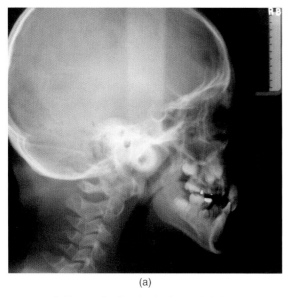
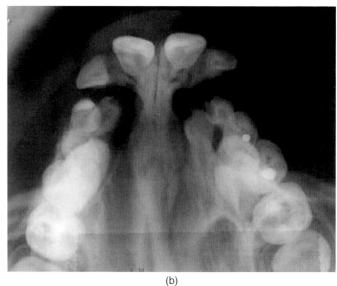

(a)
(b)

Figure 16.6 (a, b) Lateral and occlusal radiographs before treatment.

Treatment alternatives

The following treatment alternatives should be considered:

(1) Align and level the arches with a new bilateral secondary bone graft in order to gain bone for future implants.

(2) Align the premaxilla to correct the overjet and overbite, mesialize the right and left canine, and place implants distal to the canines, without any other bone surgery.

The second option seemed the safest and most rational choice for this patient.

The use of a rapid maxilar expander was recommended to normalize the transversal width. Since the patient had an important palate cleft, only one activation per day was suggested. After four weeks of activation the screw was fixed with composite and at the same time brackets on the lateral and central incisors were placed aiming at their alignment (Figure 16.7).

After 6 months, the overjet and overbite were almost normalized with the help of a utility arch (0.016″ × 0.016″ Elgiloy archwire) (Figure 16.8a). The beginning of the eruption of the upper canines can be observed on the occlusal view (Figure 16.8b).

When the upper right canine was erupted and the temporary one exfoliated, a bracket was bonded to allow it to achieve its correct position. A new surgery was performed in order to close the palatal soft tissues (Figure 16.9).

Figure 16.10 shows the situation 6 months later: the canine had reached its position and an important cleft was present on the right side. Taking into account Fontanelle's studies about moving teeth into an edentulous region, a Ni-Ti open coil spring

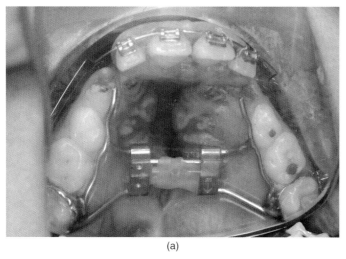
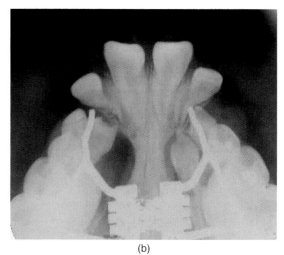

(a)
(b)

Figure 16.7 (a, b) RME in place fixed with composite with the occlusal Rx for control.

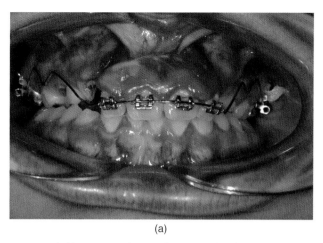
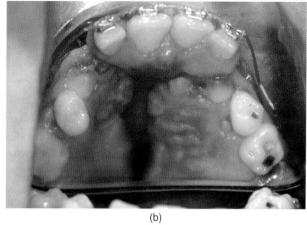

(a) (b)

Figure 16.8 (a, b) Treatment photographs at 6 months of treatment.

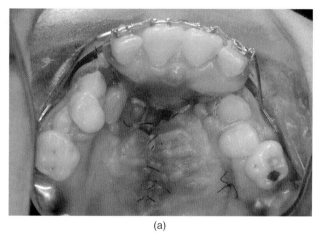
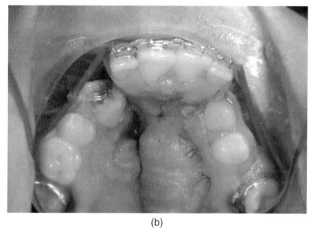

(a) (b)

Figure 16.9 (a, b) Occlusal view after the palatal surgery.

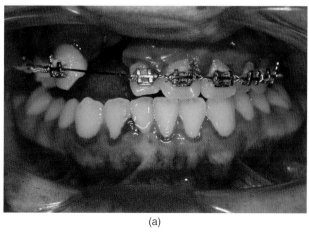
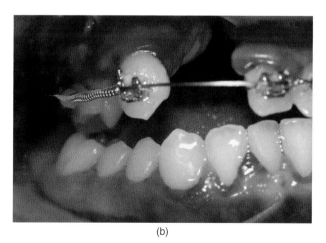

(a) (b)

Figure 16.10 (a, b) Use of a coil spring to mesialize the upper right canine.

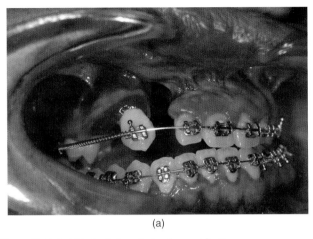
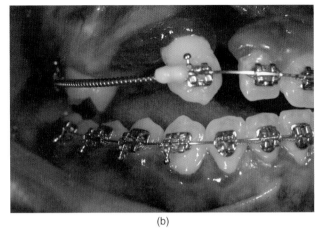

(a)   (b)

Figure 16.11 (a, b) Lateral views during the mesialization process.

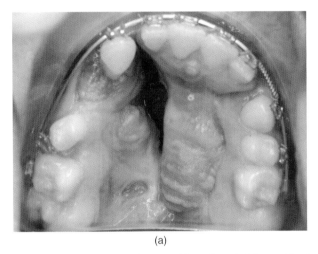
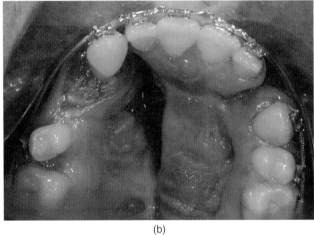

(a)   (b)

Figure 16.12 Occlusal view (a) during and (b) at the end of the mesialization progress.

was placed distal to the canine to promote its mesialization (Zachrisson, 2003) (Figure 16.10).

Figure 16.11 shows the results 7 months later. At the labial aspect the cleft is narrower than ever. The canine was mesialized through very slow and continuous forces (Figure 16.11).

The palatal view confirms the mesialization of the canine and the new bone that developed distally. This new bone presents ideal height and width for future implants (Figure 16.12).

Figure 16.13a show the occlusal Rx at this moment of the treatment (Figure 16.13a). A new soft palatal tissue surgery was performed to close the remaining cleft (Figure 16.13b).

The panoramic radiograph confirmed the mesialization of the canine on the right side. It is interesting to observe the shape of the roots of the upper lateral incisors (Figure 16.14). This approach introduces a new paradigm in treating this type of patient, since it is possible to create new bone surrounded by normal gingivoperiodontal tissues that otherwise are very difficult to obtain. No other bone graft procedure is necessary and a better prosthetic replacement of the absent teeth with good dental esthetics and function is achieved.

All the space on the right was closed (Figure 16.15). The comparison with the left side is significant. Comparing the right and left side there is no doubt over the effectiveness of this procedure. On the right side normal bone height and width to place an implant have been created. Meanwhile on the left side the cleft is still there.

Orthodontic tooth movement is a process by which the tooth is moved by the application of a force that induces bone deposition on the tension side where the periodontal ligament is stretched and new bone is formed. This process could be considered as a distraction osteogenesis of the periodontal ligament. The new bone is clearly visible distal to the right upper canine in comparison to the left side (Figure 16.16).

Rachmiel *et al.* (2014) published a very interesting case report where they reduced a wide cleft with two-stage alveolar distraction osteogenesis procedures (horizontal and vertical) accompanied by an autogenous bone grafting to the remaining alveolar defect, in the medial cleft, with very positive results.

This new treatment alternative involving dental alveolar osteogenesis can be applied in uni- or bilateral clefts in non-growing

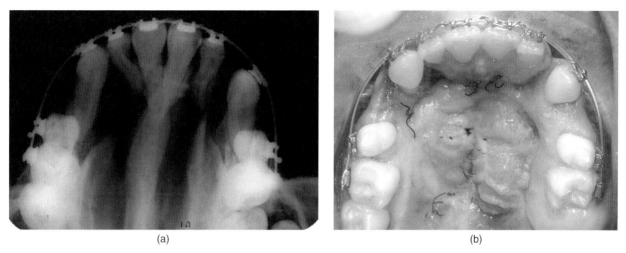

Figure 16.13 (a) Occlusal maxillar radiograph and (b) palatal view after another surgery.

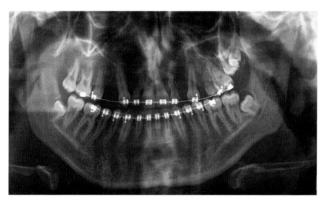

Figure 16.14 Triangular elastics (1/8 heavy) 20 hours a day were indicated to improve the Class I canine.

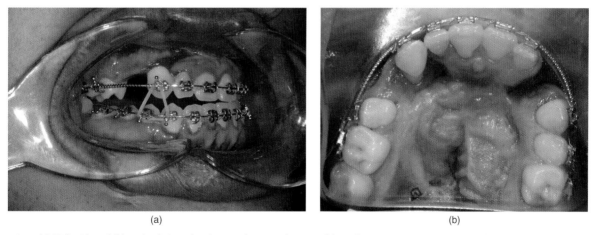

Figure 16.15 (a) Right side and (b) occlusal view after the complete mesialization of the right canine.

or growing patients without another bone graft procedure prior to implant placement. Normal width and height bone was created distally to the upper right canine (Figure 16.16). The results are significantly more predictable with higher esthetic and function. No further root resorption on the adjacent teeth was present. This procedure in cleft palate patients has not been published until now.

The canine on the right side was moved effectively with an almost normal gingival margin and periodontal support. The normalization of the gingival margin in relation to the cemento–enamel junction is important to obtain a pleasant smile. It is important to remember that its position is related to the volume of bone attached to the tooth. No corticotomy or other surgical procedures were performed.

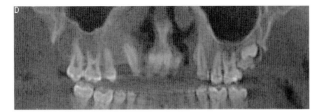

Figure 16.16 Control panoramic radiographic at this stage of the treatment.

Undoubtedly this orthodontic procedure can significantly improve both dental and functional esthetics. More longitudinal follow-up studies will be necessary.

Conclusions

The purpose of this chapter was to demonstrate the advantages of the dental alveolar distraction procedure in patients with palatal clefts (Liou *et al.*, 2000). In addition, to highlight this technique for achieving better results in tooth movement, avoiding a secondary alveolar bone grafting and gingivoperiostoplasty with or without secondary alveolar bone graft (Santiago *et al.*, 1988).

Distraction dental alveolar osteogenesis is an effective and predictable technique that can be applied to all patients at any age. One of its major advantages is the absence of new surgeries, which helps to avoid all the possible problems that could accompany it. But the most important issue is that the new bone is completely normal, with a wide area of alveolar bone on the tension side that provides sufficient buccolingual space for implant insertion. However, such repositioning has not been reported in the literature and requires complex, extensive, and time consuming tooth movement.

The key points of this treatment option are the light and controlled forces applied and the patient's motivation. The results are very predictable and have an important impact on the final prosthetic results and as a consequence on the final facial appearance.

Now a days there is an increased tendency to investigate accelerating methods for tooth movement. Among them, the piezocision technique is considered one of the most controlled.

The most interesting and important aspect in the future will be the new advances in the genetics field and how orthodontic movement can be improved and accelerated by managing the osseous turn-over. Some clinical investigations have demonstrated that this hypothesis is totally possible. This could be the answer to finding the best method to increase tooth movement with the fewest possible disadvantages. Unfortunately, to date, there are no case reports in cleft palate patients. Further results will be necessary in the near future.

References

Brägger, U., Schurch, E., Jr., Guberti, F. A., and Lang, N. P. (1985) Periodontal conditions in adolescents with cleft lip, alveolus and palate following treatment in a coordinated team approach. *J Clin Periodont* **12**:494–502.

de Almeida, A. L. P., Sonohara Gonzalez, M. K., Aguiar Greghi, S. L., *et al.* (2009) Are teeth close to the cleft more susceptible to periodontal disease? *Cleft Palate Craniofac J* **46**:161–165.

Iseri, H., Kisnisci, R., Bzizi, N., and Tuz, H. (2005) Rapid canine retraction and orthodontic treatment with dentoalveolar distraction osteogenesis. *Am J Orthod Dentofacial Orthop.* **127**(5):533–541; quiz 625.

Liou, E. J., Figueroa, A. A., and Polley, J. W. (2000) Rapid orthodontic tooth movement into newly distracted bone after mandibular distraction osteogenesis in a canine model. *Am J Orthod Dentofacial Orthop* **4**:391–398.

Rachmiel, A., Emodi, O., and Aizembud, D. (2014) Three-dimensional reconstruction of large secondary alveolar cleft by two-stage distraction. *Cleft Palate Craniofac J* **51**:36–42.

Santiago, P. E, Grayson, B. H., Cutting, C. B., *et al.* (1998) Reduced need for alveolar bone grafting by pre-surgical orthopedics and primary gingivoperiosteoplasty. *Cleft Palate Craniofac J* **35**:77–80.

Teja, Z., Persson, R., and Omnell, M. L. (1992) Periodontal status of teeth adjacent to nongrafted unilateral alveolar clefts. *Cleft Palate Craniofac J* **29**:357–362.

Yen, S. L., Yamashita, D. D., Gross, J., *et al.* (2005) Combining orthodontic tooth movement with distraction osteogenesis to close cleft spaces and improve maxillary arch form in cleft lip and palate patients. *Am J Orthod Dentofacial Orthop* **127**:224–232.

Zachrisson, B. U. (2003) Implant site development by horizontal tooth development. *World J Orthod* **4**:266–272.

CHAPTER 17

Laser treatment of cleft lip scars

Agustina Vila Echagüe
Massachusetts General Hospital, USA

Scars are usually described as hypertrophic when they are firm, raised, with excessive redness (erythematous), widening, and or stiffness (McCraw et al., 1999). Hypertrophic scars (HTS) usually remain confined to the border of the original wound, and they are associated with symptoms such as itchiness and paresthesia. The mechanism of HTS formation is not completely understood. The increase in collagen accumulation and fibroplasia may result from either exaggerated collagen synthesis or deficient matrix degradation and remodeling (Tredget et al., 1997). Hypertrophic scar (HTS) formation following cleft lip repair is relatively common; rates vary, from 1% to nearly 50% (Soltani et al., 2012).

Lasers have been used in the treatment of hypertrophic scars and keloids for over 25 years. However, clinical studies have shown that complete clearing of erythema and/or thickness of scars is not commonly achieved, usually multiple treatment sessions are required.

The pulsed dye laser (PDL) 585 nm, following Anderson's theory of selective photothermolysis (Anderson & Parrish, 1983), has been shown to provide long-standing improvement of hypertrophic and keloids scars (Alster, 1994; Dierickx et al., 1995; Nouri et al., 2012; Goldman & Fitzpatrick, 1995).

The mechanism by which the PDL achieves clinical improvement in scars includes (Nouri et al., 2012): (i) laser-induced microvasculature damage with subsequent collagen degradation via release of collagenase (Goldman & Fitzpatrick, 1995; Alster, 1994); (ii) thermal damage to collagen fibers dissipated from adjacent vessels with dissociation of disulfide bonds and collagen realignment; and (iii) increased regional mast cells, which may serve to stimulate collagen remodeling (Tsao et al., 2012).

The mechanisms of action of the CO_2 laser (10.600 nm) hypothetically include tissue ablation, immediate collagen shrinkage, and dermal collagen remodeling (Saryazdi & Mohebbi, 2012). The concept of fractional photothermolysis as described by Manstein et al. in 2004 enables the delivery of dermal coagulative injury without confluent epidermal damage. Fractional CO_2 lasers create columns of microscopic ablated epidermis and dermis after treatment which result in macroscopic epidermal regeneration, as evidenced by clinical improvement of scar and skin texture, thus decreasing the risks of scarring as well as decreasing the downtime associated with traditional ablative resurfacing (Gotkin et al., 2009).

Despite expert wound care after surgical cleft lip repair, HTS is relatively common, leaving scars with restrictive motion. To manage these complications we optimized treatment parameters for established, stiff cord hypertrophic type scars, such as post-surgical cleft lip scars, using a combination of CO_2 and a PDL laser.

The aim of this ongoing clinical study is to evaluate the efficacy of PDL + fractional CO_2 laser resurfacing to treat moderate to severe cleft lip scars.

Methods

Nine patients (ages 14–21, mean age of 16 years, skin phototypes I–IV) with cleft lip hypertrophic scars were included in this prospective study. Scars had been present for 4 to 72 months (mean duration of 18.5 months). Patients received between 2–6 laser treatments at a 4-week interval between each laser.

Scars were assigned to receive both 585-nm PDL (Vbeam Perfecta; Candela Laser Corp., Wayland, MA) and a 10.6400-nm CO_2 (CO_2Re; Syneron Candela Corp., Wayland, MA). Laser parameters for PDL treatment range from 10–14 j/cm², using

Cleft Lip and Palate Management: A Comprehensive Atlas, First Edition. Edited by Ricardo D. Bennun, Julia F. Harfin, George K. B. Sándor, and David Genecov.
© 2016 John Wiley & Sons, Inc. Published 2016 by John Wiley & Sons, Inc.

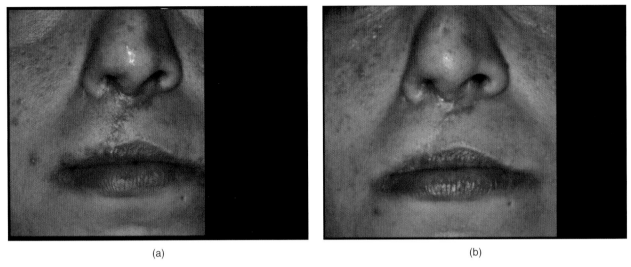

Figure 17.1 (a) Right cleft lip scar. (b) Twelve weeks after four combination PDL/Fractional CO_2 treatments.

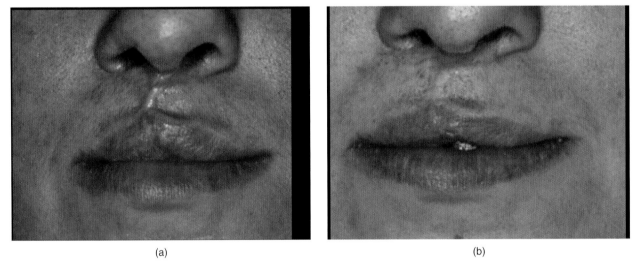

Figure 17.2 (a) Right cleft lip scar. (b) Twelve weeks after four combination PDL/Fractional CO_2 treatment

the 7 mm spot and 1.5 ms pulse duration, with 30/20DCD. For the Fractional CO_2 laser, the range was MID 156 mj 3% coverage or FUSION 156 mj/ 56 mj 3% coverage. Treatments were performed at a 3–6 week interval.

Photographic documentation and clinical evaluations were made before each treatment and four weeks after the last treatment; using the Canfield TwinFlash (Canfield Imaging Systems, Fair- field, NJ).

Results

To date, all scars showed clinical improvement after the first treatments. Scars' pliability scores, scar texture, erythema, and scar height were reduced by 50% after four treatments of combined PDL and Fractional CO_2 laser as shown in Figure 17.1 and Figure 17.2.

Scar erythema and symptoms such as pruritus also improved after each treatment session as shown in Figure 17.3 evaluated with cross-polarized photography. Average erythema scores were reduced by 52% after two sessions and by 81% after four sessions with PDL treatment in combination with Fractional CO_2.

Ongoing results for this study seem encouraging.

Conclusion

This study still requires optimization; when treating hypertrophic scars, both functional and esthetic improvement is the

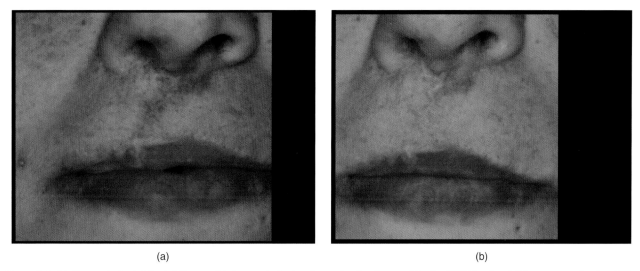

(a)   (b)

Figure 17.3 (a) Cross-polarized right cleft lip scar. (b) Cross-polarized twelve weeks after four combination PDL/Fractional CO_2 treatment showing 90% decrease in scar erythema.

ultimate goal. It is gratifying to observe the substantial improvement of hypertrophic scars after treatment with a combination of PDL and CO_2 laser.

References

Alster, T. S. (1994) Improvement of erythematous and hypertrophic scars by the 585 nm flash-lamp-pumped pulsed dye laser. *Ann Plast Surg* **32**:186–190.

Anderson, R. R. and Parrish, J. A. (1983) Selective photothermolysis: Precise microsurgery by selective absorption of pulsed radiation. *Science* **220**:524–527.

Dierickx, C., Goldman, M. P., and Fitzpatrick, R. E. (1995) Laser treatment of erthematous/hypertrophic and pigmented scars in 26 patients. *Plast Reconstr Surg* **95**:84–90.

Goldman, M. P., Fitzpatrick, R. E. (1995) Laser treatment of scars. *Dermatol Surg* **21**:685–687.

Gotkin, R. H., Sarnoff, D. S., Cannarozzo, G., *et al.* (2009) Ablative skin resurfacing with a novel microablative CO_2 laser. *J Drugs Dermatol* **8(2)**:138–144.

Manstein, D., Herron, G. S., Sink, R. K., *et al.* (2004) Fractional photothermolysis: a new concept for cutaneous remodeling using microscopic patterns of thermal injury. *Lasers Surg Med* **34**:426–438.

McCraw, J. B., McCraw, J. A., McMellin, A., *et al.* (1999) Prevention of unfavorable scars using early pulse dye laser treatments: A preliminary report. *Ann Plast Surg* **42**:7–14.

Nouri, K., Alster, T. S., Ballard, J. C., *et al.* (2012) Laser Treatment of Scars and Stria Distensae. May 21, 2012. http://emedicine.medscape.com/article/1120673-overview#showall [Accessed March 2015].

Saryazdi, S. and Mohebbi, A. (2012) Evaluation of efficacy of fractional CO_2 laser in acne scar: *J Lasers Med Sci* **3(2)**:56–60.

Soltani, A. M., Francis, C. S., Motamed, A. *et al.* (2012) Hypertrophic scarring in cleft lip repair: A comparison of incidence among ethnic groups. *Clin Epidemiol* **4**:187–191.

Tredget, E. E., Nedelec, B., Scott, P. G., and Ghahary, A. (1997) Hypertrophic scars, keloids, and contractures: The cellular and molecular-basis for therapy. *Surg Clin North Am* **77**:701–730.

Tsao, S. S., Dover, J. S., Arndt, K. A., and Kaminer, M. S. (2002) Scar management: Keloid, hypertrophic, atrophic, and acne scars. *Semin Cutan Med Surg* **21(1)**:46–75.

CHAPTER 18

3D photography in cleft patients

Virpi Harila[1,2], Tuomo Heikkinen[1,2], Ville Vuollo[1,2], George K. B. Sándor[3], and Pertti Pirttiniemi[1,2]

[1] Department of Oral Development and Orthodontics, Institute of Dentistry, University of Oulu, Finland
[2] Oulu University Hospital, Finland
[3] Tissue Engineering, University of Oulu, and Institute of Biosciences and Medical Technology, University of Tampere, Finland

Introduction

Recently, cone-beam x-rays and 3D photos have come into wider clinical use to increase the quality of treatment documentation. 3D photography can be easily performed with 3D cameras, which are, however, quite expensive today compared to traditional equipment. Despite the current cost, 3D photography is an excellent communication tool. The 3D photography method allows a more visual presentation of the treatment outcomes with better prediction of the final treatment result. The use of the 3D photography method may also diminish the need for future use of lateral cephalometry, being a non-invasive way of patient monitoring without the need for exposure to ionizing radiation. Differences in facial morphology can be evaluated in three dimensions with a 3D photo system. The benefits of the 3D method are realistic pictures, short acquisition time (1.5 millisecs), natural head posture (NHP) and it is ideal for children (Chiu & Clark,1991; Kau & Zhurov, 2005).

3D images can be used for variety of applications, for example to verify growth changes in more dimensions than with 2D photos or with lateral cephalograms. 3D photos will be used to assist in future treatment-planning decisions based upon growth. 3D photos can also be used to assess the presence and extent of craniofacial anomalies and asymmetry (Kau *et al.*, 2007; Tolleson *et al.*, 2010; Hanis *et al.*, 2010). With 3D photography it is possible to study facial differences in gender among certain age groups and during growth (Djordjevic *et al.*, 2013). The method also provides a new tool to investigate the relationship of twinning and alterations in body patterning, such as in the study of laterality and asymmetry. 3D photography may provide the resolution needed to identify and quantify specific phenotypic variations, including fine degrees of facial asymmetry. 3D photos may facilitate novel investigations of twinning, syndromic, and complex diseases (Baynam *et al.*,

2011). 3D photography is the future of cleft monitoring and represents a tremendous advance in the evolution of record quality.

Method

Any 3D model of the facial soft tissue surface is a collection of vertices, edges, and triangle faces in 3D space. Facial 3D images can consist of over 10,000 vertex points depending on the accuracy. There are numerous ways to record the facial structures in 3D. The most common ways are laser scanning and stereo-photogrammetry. In laser scanning the distance from the object is computed by means of a directional light source and detector. In stereo-photogrammetry the basic idea is to combine multiple 2D views of an object to form a 3D image. In the process of forming the facial 3D image, the grid is projected on the face and then the face is photographed from at least two different angles using at least two different cameras. Examining the grid from two different angles makes it possible to perceive the depth of the face, and 3D coordinate points for the face can be constructed. Calculating coordinate points with both these methods requires simple trigonometry and geometric principles. Nowadays measurement errors in these techniques are quite low. Errors are at maximum a half millimeter and the most recent systems provide errors below 0.1 mm. One advantage of laser scanners or 3D camera systems is the radiation-free imaging process, and in that sense they are better equipment to analyze the soft tissue than X-ray generators (Kau and Richmond, 2010).

There can be considerably more than two cameras in any one 3D imaging system. In the system used at our center, there are five camera boxes, each box containing four cameras, so that the patient can be imaged using a total of twenty cameras depending on the view required (Figure 18.1). These multiple

Cleft Lip and Palate Management: A Comprehensive Atlas, First Edition. Edited by Ricardo D. Bennun, Julia F. Harfin, George K. B. Sándor, and David Genecov.
© 2016 John Wiley & Sons, Inc. Published 2016 by John Wiley & Sons, Inc.

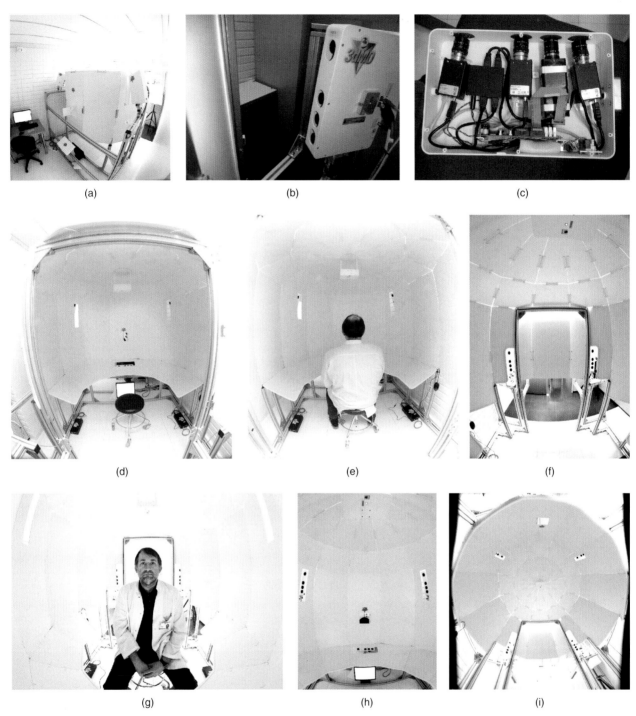

Figure 18.1 (a) 3D photography equipment for imaging of the whole head with five camera units, operator view and work station in clinical usage at Oulu University Hospital (photo by Dr. Sakari Vierola). (b) One of the five camera units with four cameras in each unit placed at key positions for 3D photography. (c) Four cameras housed inside each camera unit (photo by Dr. Sakari Vierola). (d) Inside view of white 3D photography reflection chamber with stool for the patient or parent (photo by Dr. Sakari Vierola). (e) Subject sitting facing forward in 3D photography chamber viewed from the rear of the unit (photo by Dr. Sakari Vierola). (f) View of rear aspect of 3D photography reflection chamber (photo by Dr. Sakari Vierola). (g) Subject (Dr. Tuomo Heikkinen) sitting inside 3D photography chamber viewed from the front of the unit (photo by Dr. Sakari Vierola). (h) The patient view of the front of the 3D photography unit when sitting on stool (photo by Dr. Sakari Vierola). (i) View of roof of 3D photography unit designed to capture images of skull vertex (photo by Dr. Sakari Vierola).

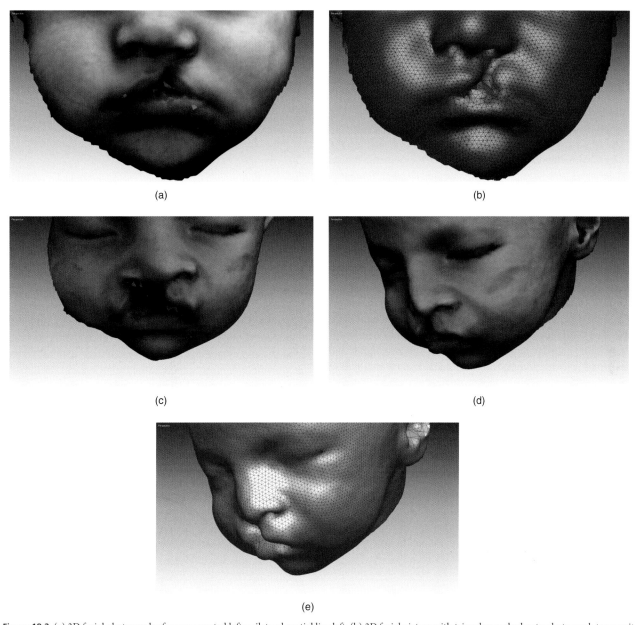

Figure 18.2 (a) 3D facial photograph of an unoperated left unilateral partial lip cleft. (b) 3D facial picture with triangles meshed onto photograph to permit volumetric facial analysis. (c) 3D facial photograph of an unoperated wide right unilateral cleft lip and palate patient. (d) 3D photograph of cleft patient in Figure 2C rotated toward the patient's right side. (e) 3D facial picture with triangles meshed onto photograph to permit measurement of facial landmarks.

cameras nodes make it possible to get a wider view of the object (Figure 18.2). Our unit is housed in a white photography reflection chamber with adjustable height and a single flash in the roof.

One can make a 3D image of the soft tissue of the whole head or body. The advantage of a stereo-photogrammetry camera compared to laser scanner is the quicker recording time. In a laser scanner the capturing of the object takes several seconds, whereas with a 3D camera it is almost as quick as with an ordinary camera. This is a great benefit especially when imaging

babies who are not able to stay calm and still for a longer period of time.

Facial 3D analysis is about making measurements based on the vertex point coordinates and the triangles that are composed by these points. The general method of examining the facial structures is analysis of landmarks, which are points that have specific geometric locations and associated biologic names. In landmark analysis the whole set of data describing the shape of facial surface is basically replaced by a few landmarks, and these coordinates are further analyzed by statistical methods.

Many studies, which deal with examining the facial 3D images of the cleft patients, use landmark analysis, for example comparing a cleft group to a control group (Figures 18.2c to 2e). Usually the number of landmarks in this kind of research is about 20 to 40 (Kau & Richmond, 2010). Of course it is possible to use more or fewer landmarks. In the study by Bugaighis *et al.* (2014), the facial, nasolabial, and nasal landmarks used were selected mainly based on previous work by Farkas (1994).

The population means can be calculated, forming an "average 3D face" with standard deviations, analyzing systematic errors, and variables such as asymmetry, dimorphism (sex differences), and growth in different parts of the face, and also the whole head can be verified. Visualization of changes can be done using graphic methods and statistical analyses using x-, y-, and z- coordinates (Kau & Richmond, 2010).

The display system needs powerful hard- and software as well as good quality tools when measuring and presenting the data. Statistical analyses may also differ from traditional analyses and require a knowledgeable statistician. Data collected from images with the 3dMD face imaging system (3dMD Inc., Atlanta, GA, USA) are highly repeatable and precise. The average error associated with the placement of landmarks is sub-millimeter and the error due to digitization and those due to the imaging system are both very low. The few measures showing a higher degree of error include those crossing the labial fissure, which are influenced by even subtle movement of the mandible. Results of studies concerning the error and precision of 3D measurements suggest that 3D anthropometric data collected using the 3dMDface System are highly reliable and, therefore, useful for evaluation of clinical dysmorphology and surgical results, analyses of genotype-phenotype correlations, and inheritance of complex phenotypes (Aldridge *et al.*, 2005).

3D photography in cleft patients

Oral clefts have many consequences for breathing, swallowing, eating, and speech, and facial asymmetry is one of the common features of oral clefts involving the lip (Bugaighis *et al.*, 2010; Garrahy, 2002; Ras *et al.*, 1994). Patients with oral clefts have different facial shapes compared to their unaffected peers. Differences vary according to the type of cleft and also the cleft repair technique used is important (Bardach, 1994). The severity of cleft is widely variable and the results of treatment are influenced by the initial deformity. Facial symmetry is a very important component in evaluating the success of surgical repair in cleft patients. Objective assessment of severity would help to guide prognosis and treatment, but most assessments are subjective. A practical and user friendly system is needed to quantify facial symmetry in three dimensions. Previously, imaging techniques have required sedation, ionizing radiation,

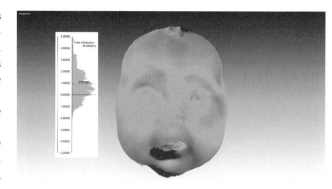

Figure 18.3 3D color map from asymmetry patient showing linear growth in various (red and blue) areas of the face, pre- and post-treatment superimpositions.

and good cooperation skills – which are difficult to achieve in infants and small children.

With the 3D photo method differences in facial asymmetry in operated cleft patients and in healthy children can be compared, as can the differences in asymmetry and growth pattern between different cleft groups (Figure 18.3). Bugaighis *et al.* (2014) introduced an indirect morphometric study applying advanced statistical tools to investigate 3D facial asymmetry occurring within and between the four main cleft groups. They concluded that a midline cleft of the soft and hard palate (CP) that does not involve the lip or alveolus, has the least effect on facial appearance and symmetry compared to other cleft types. In the study by Hood *et al.* (2003), asymmetry scores after primary repair were compared between UCLP and ULP groups. The UCLP group was more asymmetric than the ULP group, UCLP infants having greatest improvement in nasal asymmetry following primary repair. They suggested that nasal and lip asymmetry should be considered individually in cleft patients. Males in general have been found to demonstrate more asymmetry of the nose than females, when facial asymmetry is described in three dimensions in individuals with an operated complete unilateral cleft lip and palate (UCLP) (Ras *et al.*, 1994).

The reliability of a 3D photo system has been evaluated and sources of error could be technical, user dependent, or patient anatomy related. Data acquisition can be challenging in cleft patients, but it has been evaluated and found to be successful. Instead of a single measurement, utilizing the mean of multiple measurements could reduce the risk of corrupting the data during the evaluation process (Ort *et al.*, 2012). A 3D photo system is of great help in evaluating the soft tissue surface data of the face in an objective way. Three-dimensional stereophotogrammetry provides a reliable method for many anthropometric measurements of nasolabial form in infants with unrepaired and also operated unilateral cleft lip and or palate (Tse *et al.*, 2014).

Conclusions

Statistical shape analysis is a sensitive tool for the exploration of facial asymmetry in cleft patients. The assessment of the extent and the exact location of the asymmetry are challenging both to the surgeon and orthodontist and the 3D photo system provides new tools to quantify the asymmetry in three dimensions with conventional metric values. It will help to make the reconstructions of the deformed regions similar to the unaffected parts of the face. Ongoing serial follow-up with 3D photos will allow the surgeon to determine the effect of the surgical intervention on subsequent growth.

The new technology based 3D-photographic method provides tools not only for diagnosis and treatment planning, but also for the evaluation of treatment results. 3D assessment of infants with cleft lip and palate can be used to quantify improvements not only following primary surgery in three dimensions but also during and after the use of dynamic nasoalveolar molding appliances. Such monitoring will help in the validation of dynamic nasoalveolar molding protocols. With 3D photos it is also possible to collect long-term follow-up images to document whether changes in symmetry have occurred during subsequent growth. The future of 3D photography is exciting as this tool will be implemented for pre-operative diagnosis, pre-operative severity determination, for surgical planning, for the serial documentation of results, and to analyze the quality of the treatment outcomes. 3D photography will ultimately become a powerful clinical tool.

References

Aldridge, K., Boyadjiev, S. A., Capone, G. T., et al. (2005) Precision and error of three-dimensional phenotypic measures acquired from 3dMD photogrammetric images. *Am J Med Genet A* **138A**:247–253.

Bardach, J. (1994) Anthropometry in cleft lip and palate research. In: Farkas, L. G. (ed.) *Anthropometry of the Head and Face*. New York, NY: Raven Press, pp. 113–114.

Baynam, G., Claes, P., Craig, J. M., et al. (2011) Intersections of epigenetics, twinning and developmental asymmetries: insights into monogenic and complex diseases and a role for 3D facial analysis. *Twin Res Hum Genet* **14**:305–315.

Bugaighis, I., O'Higgins, P., Tiddeman, B., et al. (2010) Three-dimensional geometric morphometrics applied to the study of children with cleft lip and/or palate from the North East of England. *Eur J Orthodont* **32**:514–521.

Bugaighis, I., Mattick, C. R., Tiddeman, B., and Hobson, R. (2014) 3D asymmetry of operated children with oral clefts. *Orthod Craniofac Res* **27**:27–37.

Chiu, C. S. and Clark, R. K. (1991) Reproducibility of natural head position. *J Dent* **19**:130–131.

Djordjevic, J., Richmond, S., Zhurov, A. et al. (2013) Three-dimensional assessment of facial asymmetry during adolescent growth using laser surface scanning. *Eur J Orthodont* **35**:143–151.

Farkas, L. G. (ed.) (1994) Examination. In: *Anthropometry of the Head and Face*. New York, NY: Raven Press, pp. 3–56.

Garrahy, A. (2002) 3D assessment of dentofacial deformity in children with oral clefts. Thesis, University of Glasgow http//thesis.gla.ac.uk/1475/ [Accessed March 2015].

Hanis, S. B., Kau, C. H., Souccar, N. M., et al. (2010) Facial morphology of Finnish children with and without developmental hip dysplasia using 3D facial templates. *Orthod Craniofac Res* **13**:229–237.

Hood, C. A., Bock, M., Hosey, M. T., et al. (2003) Facial asymmetry - 3D assessment of infants with cleft lip and palate. *Int J Paediatr Dent* **13**:404–410.

Kau, C. H. and Zhurov, A. I. (2005) Natural head posture for measuring 3-dimensional facial morphology. In Middleton, J., Shrive, M. G., and Jones, M. L. (eds) *Computed Methods in Biomechanics and Biomedical Engineering-5*. Cardiff: First Numerics.

Kau, C. H., Hunter, L. M., and Hingston, E. J. (2007) A different look: 3-dimensional facial imaging of a child with Binder syndrome. *Am J Orthod Dentofac* **132**:704–709.

Kau, C. H. and Richmond, S. (eds) (2010) *Imaging for Orthodontics and Maxillofacial Surgery*. Oxford: Wiley-Blackwell.

Ort, R., Metzler, P., Kruse, A. L., et al. (2012) The reliability of a three-dimensional photo system (3DMDface-) based evaluation of the face in cleft lip infants. *Plast Surg Int* **2012**:138090 doi:10.1155/2012/138090.

Ras, F., Habets, L. L., van Ginkel, F. C., et al. (1994) Three-dimensional evaluation of facial asymmetry in cleft lip and palate. *Cleft Palate Craniofac J* **31**:116–121.

Tolleson, S. R., Kau, C. H., Lee, R. P., et al. (2010) 3D analysis of facial asymmetry in children with hip dysplasia. *Angle Orthod.* **80**: 519–524.

Tse, R., Booth, L., Keys, K., et al. (2014) Reliability of nasolabial anthropometric measures using three-dimensional stereophotogrammetry in infants with unrepaired unilateral cleft lip. *Plast Reconstr Surg* **133**:530e–542e.

Index

Cleft Lip and Palate Management: A Comprehensive Atlas, First Edition. Edited by Ricardo D. Bennun, Julia F. Harfin, George K. B. Sándor, and David Genecov.
© 2016 John Wiley & Sons, Inc. Published 2016 by John Wiley & Sons, Inc.